Insights to Performance Excellence in Health Care 2003

Also Available from ASQ Quality Press:

Improving Healthcare with Control Charts: Basic and Advanced SPC Methods and Case Studies
Raymond G. Carey

How to Use Patient Satisfaction Data to Improve Healthcare Quality
Ralph Bell, Ph.D. and Michael J. Krivch, CHE

Customer Driven Healthcare: QFD for Process Improvement and Cost Reduction
Ed Chaplin, M.D., and John Terninko, Ph.D.

How to Use Control Charts for Healthcare
D. Lynn Kelley

Measuring Quality Improvement in Healthcare: A Guide to Statistical Process Control Applications
Raymond G. Carey, Ph.D. and Robert C. Lloyd, Ph.D.

Healthcare Performance Measurement: Systems Design and Evaluation
Vahé Kazandjian

Stop Managing Costs: Designing Healthcare Organizations Around Core Business Systems
James P. Mozena, Charles E. Emerick, and Steven C. Black

From Baldrige to the Bottom Line: A Road Map for Organizational Change and Improvement
David W. Hutton

IWA-1:2001 – Quality Management Systems: Guidelines for Process Improvements in Health Service Organizations
ISO/AIAG/ASQ

To request a complimentary catalog of ASQ Quality Press publications, call 800-248-1946, or visit our Web site at http://qualitypress.asq.org.

Insights to Performance Excellence in Health Care 2003

An Inside Look at the 2003 Baldrige Award Criteria for Health Care

Mark L. Blazey
Joel H. Ettinger
Paul L. Grizzell
Linda M. Janczak

ASQ Quality Press
Milwaukee, Wisconsin

Insights to Performance Excellence in Health Care 2003: An Inside Look at the 2003
Baldrige Award Criteria for Health Care
Mark L. Blazey, Joel H. Ettinger, Paul L. Grizzell, and Linda M. Janczak

© 2003 by ASQ

10 9 8 7 6 5 4 3 2 1

ISBN 0-87389-580-0
Publisher: William A. Tony
Acquisitions Editor: Annemieke Hytinen
Project Editor: Paul O'Mara
Production Administrator: Gretchen Trautman
Special Marketing Representative: David Luth

ASQ Mission: The American Society for Quality advances individual and organizational performance excellence worldwide by providing opportunities for learning, quality improvement, and knowledge exchange.

Microsoft® is a registered trademark of Microsoft Corporation.

Attention: Bookstores, Wholesalers, Schools and Corporations: ASQ Quality Press books, videotapes, audiotapes, and software are available at quantity discounts with bulk purchases for business, educational, or instructional use. For information, please contact ASQ Quality Press at 800-248-1946, or write to ASQ Quality Press, P.O. Box 3005, Milwaukee, WI 53201-3005.

To place orders or to request a free copy of the ASQ Quality Press Publications Catalog, including ASQ membership information, call 800-248-1946. Visit our Web site at www.asq.org or qualitypress.asq.org.

Printed in the United States of America

 Printed on acid-free paper

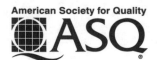

American Society for Quality

Quality Press
600 N. Plankinton Avenue
Milwaukee, Wisconsin 53203
Call toll free 800-248-1946
Fax 414-272-1734
www.asq.org
http://qualitypress.asq.org
http://standardsgroup.asq.org
E-mail: authors@asq.org

Contents

CD Files 2003 Health Care

Baldrige Studies

Criteria

NIST Files

2003 Calculating Score Summary

2003 Baldrige Application Dev

2003 Basic Overall Multiple Requirements

Baldrige Award Recipients

State and Regional Quality Award Recipients

Preface

This book was developed as a teaching text to help people from all types of organizations understand the power and benefits of integrating the Malcolm Baldrige Award Criteria into their management systems. Since it has been published as a "stand alone" book, it has guided the decisions and deliberations of people from all organizational levels as they documented their continuous improvement efforts using Baldrige Award-type management systems. Now, there is a version especially for health care based on the new Malcolm Baldrige Health Care Criteria for Performance Excellence. We know it will be a valuable tool for health care organizations, patients, stakeholders and customers, and suppliers, in assessing their continuous improvement efforts.

Two groups of readers—examiners of health care performance systems and leaders of health care organizations—can gain a competitive edge by understanding the parts of a high-performance management system, and how these parts connect and align. Our goal for this book is that readers will understand fully what each area of the system means for health care organizations and find the synergy within the seven major parts of the system: leadership; strategic planning; patients, other customers, and market focus; measurement, analysis, and knowledge management; staff focus; process management; and organizational performance results.

Organization leaders have reported that this book has been valuable as a step-by-step approach to help identify and put in place continuous improvement systems. As this progresses, improvement efforts in one area will lead to improvements in other areas. This process is similar to experiences we have all encountered as we carry out home improvement—improve one area and many other areas needing improvement become apparent. This book will help identify areas that need immediate improvement as well as areas that are less urgent but, nevertheless, vitally linked to overall improvement.

Acknowledgements from the Authors

The authors thank Karen Davison, who edited the book prior to publication, and Jessica Norris, who helped in preparing the manuscript.

Mark Blazey appreciates the help and support from his family, including his wife Karen and children, Liz and Mark, and mother, Ann. He also would like to thank the many colleagues and friends who use the Baldrige Criteria every day to improve the quality of life in schools, health care organizations, government agencies, and businesses.

Joel Ettinger acknowledges the growing number of health care workers who have and will have the passion and the conviction to improve health care quality in service to mankind. He thanks two mentors: William J. Copeland and Donald M. Berwick, M.D., who have taught him much about life, leadership, and improvement. Lastly, he expresses profound appreciation to his parents, Mark and Lil, his wife, Joan, and his children, Joshua, Jared, and Jessica—each mentors of a precious kind.

Paul Grizzell thanks Bob Hockin, who initially opened his eyes to the Baldrige Criteria, and his father, Les Grizzell, who modeled personal learning before it was a business core value. Most of all he thanks his wife, Janice, his daughter, Ashley, and his son, Nicholas, who have been incredibly patient as he has tried to implement Baldrige-based quality initiatives at home.

Linda Janczak thanks the board, medical staff, associates, and particularly the executive team of Thompson Health. She also thanks Robert Sigmund, who demonstrated the value of the written word in health care. She expresses a very special thank you to her husband, Steve, and her children, Sarah and Matthew, for their inspiration and support.

Harry Hertz, Curt Reimann, Barry Diamondstone, and the dedicated staff of the Malcolm Baldrige National Quality Award office have provided long-standing support and guidance in promoting quality excellence. The chapter on site visits, the Criteria model and integrated management systems analysis, the management and performance excellence surveys, the performance standard for leadership, the supplemental scoring guidelines, the sections concerning the potential adverse consequences of not doing what the Criteria require, and the application preparation files are used with permission of Quantum Performance Group, Inc. The core values, Criteria, selected glossary terms, award winners, and background information in this book are drawn from information in the public domain supplied by the Malcolm Baldrige National Quality Award program.

Introduction

The Malcolm Baldrige National Quality Award was established in 1998 to insert new vigor into improving the quality of products and services produced by U.S. companies. Book after book, article after article, and most telling of all, the results of business revealed that U.S. business was at risk for losing its creative and productive advantage. It appeared at a time that too many of our best-known companies were caught resting on their laurels while energetic and hungry companies—particularly from Japan and Europe—were poised to capture major segments of the emerging global marketplace. Today, the marketplace is truly global with significant growing competition emanating from many areas, such as Southeast Asia, China, and Mexico, to name just a few. The imperative of high performance by American companies is more important than ever.

During the past 15 years the health care industry has faced its own array of challenges. The downward pressure on reimbursement has been relentless. Patient expectations have increased dramatically, workforce shortages exist in key disciplines, physician satisfaction with the practice of medicine has declined, the incidence of medical errors is front-page news, and ethical issues surface with alarming frequency. In the first quarter of 2003, the world focused on health care as a global issue as a mysterious virus apparently made its way across the planet in record time threatening the global economy. This virus came to be known as Severe Acute Respiratory Syndrome (SARS). The responsibility is clear—the health care industry needs to communicate, protect, and inform the public across the planet. In the midst of these challenges the opportunity of an extraordinary robust medical research pipeline continues to produce new although often costly technology that takes the art and science of medicine to new levels of diagnostic and treatment competency. The challenges and the opportunities facing health care today touch every aspect of the industry, every corner of the globe, and every patient, customer, supplier and stakeholder.

In 1999, Congress extended to the health care industry the opportunity for self-assessment based on Criteria adapted from the highly successful Baldrige Business Criteria. The Baldrige Criteria for Performance Excellence in Health Care, modeled on manufacturing and service business excellence concepts, offers specific insight into how the leaders and stewards of health care delivery and resources can pursue and capture distinctive performance. The health services industry is populated by professionals who rank among the most trained and skilled of any industry. Yet the performance of the institutions that provide health care does not equal the potential of this talent. This book delves deeply into the understanding and use of the Baldrige framework for health care organization improvement. The adoption of this comprehensive approach to excellence will not only help guide health care through its maze of challenges and opportunities, but also secure and sustain incremental and dramatic improvement. The evidence that it will do so is just now emerging as SSM Health care became the first health care recipient of the Baldrige Award in 2002.

The Baldrige National Quality Program in 2003 presents a distinct structure and discipline for the leadership of our nation's extraordinary health care assets. The Baldrige framework, consisting of the Criteria, Core Values and Concepts, and scoring differentiators of high performance, present a powerful assessment instrument that enables leaders to understand how to achieve high performance beyond what many leaders today consider possible.

Deploying an effective management system capable of driving performance improvement in health care is an ongoing challenge. There is an intricate web of complex relationships among administration, management, physicians, trustees, labor, patients and customers, stakeholders, partners, payors, and suppliers. Despite these challenges, the best organizations demonstrate a management system that improves its work processes continuously. They measure key facets of activity and closely monitor organization performance. Leaders of these organizations set high expectations, value staff and their input, communicate clear directions, and align the work of everyone to achieve organizational goals and optimal performance. Leaders of these high performing organizations become the role models of ethical conduct and the desired culture.

The practice of medicine is complex—arguably more complex than many manufacturing processes and most service company processes. The complexity of health care presents fertile ground for errors. Reports on error rates in medicine are staggering indications of the healthcare industry's condition and potential for improvement. Just as illnesses represent a breakdown in the complex biochemical processes of life, error rates are breakdowns in the complexity of health care delivery. Both deserve our unyielding attention.

The Baldrige Criteria serves as a road map to achieve vision, mission, and clinical excellence through an empowered workforce. Insights to Performance Excellence in Health Care 2003 is a field book designed to enable health care leaders to travel these roads toward excellence. *Insights to Performance Excellence in Health Care 2003* helps leaders, performance excellence examiners, and health care practitioners clearly understand the Baldrige framework, including the Criteria, Core Values and Concepts, differentiators of high performing organizations and how the linkage of these components offers the potential for best-in-world performance.

Six types of information are provided in this book for each of the items in Categories 1 through 6:

1. The actual language of each Item, including notes (presented in the shadow box). [Author's Note: The information in these shadow boxes presents the official Baldrige Criteria and serves as the only basis for the examination. The other five types of information presented in this book for each Item (elements 2 through 6 below) provide the author's interpretation of the official Criteria requirements and should not be used as a basis for establishing additional requirements during an examination or performance review.]

2. A plain English explanation of the requirements of each Item with some suggestions about the rationale for the Item and ways to meet key requirements.

3. A summary of the requirements of each Item in flowchart form. The flowcharts capture the essence of each Item and isolate the requirements of each Item to help organizations focus on the key points the item is assessing. Note that most boxes in the flowcharts contain an item reference in brackets [ ]. This indicates that the Criteria require the action. If there is no item reference in brackets, it means the action is suggested but not required. Occasionally a reference to "[scoring guidelines]" is included in a box. This means that the authority for the requirement comes from the scoring guidelines.

4. The key linkages between each Item and the other Items. The major or primary linkages are designated using a solid arrow (⟶). The secondary linkages are designated using a dashed arrow (┅┅➤).

5. An explanation of some potential adverse consequences that an organization might face if it fails to implement processes required by each Item. (Examiners may find this analysis useful as they prepare relevant feedback concerning opportunities for improvement. However, these generic statements should be customized—based on key factors, core values, or specific circumstances facing the organization being reviewed—before using them to develop feedback comments supporting opportunities for improvements in Categories 1 through 6.)

6. Examples of effective practices that some health care organizations have developed and followed consistent with the requirements of the Item. These samples present some ideas about how to meet requirements. (Remember, examiners should not convert these sample effective practices into new organizations they are examining.)

Changes to this 2003 edition include:

• New information from the 2003 Baldrige Health Care Criteria for Performance Excellence to help leaders focus on priority opportunities for improvement and understand better the role they must play in refining their management systems and processes.

- A review guideline for examiners that highlights processes required at the Basic, Overall, and Multiple levels of scoring.

- An updated analysis of some of the adverse consequences organizations may face by failing to implement processes required by the performance excellence Criteria.

- Additional definitions to enhance understanding of key words in the Criteria and Scoring Guidelines.

- A CD that includes a full health care case study designed to help leaders envision role-model practices as part of a system of health care delivery, not a list of isolated practices.

Reading *Insights to Performance Excellence in Health Care 2003* will strengthen your understanding of the Criteria and provide insight on analyzing your organization, improving performance, and applying for the award.

THE CORE VALUES TO ACHIEVE PERFORMANCE EXCELLENCE

The Criteria are built upon a set of interrelated Core Values and Concepts, which are embedded beliefs and behaviors found in high-performing organizations. They are the foundation for integrating key business requirements within a results-oriented framework that create a basis for action and feedback.

The 2003 Core Values and Concepts follow. The text in the box presents the exact wording of the Baldrige Core Values and Concepts.

Visionary Leadership

Every system, strategy, and method for achieving excellence must be guided by visionary leadership.

- Effective leaders convey a strong sense of urgency to counter the natural resistance to change that can prevent the organization from taking the steps that these Core Values for success demand.

- Such leaders serve as enthusiastic role models, reinforcing and communicating the Core Values by their words and actions.

- Words alone are not enough.

Visionary Leadership

An organization's senior leaders (administrative and health care provider leaders) should set directions and create a patient focus, clear and visible values, and high expectations. The directions, values, and expectations should balance the needs of all your stakeholders. Your leaders should ensure the creation of strategies, systems, and methods for achieving excellence in health care, stimulating innovation, and building knowledge and capabilities. The values and strategies should help guide all activities and decisions of your organization.

Senior leaders should inspire and motivate your entire staff and should encourage all staff to contribute, to develop and learn, to be innovative, and to be creative. Senior leaders should be responsible to your organization's governance body for their actions and performance. The governance body should be responsible ultimately to all your stakeholders for the ethics, vision, actions, and performance of your organization and its senior leaders. Senior leaders should serve as role models through their ethical behavior and their personal involvement in planning, communications, coaching, development of future leaders, review of organizational performance, and staff recognition. As role models, they can reinforce ethics, values, and expectations while building leadership, commitment, and initiative throughout your organization.

Patient-Focused Excellence

This value demonstrates a passion for making the organization patient-driven. Without this, little else matters. Patients are the final judges of how well the organization did its job, and what they say counts. Patients expect immediate, accurate information and assistance. It is their perception of the service that will determine whether they remain loyal or constantly seek better providers.

The organization must focus on systematically listening to patients and other customers and acting quickly on what they say. It must build positive relationships with its patients through focusing on accessibility and management of complaints.

Dissatisfied patients must be heeded most closely, for they often deliver the most valuable information. If only satisfied and loyal patients (those who continue to use our services with us no matter what) are paying attention, the organization will be led astray. The most successful organizations keep an eye on patients and other customers who are not satisfied and work to understand their preferences and meet their demands.

Insurers and other payors influence patient choice of provider by determining which providers are included in the network. Providers with poor patient satisfaction may be excluded.

Accordingly, the health care organization that focuses on the multiple dimensions of patient satisfaction not only enhances patient loyalty, but has greater support through pay or networks.

Patient-Focused Excellence

The delivery of health care services must be patient focused. Quality and performance are the key components in determining patient satisfaction. All attributes of patient care delivery (including those not directly related to medical/clinical services) factor into the judgment of satisfaction and value. Satisfaction and value to patients are key considerations for other customers as well. Patient-focused excellence has both current and future components: understanding today's patient desires and anticipating future patient desires and health care marketplace offerings.

Value and satisfaction may be influenced by many factors during a patient's experience participating in health care. Primary among these factors is an expectation that patient safety will be ensured throughout the health care delivery process. Additional factors include a clear understanding of likely health and functional status outcomes, as well as the patient's relationship with the health care provider and ancillary staff, cost, responsiveness, and continuing care and attention. For many patients, the ability to participate in making decisions on their health care is considered an important factor. This requires patient education for an informed decision. Characteristics that differentiate one provider from another also contribute to the sense of being patient focused.

Patient-focused excellence is thus a strategic concept. It is directed toward obtaining and retaining patient loyalty, referral of new patients, and market share gain in competitive markets. Patient-focused excellence thus demands rapid and flexible response to emerging patient desires and health care marketplace requirements, and measurement of the factors that drive patient satisfaction. Patient-focused excellence also demands awareness of new technology and new modalities for delivery of health care services.

Organizational and Personal Learning

Creating a climate for organizational and personal learning is a principle responsibility of leadership. Successful organizations know that what they do today and how they do it must improve to meet future needs.

Positive reinforcement and encouragement of learning is among the highest priorities for a healthy work culture. Since many health care organization staff are required to continue their education to retain professional credentials, health care organizations have a built-in learning imperative.

In addition, staff and organizational learning are essential for establishing and maintaining competitive advantage. While some competitors may focus on improving some processes and services, those who commit to total learning at all levels are better able to meet the ever-changing needs of patients and staff.

Organizational and Personal Learning

Achieving the highest levels of performance requires a well-executed approach to organizational and personal learning. Organizational learning includes both continuous improvement of existing approaches and adaptation to change, leading to new goals and/or approaches. Learning needs to be embedded in the way your organization operates. This means that learning (1) is a regular part of daily work; (2) is practiced at personal, department/work unit, and organizational levels; (3) results in solving problems at their source ("root cause"); (4) is focused on sharing knowledge throughout your organization; and (5) is driven by opportunities to effect significant change and to do better. Sources for learning include staff ideas, health care research findings, patients' and other customers' input, best practice sharing, and benchmarking.

Organizational learning can result in (1) enhancing value to patients through new and improved patient care services; (2) developing new health care opportunities; (3) reducing errors, defects, waste, and related costs; (4) improving responsiveness and cycle time performance; (5) increasing productivity and effectiveness in the use of all resources throughout your organization; and (6) enhancing your organization's performance in building community health and fulfilling its societal responsibilities.

Staff success depends increasingly on having opportunities for personal learning and practicing new skills. Organizations invest in personal learning through education, training, and other opportunities for continuing growth. Such opportunities might include job rotation and increased pay for demonstrated knowledge and skills. On-the-job training offers a cost-effective way to train and to better link training to your organizational needs and priorities. For health care providers, personal learning includes building discipline knowledge, discipline retraining to adjust to a changing health care environment, and enhancing knowledge of measurement systems influencing outcome assessments and clinical guidelines, decision trees, or critical pathways. Education and training programs may benefit from advanced technologies, such as computer-and Internet-based learning and satellite broadcasts.

Personal learning can result in (1) more satisfied and versatile staff who stay with the organization, (2) organizational cross-functional learning, and (3) an improved environment for innovation. Thus, learning is directed not only toward better health care services but also toward being more responsive, adaptive, and efficient—giving your organization health care marketplace sustainability and performance advantages.

Valuing Staff and Partners

Compared to many industries, the staff composition of health care organizations and suppliers to health care are highly skilled and subject to continuing skill development. Health care organizations need to appreciate how valuing staff and partners who have invested time and resources to acquire skills can become even more valuable.

Leaders must acknowledge that the health care organization workforce is, generally, highly trained and capable. By focusing on their continued development, satisfaction, and well-being, the health care organization maximizes the return-on-investment of its workforce in ways that many competitors do not. High-performing organizations prepare for rapid changes by investing in their staff.

Organizational leaders that communicate, share information, and involve health care staff in decisions that affect their work produce more effective staff and better levels of service and patient care. Effective partnerships help organizations serve the best interests of patients and are necessary for health care organizations to achieve their critical success factors

Valuing Staff and Partners

An organization's success depends increasingly on the knowledge, skills, creativity, and motivation of its staff and partners.

Valuing staff means committing to their satisfaction, development, and well-being. Increasingly, this involves more flexible, high-performance work practices tailored to staff with diverse workplace and home life needs. Major challenges in the area of valuing staff include (1) demonstrating your leaders' commitment to your staff's success, (2) recognition that goes beyond the regular compensation system, (3) development and progression within your organization, (4) sharing your organization's knowledge so your staff can better serve your patients and other customers and contribute to achieving your strategic objectives, and (5) creating an environment that encourages appropriate risk taking.

Organizations need to build internal and external partnerships to better accomplish overall goals. Internal partnerships might include cooperation between health care providers and other staff, and labor-management cooperation, such as agreements with unions. Partnerships with staff might entail staff development, cross-training, or network organizations, such as high-performance work teams. Internal partnerships also might involve creating network relationships among your departments/work units to improve flexibility, responsiveness, and knowledge sharing and to develop processes that better follow patient care and needs.

External partnerships might be with customers, suppliers, business associations, third-party payors, community and social service organizations, and other health care providers. Strategic partnerships or alliances are increasingly important kinds of external partnerships. Such partnerships with other health care organizations could result in referrals or in shared facilities that are either capital intensive or require unique and scarce expertise. Also, partnerships might permit the blending of your organization's core competencies or leadership capabilities with the complementary strengths and capabilities of partners.

Successful internal and external partnerships develop longer-term objectives, thereby creating a basis for mutual investments and respect. Partners should address the key requirements for success, means for regular communication, approaches to evaluating progress, and means for adapting to changing conditions. In some cases, joint education and training could offer a cost-effective method for staff development.

Agility

Like many industries, health care is also affected by the speed of change driven by the dynamics of the Internet, urgency as health becomes a global concern effecting all aspects of international commerce and travel, daily reports of new medical discoveries and introduction of new therapies, and patients who expect immediate response to and resolution of their health care concerns. Agility is more important than ever and a key differentiator for survival in a highly competitive field.

The health care delivery design process needs to systematically accommodate the continuous flow of new discoveries and new patient demands. Health care organizations that can effectively and rapidly adopt new therapies within the context of superb patient service can achieve and sustain competitive advantage.

There is a growing expectation for instant information and treatment—patients do not want to wait to access health care, and physicians are impatient with slow health care organization analysis and decision making. The ability to be fast and flexible is crucial to meeting the needs and expectations of patients, physicians, and all staff. People make better, more consistently reliable decisions when they have information. Timely availability of accurate information is essential for agility

Agility

Success in today's health care environment demands agility—a capacity for rapid change and flexibility. All aspects of electronic communication and information transfer require and enable more rapid, flexible, and customized responses. Health care providers face ever-shorter cycles for the introduction of new/improved health care services, as well as for faster and more flexible response to patients and other customers. Major improvements in response time often require simplification of work units and processes and/or the ability for rapid changeover from one process to another. Cross-trained and empowered staff are vital assets in such a demanding environment.

Today's health care environment places a heavy burden on the timely design of health care delivery systems, disease prevention programs, health promotion programs, and effective and efficient diagnostic and treatment systems. Overall design must include the opportunity to learn for continuous organizational improvement and must value the individual needs of patients. Design also must include effective means for gauging improvement of health status—for patients and populations/communities. Beneficial changes must be introduced at the earliest appropriate opportunity.

All aspects of time performance now are more critical, and cycle time has become a key process measure. Other important benefits can be derived from this focus on time; time improvements often drive simultaneous improvements in organization, quality, cost, patient focus, and productivity.

Focus on the Future

Just as agility is a key characteristic for high-performing health care organizations, a focus on the future and a willingness to make long-term commitments must also be woven into health care organization culture. Although changes to critical factors such as reimbursement are difficult to predict, other trends, such as continued productivity of the medical research engine, the aging of the population, interest in alternative therapies, and cyberspace, among others, are clearly trends that enable health care organizations to set future directions. The dynamics of known trends and unknown circumstances are evident in all industries.

Health care organizations need to establish long-term, measurable goals and action plans to be communicated throughout the organization. In addition, the development and communication of strategy within a health care organization is one of the most powerful ways to align work, reduce unnecessary work, and get everyone pulling in the same direction. Without this alignment, fragmentation of programs and services increases. Organizational effectiveness and patient care suffer.

Focus on the Future

In today's health care environment, a focus on the future requires understanding the short- and longer-term factors that affect your organization and health care marketplace. Pursuit of health care excellence requires a strong future orientation and a willingness to make long-term commitments to key stakeholders—patients and families, staff, communities, employers, payors, health profession students, and suppliers and partners. Your organization's planning should anticipate many factors, such as changes in health care delivery systems, resource availability, patient and other stakeholder expectations, technological developments, new partnering opportunities, the evolving importance of electronic communication and information transfer, evolving regulatory requirements, community and societal expectations, and new thrusts by competitors and other organizations providing similar services. Strategic objectives and resource allocations need to accommodate these influences. A focus on the future includes developing staff and suppliers, creating opportunities for innovation, and anticipating public responsibilities.

A major long-term investment associated with health care excellence is the investment in creating and sustaining an assessment system focused on health care outcomes. This entails becoming familiar with research findings and ongoing application of assessment methods.

Managing for Innovation

Visionary leadership, agility, focusing on the future and managing for innovation are linked Core Values and Concepts in high-performing organizations. Visionary leadership encourages innovation and risk taking; agility is necessary for timely acceptance of new ideas; and successful innovation is essential to achieve future targets in the fast-moving health care industry. Innovation must be effectively integrated by management into daily work.

Effective health care organizations seek out, learn from, and build upon best practices to continually improve. Suggestions for new ideas and new ways to achieve mission need to be sought from all staff, not just a small group of planners or researchers. Innovation in the science and delivery of medicine is crucial to maintain the highest levels of success in a competitive arena.

Managing for Innovation

Innovation means making meaningful change to improve an organization's services and processes and to create new value for the organization's stakeholders. Innovation should lead your organization to new dimensions of performance. Innovation is no longer strictly the purview of health care researchers; innovation is important for all aspects of your organizational performance and all processes. Organizations should be led and managed so that innovation becomes part of the culture and is integrated into daily work.

Management by Fact

There are many opinion leaders in health care who are not shy about dominating discussion and decision making, regardless of the facts. Health care organizations that are able to sustain direction and manage complexity inherent in health care delivery do so with vigorous reliance on management by fact.

Health care organizations need to identify the facts important to determining progress in achieving mission and critical success factors, including operating and financial objectives, health care outcomes, patient/customer satisfaction, and productivity, among others.

To ensure consistently good decisions at all levels, staff reliance on facts for institutional decisions need to be as vigorous as physician reliance on clinical indicators for patient care decision making. When making decisions, ask for the facts. The inability to produce facts to support decisions should cause those involved to be more careful and thorough

Management by Fact

An effective health care service and administrative management system depends on the measurement and analysis of performance. Such measurements should derive from health care service needs and strategy, and they should provide critical data and information about key processes, outputs, and results. Many types of data and information are needed for performance management. Performance measurement should include information on health care outcomes; community health; epidemiological data; critical pathways and practice guidelines; administrative, payor, staff, cost, and financial performance; competitive comparisons; and customer satisfaction.

Analysis refers to extracting larger meaning from data and information to support evaluation, decision-making, and operational improvement. Analysis entails using data to determine trends, projections, and cause and effect that might not otherwise be evident. Analysis supports a variety of purposes, such as planning, reviewing your overall performance, improving operations, change management, and comparing your performance with competitors', similar health care organizations', or with "best practices" benchmarks.

A major consideration in performance improvement and change management involves the selection and use of performance measures or indicators. *The measures or indicators you select should best represent the factors that lead to improved health care outcomes; improved customer, operational, and financial performance; and healthier communities. A comprehensive set of measures or indicators tied to patient/customer and/or organizational performance requirements represents a clear basis for aligning all processes with your organization's goals.* Through the analysis of data from your tracking processes, your measures or indicators themselves may be evaluated and changed to better support your goals.

Social Responsibility and Community Health

Health care organizations have a unique community role. In addition to assuring that the business of delivering health care has no adverse environmental, safety, or public health effect, health care organizations also have the responsibility to improve the health of one or more communities or regions. For a health care organization, public responsibility and community health is both a declaration of citizenship and the measure of ultimate value.

Citizenship involves reinforcement of ethical practices and protection against environmental harm from hazardous wastes, radiation, and other biohazards. Role model performance to exceed compliance with regulatory requirements is desired.

Improving the health of the public, inclusive of those without insurance or access to it, is a responsibility of all health care organizations individually and working collectively in a community or region.

Social Responsibility and Community Health

A health care organization's leaders should stress responsibilities to the public, ethical behavior, and the need to foster improved community health. Leaders should be role models for your organization in focusing on ethics and the protection of public health, safety, and the environment. Protection of health, safety, and the environment includes any impact of your organization's operations. Also, organizations should emphasize resource conservation and waste reduction at the source. Planning should anticipate adverse impacts that may arise in facilities management, as well as use and disposal of radiation, chemicals, and biohazards. Effective planning should prevent problems, provide for a forthright response if problems occur, and make available information and support needed to maintain public awareness, safety, and confidence.

Organizations should not only meet all local, state, and federal laws and regulatory and accreditation requirements, but they should treat these and related requirements as opportunities for improvement "beyond mere compliance." Organizations should stress ethical behavior in all stakeholder transactions and interactions. Highly ethical conduct should be a requirement of and should be monitored by the organization's governance body. Ethical practices need to consider nondiscriminatory patient treatment policies and protection of patients' rights and privacy. Public health services and supporting the general health of the community are important citizenship responsibilities of health care organizations.

Practicing good citizenship refers to leadership in carrying out these responsibilities—within the limits of an organization's resources—and includes influencing other organizations, private and public, to partner for these purposes. For example, your organization might lead or participate in efforts to establish free clinics or indigent care programs, to increase public health awareness programs, or to foster neighborhood services for the elderly. A leadership role also could include helping to define regional or national health care issues for action by regional or national networks or associations.

Managing social responsibility requires the use of appropriate measures and leadership responsibility for those measures.

Focus on Results and Creating Value

A health care organization's ability to focus on results and its approach to creating value serve as sources of inspiration and energy for staff who appreciate knowing, in measurable terms, the impact of their work. Patients, staff, and other stakeholders want to know the value received for costs incurred. They want evidence—not from anecdotal stories, but from results.

Although there is no accepted health care industry-wide single set of standards for measuring results in outcomes, improved health of the community, or prevention of disease, there are many valid measures of results. Results are systematically used by effective leadership to set priorities for improvement and for allocation of resources. Without these results, staff must rely on intuition to make adjustments to processes and goals.

Focus on Results and Creating Value

An organization's performance measurements need to focus on key results. Results should be used to create and balance value for your key stakeholders—patients, their families, staff, the community, payors, businesses, health profession students, suppliers and partners, investors, and the public. By creating value for your key stakeholders, your organization builds loyalty and contributes to the community. To meet the sometimes conflicting and changing aims that balancing value implies organizational strategy should explicitly include key stakeholder requirements. This will help ensure that actions and plans meet differing stakeholder needs and avoid adverse impacts on any stakeholders. The use of a balanced composite of leading and lagging performance measures offers an effective means to communicate short- and longer-term priorities, monitor actual performance, and provide a clear basis for improving results.

Systems Perspective

It is important to recognize that high performance is not possible unless the entire system is optimized. All parts are necessary for success. Excellence across a health care enterprise can only be assured through understanding and implementation of a systems perspective. Enterprise-wide Performance Excellence is necessary for sustained success. Excellence in a few work areas or processes does not translate into sustainable quality or competitive advantage.

Systems perspective is defined by the Baldrige Core Values, Categories, and Items. While each, individually, is a helpful guide for improvement, together they reveal ways to improve the entire organization.

Senior leadership understanding of the system of the Baldrige framework is an important early step. Mid-level management understanding of the Baldrige framework can help breakdown unproductive and costly barriers to high performance

Systems Perspective

The Baldrige Health Care Criteria provide a systems perspective for managing your organization to achieve performance excellence. The Core Values and the seven Baldrige Categories form the building blocks and the integrating mechanism for the system. However, successful management of overall performance requires organization-specific synthesis, alignment, and integration. Synthesis means looking at your organization as a whole and builds upon key organizational requirements, including your strategic objectives and action plans. Alignment means using the key linkages among requirements given in the Baldrige Categories to ensure consistency of plans, processes, measures, and actions. Integration means the individual components of your performance management system operate in a fully interconnected manner.

These concepts are depicted in the Baldrige framework. A systems perspective includes your senior leaders' focus on strategic directions and on your patients and other customers. It means that your senior leaders monitor, respond to, and manage performance based on your organizational results. A systems perspective also includes using your measures and indicators to link your key strategies with your key processes and align your resources to improve overall performance and satisfy patients and other customers.

Thus, a systems perspective means managing your whole organization, as well as its components, to achieve success.

Insights to Performance Excellence

This section provides information for health care leaders who are transforming their organizations to achieve Performance Excellence. This section:

- Describes background for the Baldrige Performance Excellence Award Criteria

- Describes the first health care organization to achieve recognition as the recipient of the Malcolm Baldrige National Quality Award in Health Care

- Describes the Integrated Management System

- Provides practical insights and lessons learned—ideas on transition strategies to put high-performance systems in place and promote organizational change

- This section also includes suggestions about how to start down the path to systematic organizational improvement, as well as lessons learned from those who chose paths that led nowhere or proved futile despite their best efforts

BACKGROUND OF THE BALDRIGE PERFORMANCE EXCELLENCE AWARD CRITERIA

During the 1980s, many U.S. businesses suffered losses in the marketplace due to stronger international competition. For nearly 30 years, Japanese business leaders were able to improve the performance of their organizations by following the requirements of the Deming Prize Criteria. The power of the Japanese recovery from the devastation of World War II to a dominant global economic power was documented in a CBS documentary entitled, *If Japan Can, Why Can't We?* The documentary served as a catalyst for the creation of a national quality award for the United States.

It was hoped that such a program would help U.S. business leaders focus on the systems and processes that would lead them to recovery much as the Deming Prize Criteria helped Japanese business leaders earlier.

After nearly five years of work, in 1987, the U.S. Congress created the national quality award named in honor of the Secretary of the Department of Commerce, Malcolm Baldrige, who had died a few weeks earlier in a rodeo accident. The Malcolm Baldrige National Quality Award or "Baldrige Award" had one purpose: to help U.S. businesses improve their competitiveness in the global marketplace.

After much debate and discussion, the creators of the award agreed that elements of the award Criteria should not be based on theories of how organizations ought to conduct business in order to win. We had seen too many instances where organizations followed the many piecemeal theories of the management gurus that led nowhere.

Instead, the decision was made to base the U.S. national quality program award criteria on the demonstrated practices of the world's best performing companies. Rather than theories, we wanted to determine what common practices existed that enabled these organizations to achieve the highest levels of performance, productivity, customer satisfaction, and market share. We observed that the practices that enabled a company to achieve high performance in the past were no longer sufficient to ensure high performance in the present. We have since found that the practices required to achieve leadership in 1988 were different from what would be required to succeed today. Changes in the marketplace, customer requirements, advances in science and medicine, competition, worker skills and availability, and technology (to name a few) have forced organizations to change the way they manage their business in order to succeed. Accordingly, the U.S. Department of Commerce's National Institute of Standards and Technology reviews the drivers of high performance each year to be certain that the Criteria continue to be relevant and useful. Based on these analyses, the Criteria for the Malcolm Baldrige National Quality Award are validated and refined. Based on the success of the Business Criteria, public law 100-107, which created the public-private partnership of the Baldrige award, was expanded in 1999 to include health care as an eligible category for the Award.

High-Performing Health Care Organizations

High-performing health care organizations outrun their competition (or potential competition) by delivering value to patients, customers and stakeholders through an unwavering focus on them and through improved organizational capabilities. Examples of improved capabilities have occurred in all types of health care organizations, including private, government, for-profit and not-for-profit organizations. These results range from time and cost savings to patient and other customer retention and positive regard.

Many examples of significant improvements are evident from using the Baldrige-based management system and many practices have been included in the sample effective practices after each Criteria description in the book. Following is the performance description of the organization that in 2002 was the first recipient of the Baldrige Award

Sisters of Saint Mary (SSM) Health Care, Health Care Category. Based in St. Louis, MO, SSM Health Care (SSMHC) is a not-for profit Catholic health system providing primary, secondary, and tertiary health care services. The system owns, manages, and is affiliated with 21 acute care hospitals and three nursing homes in four states: Missouri, Illinois, Wisconsin, and Oklahoma. Nearly 5,000 affiliated physicians and 22,200 staff work together to provide a wide range of services, including emergency, medical/surgical, oncology, mental health, obstetric, cardiology, orthopedic, pediatric, and rehabilitative care. SSMHC delivers its health care services in inpatient, outpatient, emergency department, and ambulatory surgery settings within its acute care hospitals. Other services, which support SSMHC's core hospital business, include physician practices, residential and skilled

nursing, home care and hospice, information services, and materials management.

SSMHC generates approximately $1.7 billion annually with 22,200 staff and locations in the following states: Illinois (3), Missouri (10), Oklahoma (4), and Wisconsin (4).

Quality and performance achievements include the following:

- As part of SSMHC's "Clinical Collaborative" process, physicians work with other caregivers, administrators, and staff to make rapid improvements in clinical outcomes. Selection of clinical collaboratives occurs in alignment with system goals, such as improving patient outcomes, satisfaction, and safety.

- SSMHC has undertaken six collaboratives, involving 85 teams in 2002, up from 14 teams in 1999.

- The results for SSMHC's clinical collaboratives for patients with congestive heart failure and ischemic heart disease demonstrate levels that approach or exceed national benchmarks.

- CARE PATHWAYS®, protocols, and standing orders are used to outline a standardized plan of care for SSMHC's patients. These tools are designed with patient input and are intended to create partnerships with physicians to improve patient care.

- For the fourth consecutive year, SSMHC has maintained an investment-grade rating in the "AA Credit Rating" Category (by Standard & Poor's and Fitch). This rating is attained by fewer than 1 percent of U.S. hospitals.

- The SSMHC systemwide "Healthy Communities" initiative was launched in 1995 to leverage the system's resources with those of the communities it serves. SSMHC supports staff at all levels of the organization to participate on teams involved in identifying opportunities for community outreach. Currently, SSMHC is providing in excess of 29 percent of the previous year's operating margin to provide care to communities that are economically, physically, and socially disadvantaged.

- SSMHC's Strategic, Financial, and Human Resource Planning Process extends over a 12-month cycle and involves all of the organization's networks, entities, and departments.

- System management sets and communicates system wide goals to each entity and provides standardized forms and definitions to ensure a consistent format and alignment of plans with the system's overall goals. Department goals are further cascaded to the staff, with individual "Passports" reflecting individual goals that support the department goals. SSMHC's share of the market in the St. Louis area increased over each of the past three years to 18 percent, while three of its five competitors have lost market share.

- SSMHC has established formal and informal listening and learning tools for former and current patients and their families; surveys are customized for each of the key segments including potential patients. Tools include satisfaction surveys, market research, comment cards, a complaint management system, patient follow-up calls, and an Internet response system.

- SSMHC uses an automated system to make clinical, financial, operational, customer, and market performance information available to all of its sites. SSMHC makes data available to physician partners from any location via multiple devices, including personal computers, personal digital assistants, pagers, and fax machines. The number of connected physicians has increased steadily from 3,200 in 1999 to 7,288 in 2002.

- SSMHC uses a Continuous Quality Improvement (CQI) Process Design Model to design its key health care, support, and business processes. A CQI Process Improvement Model is used to make improvements to existing processes. Employee satisfaction data, internal customer feedback, and outcome and in-process measures are used to facilitate rapid identification and correction of potential problems.

- SSMHC tailors employee benefits to provide flexibility and respond to women employees who make up 82 percent of its workforce.

- SSMHC offers flexible work hours, work at home options, long-term care insurance, insurance coverage for legally domiciled adults, retreats, and wellness programs. Tuition assistance and student loan repayment programs are highly regarded as significant benefits differentiating SSMHC from its competitors. SSMHC's turnover rate for all staff has improved from 21 percent in 1999 to 13 percent as of August 2002.

- SSMHC has maintained a continuous focus on increasing the number of minorities in professional and managerial positions. Minorities in professional and managerial positions increased from almost 8 percent in 1997 to 9.2 percent in 2001, considerably better than the health care industry benchmark of 2 percent.

- The Team Excellence program (an award program for high-performing teams) is responsible for over $15 million in cost reductions and $103 million in revenue growth from 1996–2000.

The Integrated Management System

It is important to point out a fact that is perhaps obvious to all: in order to optimize organizational performance, organizations must actually use the principles contained in the Baldrige Criteria. It is not enough to think about them. It is not enough to have used them in the past and no longer continue to do so. It is not enough to use a part but not all of the Criteria. To leave out any part suboptimizes the performance of the organization.

Ingredients to Optimum Performance. Clearly, in today's highly competitive environment, success in the past means nothing. Desire, without disciplined and appropriate action, also means nothing. However, it is just as clear that implementing a disciplined approach to performance excellence based on the Baldrige Criteria produces high levels of performance. The key to the success of the Baldrige Criteria is the identification of the key drivers of high performance. The National Quality Award Office within the National Institute of Standards and Technology ensures that each element of the Baldrige Criteria is necessary and together they are sufficient to achieve the highest levels of performance. Many management practices of the past have proven to be "necessary" ingredients of high performance. However, when practiced in isolation, these practices by themselves have not been sufficient to achieve optimum performance. Achieving high levels of performance requires that each component of the organization's management system be optimized.

In many ways, optimizing the performance of an organization's management system is like making an award-winning cake. Too much or too little of any key ingredient sub optimizes the system. For example, a cake may require eggs, flour, sugar, butter, and cocoa. A cake also requires a certain level of heat for a certain amount of time in an oven. Too little or too much of any ingredient, including oven temperature, and the system (in this case, the cake) fails.

The same principle is true in an organization. A successful health care organization requires a strong patient and customer focus, skilled staff, efficient work and health care service processes, fact-based decision making, clear direction, and continuous improvement. Organizations that do not focus on all of these elements find that their performance suffers. Focusing on only a few of the required ingredients, such as improving work processes in admissions or training to improve staff skills, are necessary but not sufficient by themselves to drive high levels of performance.

Figure 1 contains the elements necessary and sufficient to achieve high levels of performance in any organization or part of an organization. The following principles apply to any managed enterprise, large or small.

Get Results, Be Valued. (Figure 2) In order for an organization, a team, or individual to be successful and stay in the health care service business for any length of time, it must first produce desired results. It must be valued. History has demonstrated that people, organizations, or even governments that failed to deliver value eventually went away or were overturned. Value for health care can be measured in a variety of ways, including clinical outcomes, positive patient care and cure indicators, positive referral, return on assets, profitability, reliability, and competitive awards, to name a few.

Patients and Customers—Understand and Meet Their Requirements. (Figure 3) In addition, we have learned that it makes no difference if the provider of the services believes they are valuable if the patient, customer, or user of the services believes they are not. The patient or customer is the only entity that can legitimately judge the value of the services provided. Patients and customers must make the final decision as to whether the organization, team, or government continues to stay in business. Imagine you go to a clinic for an inoculation. You sit in the waiting room and use the restroom and find that neither is clean. Upon complaining about the lack of cleanliness, the supervisor claims that the facility is cleaned daily by reliable staff and she has always been proud of the level of cleanliness of the facilities. It does not help that the supervisor finds the facilities clean. They still seem dirty to you, and unless the supervisor is willing to make improvements, you are not going to be satisfied and are

Integrated Management System

Integrated Management System

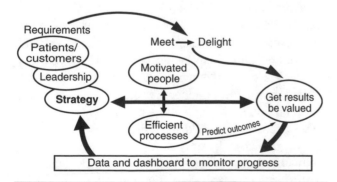

Figure 1 Integrated management system.

Figure 2 Get results, be valued.

unlikely to return. If enough patients and customers find the facilities or service offensive and do not return, the clinic goes out of business.

Accordingly, it is very important for the organization to clearly understand the requirements of its patients and customers and obtain feedback after they have an opportunity to experience its facilities or services. The failure to understand the requirements of the patients and customers may cause the organization to deliver the wrong thing, thus creating dissatisfaction, delay, or lower value. Every time an organization fails to understand and meet requirements, value suffers. In order to consistently produce value, therefore, organizations must accurately determine the requirements of its patients and customers and consistently meet or exceed those requirements. This creates the initial value chain that provides the competitive advantage for any organization or part of an organization.

To ensure that the patient or customer is satisfied, and likely to return again if services are needed, it is important to determine if appropriate value was received and to check for satisfaction. If the patient or customer is dissatisfied, you have an opportunity to correct the problem and still maintain loyalty. In any case, it is important to remember that it is the patient and customer—not the marketing department, engineering, manufacturing, or the service provider—that judges value received and determines ultimate satisfaction.

Motivated People. (Figure 4) The next part of the management system to ensure optimum performance

and value involves motivated people. In any organization or part of an organization, people do the work that produces patient and customer value and successful health care results. As described above, if the work is not focused on patient and customer requirements, they may be dissatisfied. In order to satisfy patients and customers, work may have to be redone, adding cost and suboptimizing value. In order to optimize output and value, people doing the work must have the willingness and desire to work. Disgruntled, disaffected, unwilling staff hurt productivity.

However, "motivated people" means more than simply possessing the willingness to work. People must also possess the knowledge and skills to carry out their jobs effectively. In leading-edge technologies, such as microelectronics engineering, the half-life of useful knowledge is less than one year. That means that one-half of the relevant knowledge of a microelectronics engineer becomes obsolete within 12 months. Ten years ago the half-life was 18 months, 50 percent greater. As new knowledge is created at an accelerating rate, it is more critical than ever to ensure effective training systems are in place to ensure that health care staff are up to date and can effectively apply the new knowledge.

In order to optimize output, people must also be free from bureaucratic barriers and arbitrary restrictions that inhibit work. Every time work is delayed while waiting for an unnecessary approval, cost is added, but not value. Every time work has to be redone due to the sloppy performance of a co-worker, cost is added, but not value. Every time that work has to be

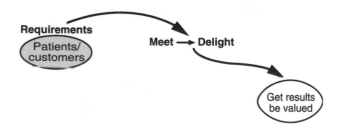

Figure 3 Patients and customers.

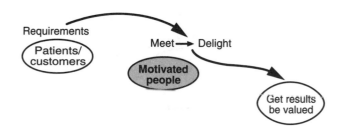

Figure 4 Motivated people.

redone because of inadequate knowledge or ability, cost is added but not value.

Remember that a single person cannot produce optimum levels of performance. However, a single person can prevent optimum levels of performance, and may not be aware that he or she is doing so. The question that should concern management is, "In your organization, how many people are disgruntled, discouraged, underskilled, or prevented from working effectively so that they suboptimize the organization's performance?"

Efficient Processes. (Figure 5) Even the most highly skilled, knowledgeable, and willing workers will fail to optimize value if asked to do stupid things. Over time, even the most efficient processes can become suboptimum and inefficient. Business process reengineering allows organizations to redesign and quickly eliminate much of the bureaucratic silliness and inefficiency that grows up over time. However, how long does it take for the newly reengineered process to lose efficiency? Even new processes must be evaluated periodically and improved or they eventually become suboptimal and obsolete. Ensuring that processes are optimal requires ongoing evaluation and refinement.

Every process in the organization has the potential for increasing or decreasing the value provided to patients and customers. Obviously, core health care service and business processes are the most important. However, frequently the core processes of an organization are disrupted because of failed support processes. For example, in scheduling patients, if services are

consistently late and patients are waiting hours for appointments and even procedures, these services will lose value, even if they are successful.

Any time an organization engages in rework, value for the customer is suboptimized. To make matters worse, if the need to engage in rework is not discovered until the service is complete, the cost of correction is higher, driving value lower. It is important, therefore, to uncover potential problems as early as possible, rather than wait for the end result to determine if the service is satisfactory. In order to uncover potential problems early we must be able to predict the outcomes of our work processes. This requires "in-process" measures. Through the use of these measures, organizations can determine if the service is likely to meet expectations. Consider these two examples:

- Example one: A customer comes to the hospital, goes to the "Wait-and-See" coffee shop, and orders a cup of coffee. The coffee is poured and delivered to the customer. The customer promptly takes a sip and informs the server that the coffee is too cold, too bitter, too weak, and has a harsh aroma. Furthermore, the customer complains that it took too long for the coffee to be served. The server, in an effort to satisfy the customer, discards the original coffee, brews a fresh pot, and delivers a new cup of coffee to the customer at no additional charge. This problem happens frequently. The "Wait-and-See" coffee shop has been forced to raise the price of coffee in order to stay in business and has noticed that fewer customers are willing to pay the higher price. Many customers have stopped coming to this coffee shop entirely. The customers that continue to buy coffee from this shop are subsidizing the sloppy performance and poor quality.

- Example two: In order to increase the likelihood that its customers will like the coffee it serves, the hospital's "In-Process-Measure" coffee shop has asked its customers key questions about the quality of coffee and service they expect. The "In-Process-Measure" coffee shop has determined through testing and surveys that its customers like coffee served hot (between 76 and

Integrated Management System

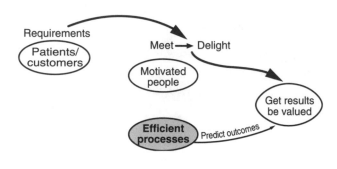

Figure 5 Efficient processes.

82 degrees Celsius); not too bitter or acidic (pH > 7.4); strong, but not too strong (75 grams of superfine grind per liter of filtered water); with a fresh aroma (is served within five minutes of brewing). By checking these measures, this coffee shop knows that nearly all customers will be satisfied with the quality and service it delivers. Since its customers like the coffee within the limits described above, no rework is required, no coffee is discarded, the price is lower, the value is higher, the store is profitable and is taking customers away from the "Wait-and-See" coffee shop.

Information and Data. (Figure 6) In-process measures help the organization and its staff make better decisions about their work. This enables them to spot problems more quickly and take actions to improve performance and correct or minimize non value-added costs. Without appropriate measures, organizations and staff must rely on intuition. They must wait for patients and customers to respond or guess at their likely satisfaction/dissatisfaction. Measures need to include those most important to patients, however. For example, patient comfort may be an important in-process measure.

One of the problems in basing decisions on intuition or best guess is that it produces highly variable outcomes. The guess of one employee is not likely to be consistent with the guess of another. Appropriate data, therefore, are critical to increase decision-making consistency and accuracy. If data are used to support decision making, organizations must develop a system to manage, collect, analyze, and display the results.

If the data that drive decision making are not accurate or reliable, effective decision making suffers. More mistakes are made, costs increase, and value is suboptimized. In the absence of data, leaders are generally unwilling to allow subordinates to substitute their intuition for that of the leader. As a result, decisions get pulled to higher and higher levels in an organization, further suboptimizing the contribution of staff who are generally closest to and know the most about the work they do. Failure to fully utilize the talents of workers, as discussed above, further reduces efficiency and morale, and suboptimizes value production.

The system described above, which includes patients and customers, motivated people, efficient processes, and a dashboard to monitor progress leading to desired results and value, applies to any managed enterprise. It applies to whole corporations as well as departments, divisions, teams, and individual work. The system applies to schools, government agencies, and health care organizations. In each case, in order to produce optimal value, the requirements of patients and customers must be understood and met. People must be motivated, possess the skill and knowledge needed to do their work, and be free from distractions in order to optimize their performance.

Leadership. (Figure 7) What makes an organization unique is the direction that top leaders set for it. Leaders must understand the requirements of patients and customers and the marketplace in deciding what direction is necessary to achieve success. However it is not enough only to understand requirements. Leaders must also understand organizational capabilities and the needs and capabilities of staff, partners, and suppliers.

Strategy. (Figure 8) Effective leaders use the process of strategy development to determine the most appropriate direction for the organization and identify the actions that must be taken to be successful in the future. Leaders use this strategy to identify the people and the processes that must be put in place to produce desired results and be valued by patients and customers.

Integrated Management System

Figure 6 Information and data.

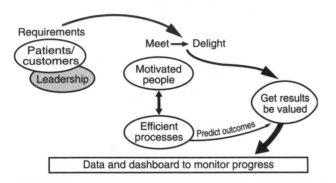

Figure 7 Leadership.

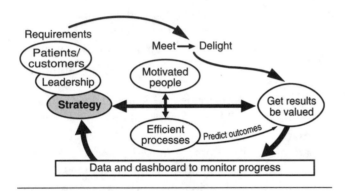

Figure 8 Strategy.

If leaders are not clear about the strategy and direction that must be taken to be successful, they force subordinates to substitute their own ideas about

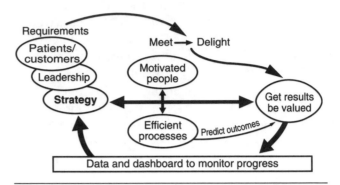

Figure 9 Integrated Management System.

the proper direction and actions. This creates chaos within an organization. People come to work and want to be successful. Without direction from the top, they will still work hard but often at cross-purposes. Unless everyone is pulling in the same direction, processes, and health care services will not be optimized and value will be reduced.

Leaders cannot eliminate a single part of this management system and still expect to produce optimum value. Each part is necessary, as shown in Figure 9.

Furthermore, studies repeatedly demonstrate that when these processes are integrated and used to run health care services, they are sufficient to achieve high levels of performance. Imagine what might happen if one or more of the pieces of the integrated management system described above were missing. The following table provides some suggestions.

MISSING ELEMENT	ADVERSE CONSEQUENCE LEADING TO SUBOPTIMUM PERFORMANCE
Systems to understand patient and customer requirements.	Designing, building, and delivering an unsatisfactory health care service. Adds delay. Increases cost due to rework.
Poor staff skills. Minimal initiative or self-direction.	Limited growth and development opportunities. Unable to keep up with changing technology. Requires close supervision. Difficulty in finding better ways to carry out work. Ultimately reduces morale, motivation, and performance.
Data about patient and customer satisfaction, key process performance, and overall organizational performance do not exist or are incomplete.	Makes it difficult to engage staff in decision making about their work. Forces decisions to be made at higher levels on the basis of intuition or guesswork. Reduces decision accuracy and increases incorrect decisions. Makes it difficult to allocate resources appropriately or determine the best use of limited resources.
Leaders do not clearly set direction, performance expectations, vision, or values.	Causes subordinates to invent their own ideas and substitute them for a common set of performance expectations, vision, and values. Creates significant inefficiencies as people throughout the organization begin the work at cross-purposes, suboptimizing organizational performance.
Plans do not contain measurable objectives and a time line for accomplishing each objective.	Leaders, managers, and staff do not know what level of performance is expected at any given time, making it difficult or impossible to effectively monitor progress. Accountability is not present.
Leaders do not make it clear that patients and customers are the key to success.	If managers and staff do not focus on patient and customer then they become internally focused. Departments, disciplines, or marketing drives the organization, not patient and customer. Patients and their requirements lose importance.
Top leaders do not encourage staff to develop and use their full potential.	Staff empowerment and well-being become optional. Some managers encourage staff participation, innovation, and creativity; most do not. The organization risks losing its best staff to competitors.
Patient and other customer comments and complaints are not encouraged. If a complaint is received, it is not resolved promptly. The root cause of complaints is not identified.	Failure to capture patient and other customer comments and complaints, identify the root causes of the complaint, and work to prevent the problem from happening again makes it difficult to learn about problems quickly and dooms the organization to repeat its failures. Failure to resolve complaints promptly increases patient and customer dissatisfaction and reduces loyalty.
Poor two-way communication exists between leaders and the organization.	Unclear top-down communication makes it difficult to ensure alignment and focus throughout the organization, reducing teamwork and increasing bureaucratic stagnation. Poor upward communication maintains organizational fragmentation and prevents problems and barriers to effective work from being discussed and resolved.

PRACTICAL INSIGHTS

Connections, and Linkages

A popular children's activity, connect the dots, helps them understand that, when properly connected, apparently random dots create a meaningful picture. In many ways, the seven categories, 19 items, and 32 areas to address in the Baldrige Criteria are like the dots that must be connected to reveal a meaningful picture. With no paths to make the web, or join the dots, staff development and work systems are not related to strategic planning; information and analysis are isolated from process management; and overall improvement efforts are disjointed, fragmented, and do not yield robust results.

Some health care organizations have improved in selected areas, such as in emergency room (ER) waiting times, operating room (OR) delays, home care registration completeness, service delivery, and billing cycle times. Often these achievements are isolated instances of success. They are not spread throughout the organization. It is through the understanding of the connections and linkages among the Baldrige Items that organization-wide impact becomes powerfully possible. This book describes the linkages for and between each item. The exciting part about having them identified is that you can look for these linkages in the organization and, if they don't exist, start building them.

Transition Strategies

Putting high-performance management systems in place is a major commitment that will not happen quickly. At the beginning, you will need a transition strategy to get you across the bridge from management by opinion or intuition to more data-driven management. The next part of this section describes one approach that has worked for many organizations in various sectors, including health care: creating a performance improvement council.

Performance Improvement Council

Identify a top-level executive leadership group of six to 10 members, inclusive of physicians and clinicians.

Each member over that number will seem to double the complexity of issues and make decision making much more cumbersome. The executive leadership group could send a message to the entire organization by naming the group the performance improvement council—reinforcing the importance of continuous performance improvement to the future success of the organization.

The performance improvement council needs to be invested and empowered as the primary policy-making body for the organization. It will spawn other performance improvement councils at lower levels to share practices and policies with staff as well as involve current and potential patients and other customers, and suppliers. The structure permeates the organization as members of the performance improvement council become area leaders for major improvement efforts and sponsors for several process or continuous improvement task teams throughout the organization. The council structure, networked and cascaded fully, can effectively align the work and optimize performance at all levels and across all functions.

Council Membership

Selecting members for the performance improvement council should be done carefully. Each member should be essential for the success of the operation, and together they must be sufficient for success. The most important member is the senior leader of the organization or unit. This person must participate actively, demonstrating the kind of leadership that all should emulate. Of particular importance is a commitment to consensus building as the modus operandi for the council. This tool, a core of performance improvement programs, is often overlooked by leadership. Clinician participation from the very beginning is essential. Choose physicians most respected by the medical staff and who are committed, articulate, and passionate about the imperative of medical excellence. Choose physicians and clinicians interested in learning and teaching. Other clinicians, such as nurses and therapists, serve this same key function in long-term care and home care operations. Other council members selected should have leadership responsibility for broad areas of the organization, such as personnel, operations planning, patients/customers, and data systems.

Council Learning and Planning

The performance improvement council needs to be extremely knowledgeable about high-performance management systems. If not, as is often the case, performance improvement council members need to be among the first in the organization to learn about continuous improvement tools and processes.

To be effective, every member of the council (and every member in the organization) must understand the Baldrige Criteria, because the Criteria describe the components of the entire management system. Participation in examiner training has proved to be an excellent way to understand the complexities of the system needed to achieve Performance Excellence. Any additional training needs to be carried out in the context of planning—that is, learn tools and use them to plan the performance improvement implementation, practices, and policies.

The performance improvement council has responsibility to:

- Develop an integrated, continuous improvement, strategic performance improvement, and health care service plan.

- Create the web (communication plan and infrastructure) to transmit performance improvement policies throughout the organization.

- Define the roles of staff, including new recognition and reward structures to cause needed behavioral changes.

- Develop a master training and development plan. Involve team representatives in planning so they can learn skills close to when they are needed. Define what is provided to whom, and when and how success will be measured.

- Launch improvement projects that will produce both short- and long-term successes. Improvement projects should be clearly defined by the performance improvement council and driven by the strategic plan. Typical improvement projects include important staff processes, such as career development, performance measurement, and diversity, as well as improving health care services.

- Develop a plan to communicate the progress and successes of the organization. Through this approach, the need for performance improvement processes is consistently communicated to all staff. Barriers to optimum performance are weakened and eliminated.

- Create champions to promote performance excellence through the categories of the Baldrige Criteria.

Category Champions

This section describes the responsibilities of category champions. The people in the appropriate administrative or clinical leadership role should each be the champion of a category. If the organization is a hospital, many category champions will be physicians. It depends on the organization—but given the dual medical-administrative structure in most health care organizations, the more the physicians serve as category champions, the better.

Organizational Leadership Champion

The *organizational leadership champion* is a senior executive who, in addition to other executive duties, works to coordinate and enhance leadership effectiveness and alignment throughout the organization. It is both a strategic and an operational activity.

From the strategic side, the champion should focus on ensuring that all senior leaders:

- Understand what is expected of them as leaders of organizational change.

- Ensure that effective governance systems are in place to protect the interests of all patient, customer, and stakeholder groups and maintain organizational integrity and ethical behavior.

- Consistently speak with one voice as a senior leadership team.

- Serve as role models of performance excellence for managers and staff at all levels of the organization.

- Set clear strategy and directions to enhance future opportunities for the organization.

- Develop future leaders (succession planning) throughout the organization.

- Create measurable performance expectations and monitor performance to achieve the key improvements and strategic objectives of the organization. This means that necessary data and analyses must be coordinated to ensure appropriate information is available for the champion and the entire senior leadership team.

From the operational side, the champion should work to identify and eliminate both individual and system deficiencies, territorial conflicts, and knowledge shortfalls that limit a leader's ability to meet expectations and goals consistently.

The champion should be the focal point in the organization to ensure all parts of the organization have systematic processes in place so they fully understand leadership and management requirements.

A process should exist to monitor ongoing initiatives to ensure leaders effectively set and communicate organizational values to staff.

- They must demonstrate that they focus on delivering value to patients and customers and other stakeholders.

- They must aggressively reinforce an environment that promotes empowerment and innovation throughout the workforce. This may involve reviewing policies, systems, work processes, and the use of resources—ensuring sufficient data are available to assist in manager and staff decision making.

- They should review (conduct independent audits) ethical and legal behavior of all leaders and managers and hold them accountable for their actions.

The champion should coordinate the activities involving the review of organizational performance and capabilities.

- Key performance measures should be defined.

- Systems to review organizational success, performance, and progress relative to goals should be in place.

- Performance review findings should be used to identify priorities for improvement. Those priorities should be communicated to all units that have responsibilities for making the improvements, including suppliers.

- Performance review findings, together with staff feedback, should be used systematically to assess and improve senior leadership (including the chief executive) effectiveness and the effectiveness of managers throughout the leadership system.

Finally, the champion must work as part of the senior leadership team to help coordinate all facets of the management system to drive high performance. This involves teaching the team about the requirements of effective and consistent leadership at all levels and its impact on organizational performance. The senior leader of the organization usually serves as the Organizational Leadership Champion and leads this council.

Strategic Planning Champion

The *strategic planning champion* is a senior executive who, in addition to other executive duties, works to coordinate and enhance strategic planning and action plan alignment throughout the organization. It is both a strategic and an operational activity.

From the strategic side, the champion should ensure that the focus of strategy development is on sustained competitive leadership, which usually depends on achieving revenue growth, as well as consistently improving operational effectiveness. The Strategic Planning Champion should help the senior leadership team acquire a view of the future and provide clear strategic guidance to the organization through goals, objectives, action plans, and measures.

From the operational side, the champion should work to ensure sufficient data are available regarding:

- The organization's operational and human resource strengths and weaknesses

- External risks and threats that may arise from competitors, supplier weaknesses, regulatory changes, economic conditions, and financial, ethical, and societal risks

- The competitive environment and other challenges that might affect future direction

The champion should be the focal point in the organization to ensure all parts of the organization have systematic processes in place so they fully understand the implications of strategy on their daily work.

The champion should ensure that strategy is patient-, customer- and market-focused and is actually used to guide ongoing decision making and resource allocation at all levels of the organization.

- A process should exist to convert strategy into actions at each level of the organization, which are aligned to achieve goals necessary for business success.

- Every employee should understand his or her role in carrying out actions to achieve the organization's goals.

The champion should coordinate the activities involving strategy development and deployment to:

- Acquire and use various types of forecasts, projections, scenarios, or other techniques to understand the plausible range of future options.

- Determine how the projected performance of competitors is likely to compare with the projected performance of the organization in the same time frame in order to set goals to insure competitive advantage.

- Define the expected path along which growth and performance are likely to take for strategic objective. Timelines of projected future performance should match the frequency of organizational performance reviews.

- Determine what capabilities must be developed within the organization to achieve strategic goals and coordinate with other members of the senior leadership team and category champions to ensure those capabilities are in place.

- Determine what changes in health care services might be needed as a part of strategic positioning and direction.

- Ensure a system is in place to develop action plans that address strategic goals and objectives. Ensure those action plans are understood throughout the organization, as appropriate.

- Ensure a system is in place to identify the human resource requirements necessary to achieve strategic goals and objectives. This may include training, support services for staff, reorganization, and new recruitment, to name a few.

- Ensure a system is in place to allocate resources throughout the organization sufficient to accomplish the action plans.

- Coordinate with the leadership system during performance reviews to help ensure priorities for improvement and innovation at different levels throughout the organization are aligned with strategy and action plans.

- Ensure the process for strategic planning, plan deployment, the development of action plans, and the alignment of resources to support actions is systematically evaluated and improved with each cycle. Also evaluate and improve the effectiveness of determining the projected performance of competitors for use in goal setting.

Finally, the champion must work as a contributing member of the senior leadership team to help coordinate all facets of the management system to drive high performance. This involves teaching the team about the requirements of strategic planning and its impact on organizational performance.

Patient and Customer Value Champion

The *patient and customer value champion* is a senior executive who, in addition to other executive duties, will coordinate and enhance customer satisfaction, relations, and loyalty throughout the organization. It is both a strategic and an operational activity.

From the strategic side, the champion should focus on ensuring that the drivers of patient and customer satisfaction, retention, and related market share (which are key factors in competitiveness, profitability, and health care success) are considered fully in the strategic planning process. This means that necessary data and analyses must be coordinated to ensure appropriate information is available for the executive planning councils.

From the operational side, the champion should work to identify and eliminate system deficiencies, territorial conflicts, and knowledge shortfalls that limit the organization's ability to meet patient and customer satisfaction, repeat business, and loyalty goals consistently.

The champion should be the focal point in the organization to ensure all parts of the organization have systematic processes in place so they fully understand key patient-, customer-, market-, and operational-requirements as input to customer satisfaction and market goals.

A process should exist to monitor ongoing initiatives to ensure they are aligned with the customer aspects of the strategic direction. This may involve:

- Reviewing policies, systems, work processes, the use of resources, and the availability of staff who are knowledgeable and focus on customer relations and loyalty

- Ensuring sufficient data are available to assist in decision making about patient and customer issues

- Ensuring that strategies and actions relating to customer issues are aligned at all levels of reorganization from the executives to the work unit or individual job level

The champion should coordinate the activities involving understanding customer requirements as well as managing the interaction with patients and customers, including how the organization determines patient and customer satisfaction and satisfaction relative to competitors. (Satisfaction relative to competitors and the factors that lead to customer preference are of increasing importance to managing in a competitive environment.)

- The champion should also examine the means by which patients and customers have access to seek information and assistance, or to comment and complain.

- The champion should coordinate the definition of patient and customer contact requirements (sometimes called customer service standards) and the deployment of those requirements to all points and people in the organization that have contact with patients and customers.

- The champion should ensure that systems exist to respond quickly and resolve complaints promptly to recover patient and customer confidence that might otherwise be lost.

- The champion should ensure that staff are responsible for the design and delivery of services and receive information about patient and customer complaints so they may eliminate the causes of these complaints.

- The champion should work with appropriate line managers to help set priorities for improvement projects based on the potential impact of the cost of complaints and the impact of patient and customer dissatisfaction and attrition on the organization.

- The champion should be charged with coordinating activities to build loyalty and positive referral, as well as evaluating and improving customer relationship-building processes throughout the organization.

Finally, the champion must work as a contributing member of the senior leadership team to help coordinate all facets of the management system to drive high performance. This involves teaching the team about the requirements of patient, customer and market focus and its impact on organizational performance.

Analysis and Knowledge Management Champion

The *analysis and knowledge management champion* is an executive-level person who, in addition to other executive duties, will coordinate and enhance information, analysis, and knowledge management systems throughout the organization to ensure that they meet the decision-making needs of managers, staff, patients, customers, and suppliers. It is both a strategic and an operational activity.

From the strategic side, information and analyses and the resulting knowledge can provide a competitive advantage. The champion should focus on ensuring, to the extent possible, that timely and accurate information and analyses are available to enhance knowledge acquisition and the development and delivery of new and existing products and services to meet ongoing and emerging patient and customer needs.

From the operational side, the champion should work to ensure that information and analyses are available throughout the organization to aid in decision making at all levels. This means coordinating with all other champions to ensure data are available for day-to-day review and decision making at all levels for their areas of responsibility.

The analysis and knowledge management champion has responsibility for both information infrastructure and ensuring the appropriate use of data for decision making. The champion should coordinate activities throughout the organization involving data collection, accuracy, analysis, retrieval, and use for decision making. The champion should ensure:

- Complete data are available and aligned to strategic goals, objectives, and action plans to ensure performance against these goals, objectives, and action plans can be effectively monitored.

- Systems are in place to collect and use comparative data and information to support strategy development, goal setting, and performance improvement.

Staff Focus Champion

The *staff focus champion* has responsibility for ensuring that staff (including managers and supervisors at all levels; permanent, temporary, and part-time personnel; and contract staff and volunteers supervised by the organization) needs are met to enable them to contribute fully to the organization's goals and objectives. The champion should ensure:

- Work and jobs are structured to promote cooperation, collaboration, individual initiative, innovation, and flexibility.

- An effective system exists to provide accurate feedback about staff performance and to enhance their performance. This includes systems to identify skill gaps and recruit or reassign staff to close those gaps, as well as ensuring that fair work practices are followed within the organization. This may also include evaluating managers and enhancing their ability to provide accurate feedback and effective coaching to improve staff performance.

- Compensation, recognition, and rewards are aligned to support high-performance objectives of the organization (contained in strategic plans and reported in the balanced scorecard or health care results report card).

- Education and training support health care objectives and build staff knowledge, skills, and capabilities to enhance staff career progression and performance. This includes ensuring staff understand tools and techniques of performance measurement, performance improvement, quality control methods, and benchmarking. This

also includes ensuring that managers and supervisors reinforce knowledge and skills on the job.

- The work environment is safe, with performance measures and targets for each key factor affecting staff safety.

- Factors that affect staff well-being, satisfaction, and motivation are routinely measured and actions are taken promptly to improve conditions that adversely affect morale, motivation, productivity, and other related health care results.

Finally, the champion must work as part of an organizationwide council to help coordinate all facets of the management system to drive high performance.

Process Management Champion

The *process management champion* is an executive-level person who, in addition to other executive duties, will coordinate and enhance all aspects of the organization's systems to manage and improve work processes to meet the organization's strategic objectives. This includes activities and processes to create value for patients and customers and other stakeholders and involves customer-focused design, product and service delivery, as well as internal support services. It is both a strategic and operational activity.

From the strategic side, rapid and accurate design, development, and delivery of health care services creates a competitive advantage in the marketplace.

From the operational side, the champion should work to ensure all key work processes are examined and optimized to achieve higher levels of performance, reduce cycle time and costs, and subsequently add to organizational profitability.

The process management champion has responsibility for creating a process management orientation within the organization. Since all work is a process, the Process Management Champion must ensure that the process owners (including processes owned by other champions) systematically examine, improve, and execute their processes consistently. The champion should ensure:

- Systematic continuous improvement activities are embedded in all processes, which lead to ongoing refinements.

- Initial and ongoing patient and customer requirements are incorporated into all health care service designs and delivery systems, and processes.

This includes core development processes as well as key health care (such as research and development, asset management, technology acquisition, and supply chain management) and internal support processes (such as finance and accounting, facilities management, administration, procurement, and personnel).

- Design and delivery processes are structured and analyzed to reduce cycle time; increase the use of learning from past projects or other parts of the organization; reduce costs; increase the use of new technology and other effectiveness or efficiency factors; and ensure all services meet performance requirements.

Finally, the champion must work as part of an organizationwide council to help coordinate all facets of the management system to drive high performance.

Results Champion

The *results champion* is an executive-level person who, in addition to other executive duties, will coordinate the display of the organization's business results. This champion has substantially different work than the champions for Categories 1 through 6. No actions leading to or resulting from the performance outcome data are championed by the Organizational Results Champion. Those actions are driven by the Category 1 through 6 champions because they have responsibility for taking action to implement and deploy procedures necessary to produce the business results. For example, the Analysis and Knowledge Management Champion (Category 4) is responsible for collecting data that reflect all areas of strategic importance leading to business results. The Analysis and Knowledge Management champion is also responsible for ensuring data accuracy and reliability.

The results champion is responsible, however, for ensuring that the organization is able to display all organizational results required by Category 7 to provide evidence of the organization's performance and improvement in key business areas and facilitate monitoring by leaders. These include health care results, patient and other customer satisfaction, financial and marketplace performance, staff results, operational performance and governance, and social responsibility results.

Results must be displayed by appropriate segment and group, such as different patient and customer groups, market segments, staff groups, or supplier groups. Appropriate comparison data must be included in the organizational results display to judge the relative "goodness" or "strength" of the results achieved. These results are used by senior leaders to monitor organizational performance.

Finally, the results champion must work as part of an organizationwide council to help coordinate all facets of the management system to drive high performance. For example, if the organization is not collecting data necessary for inclusion in the business results report card, the results champion coordinates work with the other champions on the council to ensure those data are available, used for decision making, and included in appropriate reports.

The Critical Skills

A uniform message, set of skills or core competencies, and constancy of purpose are critical to success. Core training should provide all staff with the knowledge and skills on which to build a learning organization that continually gets better. Such training typically includes team building, leadership skills, consensus building, communications, and effective meeting management. These are necessary for teams to solve critical problems.

Another important core skill involves using a common process to define patient and customer requirements accurately, determining the ability to meet those requirements, measure success, and determine the extent to which patients and customers—internal and external—are satisfied. When a problem arises, staff must be able to define the problem correctly, isolate the root causes, generate and select the best solution to eliminate the root causes, and implement the best solution.

It is also important to be able to understand data and make decisions based on facts, not merely intuition or feelings. Therefore, familiarity with tools to analyze work processes and performance data is important. With these tools, work processes can be analyzed and vastly improved. Reducing unnecessary steps in work processes, increasing process consistency, reducing variability, and reducing cycle time are powerful ways to improve quality and reduce cost simultaneously.

Courses in techniques to acquire comparison and benchmarking data, work process improvement and reengineering, supplier partnerships and certification, role modeling for leaders, strategic planning, team building, and enhancing patient/customer satisfaction and loyalty will help managers and staff increase their effectiveness.

Leadership Qualities and Skills of the Health Care CEO

What qualities and skills must the health care CEO possess to take the organization on the Performance Excellence superhighway? We are often asked for characteristics of a CEO that can bring about the change needed for Performance Excellence. The following skills, attitudes, and character traits are our requirements:

- Has an unending positive attitude, positive approach, and an overall positive outlook

- Is perpetually visionary

- Has a high tolerance for ambiguity

- Is flexible and understands that a plan is just a plan and can be changed

- Has the ability to let go so empowerment can happen

- Inspires confidence in others

- Possesses self-differentiation from the "united front" thinking

- Does not have a personal agenda but is able to always attend to the organization's agenda

- Understands the use of power and treats it with respect

- Keeps the focus and keeps it around the vision

- Is committed to the development of others

- Knows how to coach as opposed to supervise

- Understands the value of being a steward of the organization's mission

- Functions in an electronic age and is able to integrate that with the quality concepts

- Is able to orchestrate change

- Has a sense of curiosity and knows how to foster it in others

- Is able to communicate at all levels so that others understand

- Has the courage to do the unpleasant tasks

- Is not afraid to learn

- Is not afraid to take risks

- Knows the meaning of community—common-unity—and is able to connect with the community

- Is able to develop meaningful relationships

- Demonstrates a caring attitude and knows how to foster the healing process

- Can navigate the health care industry and the political landscape

- Understands organizational structure and how to enhance board involvement with the organization

- Has an effective understanding of the practice of medicine and is passionate about its potential

- Understands the challenges and pressures faced by physicians and is able to guide and inspire them to achieve their potential as a customer, employee, and/or business partner of the institution

- Is highly visible throughout the organization and recognizes that more is learned making rounds than by any other endeavor

THE IMPERATIVE FOR PERFORMANCE EXCELLENCE IN HEALTH CARE

Health Care: The Current State

Donald M. Berwick, M.D., President of the Institute for Healthcare Improvement, has advised that, "Our challenge is to have the courage to name boldly the problems we have, which are many, at the size they occupy, which is immense. The timing of incremental improvement, if not coming to a close, is needing the additional energy of fundamental changes."

The readers of this book are people who devote their careers to the health care services industry. This industry was once cherished for its commitment to healing. Physicians were leaders in the community. Nurses were admired for doing angelic work. It is now too often perception, and sometimes the reality, that this is no longer the case. It is time for the health care industry, blessed with talent and resources, to do the work necessary to recapture the image and confidence of the people it serves.

Health care delivery is dependent on knowledge, compassion, process, and technology. Today, the health care industry is blessed with remarkable talent and expertise and many of our institutions possess significant resources to support the practice of health. Yet, health care organizations continue in various forms of disarray. Financial performance in even some of our better-known organizations remains weak. In some communities there is significant over-capacity, and on others too little capacity, causing long delays in receipt of emergency care. Bond ratings of many health organizations have suffered three years of downgrading. Corporate scandals, not unlike highly publicized failures in manufacturing and service industries, have plagued the health care industry as well. Patients are increasingly demanding and increasingly dissatisfied.

A study by the Institute for Healthcare Improvement found only 15 percent of physicians surveyed believed their work environment is good to excellent. Workforce shortages in key disciplines challenge institutions to provide fully competent health care and reduces workforce morale.

Millions of people have no or unequal access to care, although the per capita expense for health care in United States is 30 percent higher than the next most expensive country. The high cost of health care services, often the burden of employers, has again accelerated well beyond other increases in the cost of living. States across the nation are finding it increasingly difficult to support their share of health care expenses for Medicaid and other health care programs facing billions of dollars of funding deficits in a declining economy.

Injuries to patients by avoidable adverse events and errors have gained the attention of the public and much work remains to fully redress it. The variation in the practice of medicine from one organization to the next or from one clinician to the next cannot be justified by science. Evidence-based medicine research has demonstrated that certain diagnostic and treatment courses are more effective than others. Yet the care delivered in one emergency room for myocardial infarction or pneumonia differs from the next emergency room. The care provided at 4 a.m. in the same emergency room may differ from the care at 9 a.m. A patient may not get the same quality care if his/her doctor is on vacation. The variation quality is significant and unsupportable.

Despite this litany of challenges, there is much cause for optimism. The health care industry in America is blessed with extraordinary resources of talent and funding. The principal problem is that the leadership of our health care organizations has not yet taken effective action to maximize the potential value of either the talent or the revenue.

It is time for the leaders, professionals, and staff that do the hard work of health care to become revered by the people served. The opportunity exists to do it. The Baldrige framework offers the most effective road map. The challenge is up to you.

Health Care 2003 and Beyond: The Future

Despite these dilemmas, there is good reason to be cautiously optimistic about the future course of the business of health care services. Health care in the United States is still, in many ways, considered the world-class standard. It is sought after by foreign nationals able to seek care beyond that available in their country. The potential to "trade" health care via the Internet will be clearer as the e-commerce industry moves through its adjustment cycles. The opportunity for a global presence in health care is promising. In addition to the research engine, the industry is blessed with an enviable pool of highly skilled talent. Continued learning is expected and accepted. Demand for the services of health care providers will grow as the population ages. The product pipeline increases with new health care services derived from research, gene mapping, and more.

If properly managed, the future opportunities are endless. However, there is an urgent need to improve how health care is provided today. Health care leaders must understand and take action on the imperative for Performance Excellence. Senior leaders of health care organizations must ensure that:

- Their system of leadership is effective and up to the challenge.

- The strategic planning process works to identify opportunities to succeed and to meet stretch targets.

- The strategic plans are converted to action plans and used to align work throughout the organization.

- Market data are valid and segmented for precise design and marketing of services that will sell.

- Patients and families have easy access and patient/customer satisfaction determination is accurate for further decision making and resource commitment.

- The information system is based on user needs and produces actionable information for decision makers and for the daily delivery of health care.

- Job responsibilities are designed to meet the changing dynamics of health care delivery and needed skills are secured for new initiatives.

- New services offered to patients and customers are designed systematically throughout the organization with patient/customer input and testing prior to making final resource implementation decisions.

- Cost cutting efforts will result in increased productivity and not just be short-lived cost reductions that demoralize staff.

- Business partners—or, increasingly, joint venture partners—are themselves competent and aligned with the needs/objectives of the organization.

- The performance results, key to critical success factors, are tracked, trended, compared to the competition and best-in-industry, and used to further improve everywhere.

By taking these actions and committing to improve performance at every level, we can expect the following types of outcomes:

- Zero adverse drug events in all patient care areas

- Fewer complaints

- Fewer patient accidents or falls

- Reduced OR waiting times, resulting in increased OR throughput and increased revenue, with no measurable increase in adverse outcomes

- Access to care available 24/7/365 without long waits, obtrusive non-value-added permission, unnecessary forms, and restrictions on getting needed health care expertise

- Reduced avoidable morbidity or complication rates

- Reduced nosocomial infection rates

- 100 percent of lab and X-ray reports on the chart or available for decision making by clinicians

- No lost medical records

- Medications administered when prescribed and not according to change in personnel shifts

- Increased patient compliance with home care services

- Increased patient, payor, and physician satisfaction

- Reduced patient waiting times everywhere

- Reduced accounts receivable days outstanding

- Reduced waste of supplies and food

- More rapid patient return to normal life routine

All health care professionals are familiar with clinical quality. They focus on this every day to assure that the best clinical outcome is possible. The Joint Commission on Accreditation of Healthcare Organizations (JCAHO) has been requiring clinical quality for years. Managers and physicians monitor elements of care and report any untoward events on a regular schedule. However, the other side of the excellence quest is often overlooked by health care management—and that is service excellence.

Health care providers are often so preoccupied with the clinical side that they miss what patients/customers call the human or personal side of health care delivery. Service excellence is that personal side.

To be successful in this area means exceeding patient and customer expectations. A positive and nurturing environment enhances the healing process. In the best health care organizations, excellence means service performance as well as clinical performance. Health care leaders identify process improvement opportunities and train the workforce so that excellence is nurtured and deployed throughout the organization. Excellence in service is possible only with effective decision making at all levels, including the front line. This is the challenge of leadership—the spirit of health care—and it starts at the top.

It is up to the CEO to lead the way. This cannot be emphasized enough. The CEO sets the standard. Every ship has its captain who charts the course and sets the sails. Developing a framework for excellence is charting that course. Educating and instilling the legacy of caring is setting the sail. Now the course is set, the crew is in line, and the destination is in sight. To bring it all home is not an easy task. It takes a commitment that needs to be continually reinforced.

Computers, fax machines, cell phones, e-mail, voice mail, regulations, telemedicine, and more have distanced health care workers from patients and customers, both external (the patient) and internal (the health care associate). Health care is "Big Business." Unfortunately, many often are caught up in the stress of it all. There is a great deal of stress as the organizational change ramps up. For these reasons, as well as to hang onto the personal caring side, there is a need to "bring the spirit back!"

A Case Study:

Moving the Organization Forward

Community Health System (CHS) is a small health care system in upstate New York. With seven organizations and very diverse agendas, CHS leaders asked the question: "How does one move seven corporations in the same direction at the same time?" The answer and the challenge was to empower the workforce.

At CHS, the employees were called "associates." The word associate means partner, and the associates truly are partners. It is through developing partnerships that performance excellence is achieved. Top management set the example. The top level led the organization through the massive change effort that transformed the organization into a team of involved, committed, and dedicated associates. This commitment is the true test of leadership, not the management "principles" leaders are taught.

The associates are the most important component in health care. They are the organization's most valuable resource. Everything happens because of them. That is why management is there—to give them all the tools, knowledge, and skills they need to deliver the excellence that the customer expects and deserves. CHS found a direct correlation between associate satisfaction and customer satisfaction

CEOs and top leaders set the example at CHS. The CEO set the vision in partnership with the board, medical staff, and management and translated that vision into reality. The CEO kept the organization focused on the vision throughout the change process. There was and always will be significant resistance and "noise" while an organization is changing. Having a focus to reference continually was very important. It kept the organization on the right path. That is why a framework for Performance Excellence was a great tool for the CEO and CHS.

The first step in building Performance Excellence was creating a framework within which all can work. It was definitely a building process that took time. It was a process that occurred with continual nurturing, "grain by grain, a loaf—stone by stone, a castle" (a Yugoslavian proverb). A framework defined and promoted the corporate health care culture. Most importantly, it provided a structure through which the associates could be successful in their role. The framework also integrated management practices and laid the groundwork for that success. Previously, management was often fragmented and pulled in different directions depending on the vice president's or department manager's perception of priorities. The framework clearly defined the direction of the whole organization. Managers followed organizationwide goals in making decisions about priorities. It was also a structure for rewarding the associates for performance improvement actions that furthered the organizational direction.

The framework was the basis and the key to empowerment. It allowed everyone in the organization to change and make decisions without fear. It clearly demonstrated that there were certain decisions that belonged to management alone; there were certain decisions that the associates could make for themselves without management; and there were decisions that were made together. The framework fit the organizational philosophy. At CHS, the framework included the vision, mission, values, key results areas, and strategic plan, including corporate goals and work plans.

The values were a major part of the framework. At CHS, the values of commitment, action, respect, excellence, and service (CARES) were the core of the framework. The managers and associates determined the true values of the organization. Senior management led the roll-out campaign. The associates embraced the values quickly and with excitement. As long as associates made decisions at the front line within the boundaries of the framework, it was the right decision. It was the associates' actions in excellence that brought the framework to life. At Community Health System, the framework was and is The Community Health System Way—the way to excellence.

It was very important that the framework was used every day and in every way possible. In doing so it continued to be deployed throughout the system. The values were used as the basis of rewards and recognition. The manner in which the organization communicated was grounded in the framework. It was most important for the CEO, senior management, and middle management to continually teach, use, and reinforce the framework. The CEO had regular sessions to strengthen this culture. Quarterly, "CHS Way" sessions communicated what was happening, and a Community Health System Way newsletter taught aspects of the framework that reinforced the corporate culture.

Commitment and Responsibility

To ensure that the organization believed and understood that its leaders supported the framework, the commitment by the leadership of the organization was critical. Leaders took actions that supported commitments, clearly understood the expectations and the process, and took responsibility for implementation. At CHS, the commitment took the form of everyone signing a group commitment statement. The group commitment statement was very effective in that the team bonded together in the new corporate culture.

The Board of Directors were committed and understood the process improvement initiative.

In health care organizations, investments are typically made in equipment like ultrasound and CT scanners. It was just as important, if not more so, for CHS to invest in human resources. Deploying Performance Excellence was that investment. There was a return on investment methodology for human resource investments that clearly demonstrated to the board the value of that investment.

CHS associates care and believe in caring because it is the legacy that was established when the health care organization was founded. That is the legacy they continue to pursue. It is up to management to instill in the associates the belief, the expectation, and the desire to deliver on the promise of excellence and caring. Many people do not think that caring is OK. In health care, it is the caring that sets us apart. It is the caring that brings meaning to life and that is what we strive for in excellence.

At CHS, like any health care organization, the medical staff was a very important group to include in the process. They were an integral part of the team and needed to understand the difference between clinical excellence and service excellence. When CHS first introduced Performance Excellence initiatives, there was little preparation with the medical staff. As a result, significant resistance occurred. Educating the medical staff on the processes, terminology, and nuances of Performance Excellence not only brought them on board with the rest of the organization, but also assisted them in their own practices. Physician office practices that functioned in a Performance Excellence mode reinforced the effort of the health system.

Managers needed to understand clearly what was expected. There were many approaches to this, the first of which was education. Educating leaders was beneficial because it clearly defined the expectation and standards of excellence. It provided a common language and methodology and it standardized the knowledge base so that all managers were on the same level. Usually a series of off-site, educational sessions worked well. Sometimes it was more effective to have a person from outside the organization deliver the session. In either case, major involvement of senior management was necessary. Education incorporated system change in the intervals between the educational sessions. At the conclusion of the sessions, "successful graduates" were set apart through a recognized graduation of managers who met specific target criteria. Managers who were unable to make the transition did not "graduate." Another method of setting clear expectations for management was to just "do it" and let everyone know the expectations. As an example, CHS's Leadership Expectations included:

• A Passion for Excellence

• Live, Eat, and Breathe the CARES Values

• Recognize and Support Each Other

• Recognize Associates, Let Them Know the Value They Bring

• Ensure the Delivery of Excellence in Care and Service

• Always, Always Create a Positive Environment

• Lead Change with Innovative and Responsive Action

Responsive action was emphasized. Responsibility was defined as the ability to respond in a situation or "respond–ability." So the managers and the associates had the knowledge, the equipment, and the environment to respond to a situation to bring about excellence.

Middle management can never be underestimated. Educate, educate, educate is the constant here. Middle management turns over more quickly than upper management, therefore it is necessary to make sure the orientation, the knowledge base, and the supports are in place to keep them going. Senior management needs to believe that they are there for the middle managers, that they live the corporate values, and that they demonstrate the organizational beliefs in everyday operations. If they do not, the associates immediately recognize this and react accordingly. Management was in place for the associates, to provide all the tools needed to deliver excellence at the front line. Management let associates know that they were there for them. The CEO and managers knew the associates made a difference, no matter what their position, and communicated to associates in a way that they understood. Leaders asked for feedback. Management's responsibility was to listen to the associates' feedback, act on their recommendations, and let them know that they did.

After the Culture was Set

Once trust is built, then expectations are clear and the framework is understood by all. That was the time for CHS to outline the methodology for process improvement. After the culture is in place, the quality process improvement system is put into action by everyone working together to achieve excellence. Success does not occur until the excellence process is absorbed and it takes all associates to make that happen. Deployment to the front line was the most important goal. Then the cycle of improvement began again.

There are many different methods that organizations use for process improvement circles. The method of process improvement needs to fit with the organization's process. In health care, the clinical monitoring tends to be complex; therefore, the simpler the process for service excellence, the better. At CHS, a very simple four-step problem solving process was used. It started with the assistance of Clay Sherman, author of "Creating the New American Hospital." His concept is to develop "Do It Groups" (DIGs). The four steps are: Define the task, Outline your options, Implement the solutions, and Track the results; or simply Plan, Act, Do, Results.

Any associate who has a process improvement idea, as long as it is in line with the framework and does not have to do with policy, wages and benefits, can begin the process of implementation. The implementation is in the form of small groups. Associates who are interested in the same process improvement idea work together to plan and make the idea a reality. If the idea is within the realm of the associate's responsibility, then the associate can go ahead and "just do it." These are called "JDIs." The education of associates in the use of quality tools is done at the time a process is introduced.

CHS provided the tools, assistance, and structure that the associates needed for the implementation of their ideas. This was done by teaching the managers and having the managers, in turn, teach the associates. The education department also taught the associates. At CHS, they made this a fun process by making a file box into "The Community Health System Tool Kit."

This included a quick reference manual as well as all the forms and directions for the quality improvement tools. To make sure everyone had fun with this, an autographed picture of Tim "The Tool Man" Taylor and his partner, Al, were placed in the front of the tool kit.

Bringing the Spirit Back

There are many ways to bring the spirit back to health care. One is recognition and rewards. Not everyone is comfortable with recognition but they certainly feel good after the recognition is given. It can be done as a simple thank you or a grand celebration. At CHS, it was helpful to find out what the associates found meaningful in the areas of recognition and rewards. After some controversy, CHS discovered the best way to reach the associates in this area. Then CHS implemented their findings. So often, previously, information had been requested and it was not taken seriously or there was no follow-up.

A form of recognition that CHS used (and continues to use) was a "Caresgram." It was given by any associate to any associate to thank or recognize them for living the CARES values. Attached was a bag of M&Ms, a pack of flower seeds, or a coupon for a free ice cream sundae. This was presented by the vice president or the department leader in front of as many associates as possible to announce that this person had contributed to "The CHS Way."

To incorporate fun into the culture, there was a group of associates dedicated to helping the organization have fun. The Socialization Action Committee, or SAC, was open to all associates. They gave the extra time and effort to bring fun, games, and parties to lighten the stress level. From chili contests to carnivals, socialization activities allowed the organization to change quickly while maintaining a positive and caring environment.

The importance of a positive organizational climate —the spirit—cannot be overstated. It is key to Performance Excellence. Associates who are not happy and satisfied in their work environment lead to dissatisfied and unhappy patients and customers. A positive climate is generated by positive leadership. Like key result areas for the organization, CHS developed key leadership areas. They were fun, productive, positive, and together. They were simple and straightforward areas of performance results for all management. Integrating the principles of Performance Excellence into the spirit of the organization brought about lasting change at CHS.

Beyond the Comfort Zone

Lasting change is both an evolutionary and revolutionary process. Excellence may happen today, but not tomorrow. Performance improvement process efforts need to happen every day once the journey begins. In order to track results of this journey, CHS found feedback was necessary. In order to get feedback, CHS first had to request it. Surveys were a very popular technique. For immediate feedback, customer feedback cards were distributed at the time of a customer visit or a few days after the visit. This was a fairly successful technique.

Another way CHS received feedback for organizational excellence was applying for an excellence standards-based quality award. These include The Malcolm Baldrige National Award or a state award. The patient care delivery corporations of Community Health System applied for a state award for excellence. This program was based on the Baldrige Criteria. Processes such as this, as well as any feedback process, took the organization outside its comfort zone.

Everyone's comfort zone was affected, starting with the executive team. CHS found that there was resistance from the senior management team, bolstered by middle management. Senior leadership's buy-in was made up-front, before the commitment was made to engage in the excellence award process. CHS found the commitment to the feedback process needed to be as strong as the commitment to the excellence process. This process is not for the "faint of heart." It takes courage and determination. The organization needs to be open and ready to receive and act on the information delivered in the review process. The organization also needs to realize the processes it has in place and how to readily access all the information related to the standards.

The award application required a coordinated effort throughout the organization. The application process was labor intensive. After writing the first application in-house, CHS hired a writer the second and third time around. It took several applications to understand and refine the process. They found this was an ongoing journey that never ended.

To prepare for the feedback report, CHS informed all associates that assisting in the performance excellence process was a learning experience. Even management needed to focus on process improvement. This reinforcement of management accountability was a wonderful example to all associates. It was also an accountability "wake-up call" for management. Communication needed to take place at all levels, all the time. Communication cannot take place overdone. Once an idea or a process was communicated, it was repeated three or four more times to make sure everyone heard it.

Another issue CHS dealt with was that many of the associates thought they were applying for the award for management recognition since the award and certification focused on management and leadership components. A CHS Way session explained to all associates that the award process was designed to help identify ways to achieve the mission better, not to win a prize. It was also explained that "the organization" was not bricks and mortar, but rather consisted of the associates and what they delivered. Through the award assessment process, the organization received unbiased external feedback for improving the Performance Excellence process. It also underwent a massive learning and self-discovery process when it compared its own performance to national and/or state excellence standards. Therefore, it was clear to all associates that the award process supported the organization framework, particularly the mission of serving the people of the community.

The organization assessment is very time consuming. It is important to keep the focus on the purpose. Keeping everyone focused on the culture of Performance Excellence is the role of management. The language of the application and criteria is not familiar to health care. This was particularly true before Baldrige was authorized to include an award for health care. Therefore, interpretation is necessary to make the linkages to familiar language. It is not always easy to hear some of the feedback. It is important for management not to take the report personally, but to consider it a step in the improvement process.

The Journey

Albert Einstein once said, "The significant problems we face cannot be solved by the same level of thinking that created them." The environment that exists in health care reflects what we create. If staff believe a patient is helpless and cannot participate in their own healing process, then the patient will not heal. If staff believe that the workforce cannot achieve greatness, then they will not. Beliefs create the environment, and CHS needed to change its beliefs in order to achieve Performance Excellence. Leadership set the vision and the new belief system in order to change the organizational culture. Actions followed thought. Change the thinking, then the behavior will change. "Risk taking," or more positively stated, "opportunity taking" initiates the journey.

Changing the words changes thinking as well. For instance, CHS went on "advances" rather than retreats. That meant they believed that they were going forward in their planning efforts rather than falling back. As mentioned previously in this text, associates, respond–ability, and opportunity taking were all examples of changes in thinking. CHS believed that Performance Excellence was the way to deliver the mission. This is why the journey started with commitment.

The journey to Performance Excellence thrives in a flexible culture. CHS dealt with change in a positive way and did it rapidly. The more open and flexible the corporate culture was to the idea of change, the more successful it became. CHS could not have achieved excellence without a positive organizational climate.

Instead of managing quality programs, CHS needed to manage with quality. Quality was everything. Staff were very familiar with monitoring elements of care and treatment outcomes. It became necessary to think of everything as related to quality. The CEO, like all department leaders, reports semiannually to the Quality Improvement Committee of the board. In that way, management of the organization was a measure of quality.

The rigors of this journey needed to be planned and tracked. The strategic plan did not sit on the shelf collecting dust. At CHS, it began with everyone's buy-in at the department level. All corporate and departmental goals and action plans were tied to the systemwide strategic imperatives. This uniform direction setting led the organization every day in every meaningful activity. This was electronically monitored in a systemwide database. The CEO knew exactly what was happening throughout the organization with a touch of the keyboard.

Once an organization has achieved excellence, and it is obvious when it has, there is no turning back. The quality journey has begun. The associates know it, the community knows it, and the regulatory agencies know it. Excellence is achieved day by day. Everyone in the organization achieves excellence. That is why the deployment to all levels of the organization is so important. The twist is that even if an organization achieves excellence today, that may not be the case tomorrow unless everyone continues the commitment and delivers on that commitment.

Going Beyond

One of CHS's nurses once said that this was "an instant potato generation." It was an apt description of what society has come to expect. Americans have instant food, instant service, cell phones, and fax machines so all can respond immediately. It is not surprising that patients and customers expect an immediate response to their needs, with the best possible outcomes in care and service. To meet and reach beyond the expectations, CHS needed to reach beyond the four walls of the health care building. It needed to reach out to the community of people they served, by getting to know them, their health status, and their expectations of the health care experience. Discovering this information and making the linkage back to the improvement process connected CHS to its community. In this way, it benefited the community—which is the intent of its mission.

The mission to benefit the community led CHS to be an active partner in various community support programs involving education, clinics, developing relationships with schools and police to enhance healthful life styles, and linking with other health care providers. For example, one program that CHS developed was the Community Health System Grants. The Community Health System Foundation set aside money in a community grant fund. The foundation offered grants to partnering organizations in the community that created programs and services that supported the mission of Community Health System and its corporations. The community benefit went far beyond the expected.

The poor and the underserved are groups that are often overlooked. Sometimes health care gets immersed in managed care, reimbursement, and regulation and this group is often forgotten. CHS used a community benefits analysis to assist in identifying not only this population, but also the specific disease processes that were affecting the community. CHS focused on these areas. The health system then encompassed all people, including those often overlooked, when it designed delivery of new programs to address specific health needs.

New Life

The commitment to Performance Excellence set CHS on the quality journey, bringing a new level to its organizational quality of life. It was like opening the windows and doors of the corporation so that fresh air and fresh ideas moved through it like the wind. With the seeds of change planted, the organization flourished with new life. It moved from an old stress-inducing philosophy to an organizational climate of fun and leadership. The procrastination faded and in its place empowered associates took positive action for positive results. The negative energy that fostered pain became a positive healing environment with associates taking pride in service. Previous territorializing was transformed into an integrated health care delivery system that worked together with the community.

Once the journey started, there was no return. The organization experienced excellence and knew the difference. Patients and customers felt the difference in attitude. They knew that Performance Excellence was available. Why settle for anything less? Bringing new light and life through Performance Excellence rewarded, nourished, and brought the spirit back.

LEADING THE CHANGE TO HIGH PERFORMANCE

Changing organizational culture is not easy and requires dedicated and unwavering consistency in support of the "new way" or "desired way" of behaving and believing. The following actions are usually critical to change culture in an organization:

- *Establish clear goals and a clear direction.* Explain clearly what will be required and how the new requirements are different from the old. If you do not know what new behaviors are required, find out. Talk to those leaders who have successfully engineered this kind of improvement in the past. Leaders who are not clear invite confusion and inaction.

- *Show unwavering commitment.* Leaders are pivotal to the success of the enterprise—staff are watching them closely. Don't blink in the face of setbacks—quitting is easy and doing so will make staff more cynical and demoralized. When leadership commitment and support is seen as tentative, staff and other subordinates will perceive the changes as "optional," take-or-leave suggestions. Considering the profound ability most people have to resist change, this creates more support for doing nothing.

- *Prove you will change.* If leaders do not "walk the talk," thus demonstrating their eagerness to operate differently, others once again conclude that the leaders are not serious and the new requirements are optional.

- *Keep the energy level high and focused on both process improvements and better performance outcomes.* Select improvements that are easy as well as difficult. Small successes are needed to keep the energy and support for Performance Excellence high. Larger improvement projects take longer to carry out, but usually bring greater benefit. Celebrate process improvements as well as better performance outcomes.

- *Encourage people to challenge the status quo* when doing so is consistent with enhancing customer value and organizational goals. Do not tolerate system craziness, but do break old bureaucratic rules and policies that prevent or inhibit work toward goals. Free your people from bureaucratic silliness and you will find great energy and support from staff.

- *Change rewards to make them consistent with goals and objectives.* Make following the new culture and achieving goals worthwhile by rewarding desired behaviors and making the continued use of the old ones unpleasant. All staff must understand that the rewards are issued for behaving in a certain way and for achieving desired results. Rewards, including compensation and incentives, should not be considered an entitlement of employment. It is important to test the effectiveness of rewards and recognition. Remember, just because you value a reward does not mean that staff will do the same.

- *Measure progress.* What gets measured gets done. When leaders use measurements to track progress, people think they are serious about tracking and improving. If you do not bother measuring, staff productivity is usually lower. In addition, measurements help identify those who should be rewarded and those who should not. Finally, keep measurements simple and efficient. Do not allow the process of measurement to divert energy and focus. Stop collecting data that no longer supports effective decision making.

- *Communicate, communicate, communicate.* Communication cannot replace an inspiring vision and sound goals, but poor communication can scuttle them. People must understand the logic and rationale behind the vision and goals. Leaders must tell them what is coming, how they will be affected, and what is expected of them. Remember to take every opportunity to communicate your desires—once is not enough. The opponents of change will work nonstop to undermine the new goal, vision, and culture—communicate consistently to overcome this resistance. Leaders who do not communicate effectively invite the rumor mill to fill in the blank spaces. Bad news, rumors, and outright lies frequently fill the communication gap leaders might inadvertently leave.

- *Involve everyone.* People who do not actively support change, oppose it—perhaps inadvertently. Insist on full involvement and define a role for everyone. Find ways to make everyone accountable for transforming the culture and improving performance. Remember that if a manager fails to support the changes needed to improve performance, it is probably a good idea to encourage that person to find other work—preferably with a competitor.

- *Start fast, then go faster.* Slow progress, which the opponents of change like to see, creates a self-fulfilling prophecy—that the proposed changes will not be effective. However, speed creates a sense of urgency that helps overcome organizational inertia, achieve stunning results, and defeat the gloom and pessimism of naysayers.

Remember to remain steadfast in support, walk the talk, involve everyone, communicate, achieve quick results, measure, and reward progress.

Improve Performance, Efficiency, and Timeliness

What does it mean?

- It includes, but is not limited to, process identification, analysis, and ongoing improvement. Define and measure process cycle time and defects and reduce them consistently.

What is the manager's responsibility?

Set an example—ask for data/measurements on cycle time and defects.

- Make time available
- Make training available
- Ensure that records of discipline exist
- Charter teams
- Set low goals, get low performance
- If you do not tell staff what you expect, do not be surprised if they do not get where you want them to go

Create a Participative, Cooperative Workplace

What does it mean?

- It includes, but is not limited to, setting boundary conditions and relevant goals, moving decisions to the lowest possible level, using work teams for planning and process improvement, and creating a "family-friendly" work environ-

ment. Leaders motivate people; provide training for managers and staff; encourage the development of self-directed work teams; delegate authority and decision making downward; empower people to focus on achieving mission and vision; value diversity; provide open communication in all directions; and measure and improve staff well-being, motivation, and satisfaction.

What is the manager's responsibility?

- Coach and counsel, rather than control
- Encourage participation with the goal of achieving better decision quality—make better use of staff
- Create and build a highly motivated and satisfied workforce

Planning Action

Based on vision and results from the previous year, every organization clarifies direction through planning and the deployment of the plan to guide daily action. Leaders are responsible for:

- Identifying improvement opportunities in their units and identifying the key actions needed to achieve the improvements
- Identifying who will lead the improvements and chartering teams to do so
- Identifying unit and individual performance objectives to achieve desired performance levels and targets at all levels of the organization

Taking Action

- All leaders have a responsibility for communicating the mission, vision, goals, and improvement targets to all staff.
- It is very important that leaders and staff understand and agree fully with the planned objectives. The plan deployment process cascades from top management to all locations and levels of the organization. Top managers do not micromanage the process. This means that the top leaders

determine the objective or target and an action officer determines the means. This then sets the target for the next level to determine means. Figure 10 provides one example of this effect.

Personal Management Effectiveness—The Use of Upward Evaluations

Formal upward evaluations have been used for over 50 years to help assess job performance. As organizations become committed to improving labor relations and manager effectiveness, upward evaluation has become a widely used tool that more and more leaders value.

Three reasons why upward feedback is beneficial include:

1. *Validity.* Subordinates interact regularly with their managers and have a unique vantage from which to assess manager style.

2. *Reliability.* Numerous subordinates provide the best chance for reliable data.

3. *Involvement and Morale.* Asking people to comment on the effectiveness and style of their managers boosts morale and sends a clear message that the organization is serious about increasing staff involvement.

Before managers can effectively change the way they manage, they should gather facts about their current style. They need to know what aspects of their style are considered strong and should not be changed. The starting point for improving management style, therefore, is an honest assessment of the manager's current behavior by his or her subordinates, peers, and supervisors.

The Feedback Process

1. Leaders solicit feedback on how they perform against specific behaviors that are characteristic of an effective manager.

2. They use this information to plan personal improvement strategies.

3. They share the results of the survey with their staff and discuss improvement actions.

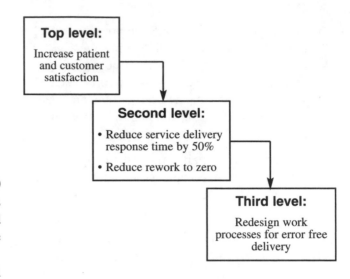

Figure 10 Deploying strategic objectives.

4. They make improvements as planned and start the process again next year.

Figure 11 maps the process that enables staff to help their manager understand how he or she is perceived, as well as identify areas of strength on which the manager can build. However, some important procedures should be in place to prevent improper use of the tool.

- Feedback should always be used and interpreted in the spirit of continuous personal improvement. Personally identifiable results should go only to the manager who was rated and should not be used as a basis for performance ratings, promotion, assignments, or pay adjustments (unless, of course, the manager refuses to work to improve).

- Anonymity for those completing questionnaires should be carefully protected. No one other than the staff should see the actual completed questionnaire. To further protect anonymity, questionnaires should not be summarized and reported to the manager in cases where fewer than three to five staff completed the questionnaire.

- Personally identifiable results should be provided only to the manager named on the questionnaire. When the managers receive the results, they review their own ratings to determine their

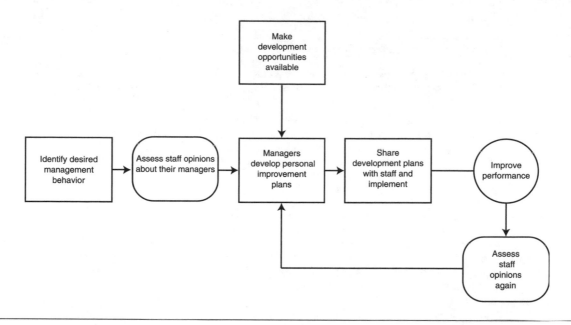

Figure 11 Management feedback process.

strengths and opportunities for improvement. Then they take steps to improve.

The Management Effectiveness Survey (Figures 12 and 13) can provide information that might help leaders and managers at all levels determine areas to address in order to strengthen their personal effectiveness. It represents one set of questions to examine leadership communication, openness, and effectiveness. Certainly other questions may be asked as circumstances change. In fact, in order to determine if any survey is asking the correct questions, the survey itself should be evaluated. This can be done by using open-ended questions and asking the staff to identify other issues that are of concern to them and should be included in the survey. Also ask if some of the questions are not relevant or important and should be eliminated. Then adjust the survey accordingly.

In addition to aggregating scores from staff, it is also useful to compare the perceptions of managers with the perception of the leader or manager who is the target of the assessment. Many times staff identify a specific weakness that the leader believes is much stronger. These differences, together with key areas where both parties agree that a weakness exists, could be targeted for specific improvement. By aggregating the assessment data for all managers and making the overall results available to individuals, they can determine how their stage of development compares with other managers in the office.

MANAGEMENT EFFECTIVENESS SURVEY

The following questionnaire lists some key indicators to help you assess your manager's style in several key areas. Enter 1 for strongly disagree, 2 for disagree, 3 for agree, and 4 for strongly agree. If you cannot answer a question, leave it blank.

General

1. My manager keeps me well informed about what is going on in the office.   1 2 3 4
2. My manager clearly and accurately explains the reasons for decisions that affect my work. 1 2 3 4
3. I am satisfied with my involvement in decisions that affect my work.   1 2 3 4
4. My manager delegates the right amount of responsibility to me and does not micromanage.   1 2 3 4
5. My manager gives me honest feedback on my performance.   1 2 3 4
6. I have confidence in my manager's decisions.   1 2 3 4
7. My manager has the knowledge he/she needs to be effective.   1 2 3 4
8. I can depend on my manager to honor the commitments he/she makes to me.   1 2 3 4
9. My manager treats people fairly and with dignity and respect.   1 2 3 4
10. My manager is straightforward and honest with me.   1 2 3 4
11. My manager is committed to resolving the concerns that may be identified in this survey and has made improvements based on past surveys (if applicable).   1 2 3 4
12. My manager strongly supports doing the right thing for the patient, customer and all other stakeholders.   1 2 3 4
13. The communication process in my unit is effective. I always understand what is being communicated. (Unit refers to the level in the office your manager heads.)   1 2 3 4
14. In my unit, there is an environment of openness and trust.   1 2 3 4
15. I feel free to speak up when I disagree with a decision.   1 2 3 4
16. I feel I can elevate issues to higher-level managers without fear of reprisal.   1 2 3 4
17. The people I work with cooperate to get the job done.   1 2 3 4
18. In my unit, we are simplifying the way we do our work.   1 2 3 4
19. We have an effective process for preparing people to fill open positions.   1 2 3 4
20. All staff have fair advancement opportunities based on skills and abilities. Diversity of ideas is valued.   1 2 3 4

Effective Management Practices

My manager frequently…

21. provides me with honest feedback on my performance.   1 2 3 4
22. encourages me to monitor my own efforts.   1 2 3 4
23. encourages me to make suggestions to improve work processes.   1 2 3 4
24. ensures I have the information I need to do my job.   1 2 3 4
25. defines his/her requirements of me in clear, measurable terms.   1 2 3 4
26. acts as a positive role model for performance excellence.   1 2 3 4
27. ensures that organizational goals and objectives are understood at all levels.   1 2 3 4
28. favors facts before making decisions affecting our patients and customers, staff, partners, and organization.   1 2 3 4
29. identifies and removes barriers to alleviate work-related problems.   1 2 3 4
30. encourages people in our unit to work as a team.   1 2 3 4
31. informs us regularly about the state of the health care organization.   1 2 3 4
32. encourages me to ask questions and creates an environment of openness and trust.   1 2 3 4
33. behaves in ways that demonstrate respect for others.   1 2 3 4
34. ensures regularly scheduled reviews of progress toward goals.   1 2 3 4
35. monitors my progress and compares against benchmarks.   1 2 3 4
36. ensures that rewards and recognition is fairly applied and closely tied to strategic goals, objectives, and required actions plans.   1 2 3 4
37. sets work goals based on strategic objectives and patient/customer requirements.   1 2 3 4
38. runs effective meetings.   1 2 3 4
39. uses a disciplined, fact-based process to make health care and operational decisions and solve problems.   1 2 3 4
40. treats performance excellence as a basic operating principle.   1 2 3 4

Please list on the back of this form additional questions that the survey should ask about your manager. Also tell us which questions already on the survey are not very important and should be removed. In this way we can improve the effectiveness of the survey and better identify areas most needing improvement.

Figure 12 Sample management effectiveness survey partially scored.

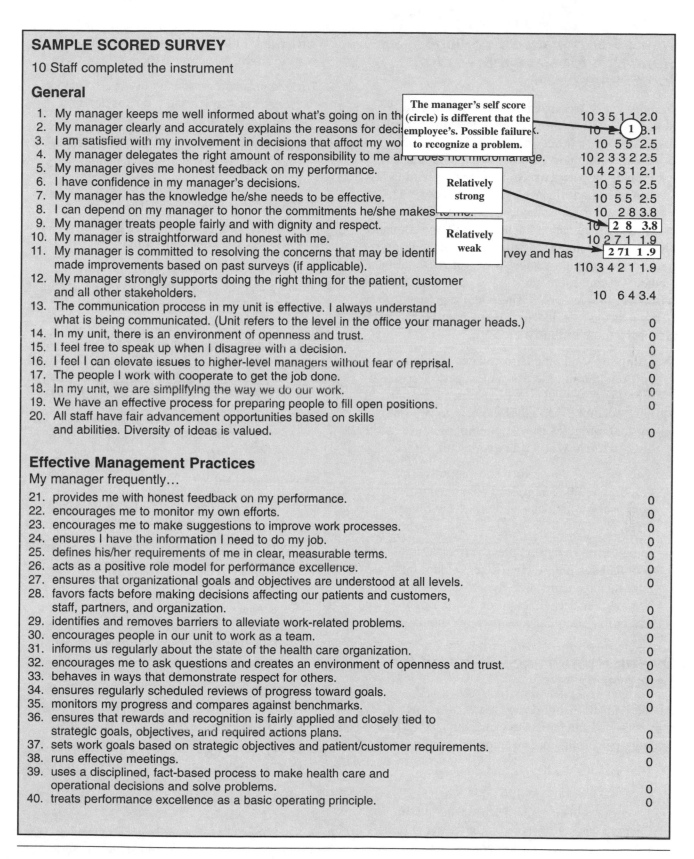

SAMPLE SCORED SURVEY

10 Staff completed the instrument

General

1. My manager keeps me well informed about what's going on in th...   10 3 5 1 1 2.0
2. My manager clearly and accurately explains the reasons for deci...   10 2 ① 3.1
3. I am satisfied with my involvement in decisions that affect my wo...   10 5 5 2.5
4. My manager delegates the right amount of responsibility to me and does not micromanage.   10 2 3 3 2 2.5
5. My manager gives me honest feedback on my performance.   10 4 2 3 1 2.1
6. I have confidence in my manager's decisions.   10 5 5 2.5
7. My manager has the knowledge he/she needs to be effective.   10 5 5 2.5
8. I can depend on my manager to honor the commitments he/she makes to me.   10 2 8 3.8
9. My manager treats people fairly and with dignity and respect.   10 2 8 3.8
10. My manager is straightforward and honest with me.   10 2 7 1 1.9
11. My manager is committed to resolving the concerns that may be identif... rvey and has made improvements based on past surveys (if applicable).   2 71 1.9   110 3 4 2 1 1.9
12. My manager strongly supports doing the right thing for the patient, customer and all other stakeholders.   10 6 4 3.4
13. The communication process in my unit is effective. I always understand what is being communicated. (Unit refers to the level in the office your manager heads.)   0
14. In my unit, there is an environment of openness and trust.   0
15. I feel free to speak up when I disagree with a decision.   0
16. I feel I can elevate issues to higher-level managers without fear of reprisal.   0
17. The people I work with cooperate to get the job done.   0
18. In my unit, we are simplifying the way we do our work.   0
19. We have an effective process for preparing people to fill open positions.   0
20. All staff have fair advancement opportunities based on skills and abilities. Diversity of ideas is valued.   0

Effective Management Practices

My manager frequently…

21. provides me with honest feedback on my performance.   0
22. encourages me to monitor my own efforts.   0
23. encourages me to make suggestions to improve work processes.   0
24. ensures I have the information I need to do my job.   0
25. defines his/her requirements of me in clear, measurable terms.   0
26. acts as a positive role model for performance excellence.   0
27. ensures that organizational goals and objectives are understood at all levels.   0
28. favors facts before making decisions affecting our patients and customers, staff, partners, and organization.   0
29. identifies and removes barriers to alleviate work-related problems.   0
30. encourages people in our unit to work as a team.   0
31. informs us regularly about the state of the health care organization.   0
32. encourages me to ask questions and creates an environment of openness and trust.   0
33. behaves in ways that demonstrate respect for others.   0
34. ensures regularly scheduled reviews of progress toward goals.   0
35. monitors my progress and compares against benchmarks.   0
36. ensures that rewards and recognition is fairly applied and closely tied to strategic goals, objectives, and required actions plans.   0
37. sets work goals based on strategic objectives and patient/customer requirements.   0
38. runs effective meetings.   0
39. uses a disciplined, fact-based process to make health care and operational decisions and solve problems.   0
40. treats performance excellence as a basic operating principle.   0

Callout: **The manager's self score (circle) is different that the employee's. Possible failure to recognize a problem.**

Callout: **Relatively strong**

Callout: **Relatively weak**

Figure 13 Sample management effectiveness survey partially scored.

Create Performance Excellence Standards for Managers—A Key Job Element

Virtually every organization has the ability to determine what performance requirements are critical for the success of staff and managers. These critical performance requirements are usually included as a key requirement in performance plans and appraisals. By declaring that performance excellence is critical to the success of the organization, a specific key performance requirement can be included in the performance plan (sometimes these are called personal commitment plans, personal improvement plans, or personal management objectives, to name a few) and evaluation of managers and leaders. Using this approach, every manager and supervisor begins to take performance excellence more seriously.

- Using the following performance standards as an example, in order for a manager to receive a rating at a particular level, that manager must have accomplished all of the activities described for that rating level. If all are not met, the rating goes to the lowest level at which all are met.

- The writer of the performance appraisal must cite measurable examples in the performance appraisal for actions listed under the rating level.

- Supervising reviewers must verify that these actions have indeed been taken. Under this system, managers are strongly encouraged to keep accurate records of activities which might exemplify compliance with these standards.

Overall Performance Standard for Leadership

The individual visibly demonstrates adherence to the high personal standards and characteristics of leaders in a high-performing organization. The individual:

- Understands the health care processes of the unit.

- Is patient and customer focused and driven. Demonstrates a firm commitment to the principles of patient and customer satisfaction.

Understands their requirements and consistently works to meet and exceed them.

- Understands and personally uses performance excellence principles and tools for decision making and planning.

  – Favors the use of data and facts to drive decisions and ensures that staff and subordinate managers do the same.

  – Ensures that organizational goals are converted to appropriate actions to align work within his or her organizational unit.

  – Measures and monitors progress toward achieving the goals within his or her organizational unit.

- Demonstrates a firm commitment to the principles of staff empowerment, well-being, and satisfaction.

  – Promotes flexibility and individual initiative.

  – Encourages and supports the personal and professional development of self and staff.

  – Supports effective training and reinforces the use of new skills on the job.

  – Ensures compensation is aligned to support health care strategies and actions.

  – Rewards and recognizes staff who incorporate the principles of performance excellence in their day-to-day work.

  – Fosters an atmosphere of open, honest communication and knowledge sharing among staff and health care units throughout the organization.

- Rigorously drives the systematic, continuous improvement of all work processes, including his or her personal effectiveness as a leader.

- Achieves consistently improving performance outcomes in customer satisfaction; staff well-being, motivation, and satisfaction; operational excellence; and financial (cost/budget) performance.

Rating Number 1: Performance is unsatisfactory. The individual frequently fails to meet the performance standard for leadership.

- Does not fully understand the health care processes of the unit.

- Consistently disregards the needs of patients and customers.

- Does not understand and has not taken steps to implement Performance Excellence (may even work against the changes needed).

  - Intuition tends to dominate decision making, not data or facts.

  - Organizational goals and actions are not aligned to actions within his or her unit.

  - May measure and monitor some performance outcomes (such as budget tracking) but most measures are not aligned to organizational goals.

- Does not effectively promote staff well-being, motivation, and morale.

  - Tends to micromanage—does not delegate decision-making authority to the lower levels except as directly instructed to do so.

  - Rarely listens to staff or cares what they think.

  - Does not consistently promote flexibility and individual initiative.

  - Does not consistently encourage and support the personal and professional development of self and staff.

  - May send staff to training but does not consistently reinforce the use of new skills on the job.

  - Has not taken effective steps to ensure compensation and other rewards or recognition are aligned to support health care strategies and actions.

  - Reward and recognition is not aligned to support organizational goals or the principles of performance excellence or patient and customer satisfaction.

- Does not communicate effectively or foster an atmosphere of knowledge sharing among staff and health care units.

- Does not regularly assess or improve work processes, including his or her personal effectiveness as a leader.

- Does not achieve consistently improving performance outcomes in customer satisfaction; staff well-being, motivation, and satisfaction; operational excellence; and financial (cost/budget) performance.

Rating Number 2: Performance is minimally acceptable. Individual occasionally fails to meet the performance standard for leadership. Performs higher than indicated by level one but less than level three.

Rating Number 3: Performance is acceptable. Individual basically meets the performance standard for leadership.

- Is considered to be a capable leader.

- Understands the key health care processes of the unit.

- Is customer driven and promotes customer-focused values throughout his or her unit.

  - Demonstrates a commitment to the principles of patient and customer satisfaction.

  - Develops systems to understand patient and customer requirements, strengthen relationships, resolve problems and prevent them from happening again, and obtain information about patient and customer satisfaction and dissatisfaction.

- Personally uses many Performance Excellence principles and tools for decision making and planning.

- Visibly supports performance excellence within the organization. Usually uses data and facts to drive decisions and ensure that many staff and subordinate managers do the same.

- Ensures that key organizational goals are converted to appropriate actions to align most work within his or her organizational unit. Most goals and actions have defined measures of progress and timelines for achieving desired results.

- Demonstrates some commitment to the principles of staff empowerment, well-being, and satisfaction. Is well-regarded by staff for:

  - Involving the workforce in identifying improvement opportunities and developing improvement plans.

  - Valuing staff input on work-related matters.

  - Promoting flexibility and individual initiative and ensuring that many subordinate managers do the same.

  - Encouraging and supporting the personal and professional development of self and staff.

  - Supporting effective training and reinforcing the use of new skills on the job.

  - Ensuring compensation is aligned to support health care strategies and actions.

  - Rewarding and recognizing staff who incorporate the principles of performance excellence in their day-to-day work.

- Fosters an atmosphere of open, honest communication and knowledge sharing among staff and health care units throughout the organization.

- Visibly drives continuous improvement of many work processes, including his or her personal effectiveness as a leader.

- Achieves consistently improving performance outcomes in customer satisfaction; staff well-being, motivation, and satisfaction; operational excellence; and financial (cost/budget) performance.

- The levels of performance outcomes are better than average when compared with organizations providing similar programs, products, or services.

Rating Number 4: Individual occasionally exceeds the performance standard for leadership. Performs higher than indicated by level three but less than level five. Performance is very good.

Rating Number 5: Individual consistently exceeds the performance standard for leadership. *Is considered a role model for leadership.* Performance is superior.

- Understands the health care processes of the unit in great detail.

- Is customer driven and actively promotes customer-focused values throughout his or her unit.

  - Demonstrates a firm commitment to the principles of patient and customer satisfaction.

  - Develops effective systems to understand customer requirements, strengthen loyalty and patient and customer relationships, resolve patient and customer problems immediately and prevent them from happening again, and obtain timely information about patient and customer satisfaction and dissatisfaction.

  - Advocates the needs of patients and customers through the collection and use of information on patient and customer satisfaction, dissatisfaction, and product performance.

- Personally uses Performance Excellence principles and tools for decision making and planning.

  - Serves as a Performance Excellence champion within the organization and as a resource within the work unit, providing guidance, counsel, and instruction in performance excellence tools, processes, and principles.

  - Is a role model for using data and facts to drive decisions and ensures that staff and subordinate managers do the same.

  - Ensures that all organizational goals are converted to appropriate actions to align work within his or her organizational unit.

  - Each goal and action has defined measures of progress and timelines for achieving desired results.

- Demonstrates a firm commitment to the principles of staff empowerment, well-being, and satisfaction. Is highly regarded by staff for:

  - Involving the workforce in setting standards of performance, identifying improvement opportunities, and developing improvement plans.

  - Seeking and valuing staff input on work-related matters.

– Promoting flexibility and individual initiative and ensuring that subordinate managers do the same.

– Encouraging and supporting the personal and professional development of self and staff.

– Supporting effective training and reinforcing the use of new skills on the job.

– Ensuring compensation is aligned to support health care strategies and actions.

– Rewarding and recognizing staff who incorporate the principles of performance excellence in their day-to-day work.

• Fosters an atmosphere of open, honest communication and knowledge sharing among staff and health care units throughout the organization.

– Checks the effectiveness of nearly all communication and makes changes to improve.

• Rigorously drives the systematic, continuous improvement of all work processes, including his or her personal effectiveness as a leader.

– Develops personal action plan and always incorporates results of 360-degree feedback to continuously improve his/her leadership effectiveness and ensures subordinate managers do the same.

• Achieves consistently improving performance outcomes in patient and customer satisfaction; staff well-being, motivation, and satisfaction; operational excellence; and financial (cost/budget) performance.

– The levels of performance outcomes are among the highest in the organization and are also high when compared with organizations providing similar programs or services.

The following tables display the performance excellence ratings side by side to make it easier to see the progression from poor (1) to excellent (5).

Performance Excellence Standards Table

Level 1	Level 2	Level 3	Level 4	Level 5
Performance is unsatisfactory: Individual frequently fails to meet the performance standard for leadership. Is considered a poor leader.	Better than level 1 and some of level 3.	**Performance is acceptable:** Individual basically meets the performance standard for leadership. Is considered to be a capable leader.	All of level 3 and some of level 5.	**Performance is superior: Individual consistently exceeds the performance standard for leadership. Is considered a role model for leadership.**
• Does not fully understand the key health care processes of the unit.		• Understands the key health care processes of the unit.		• Understands the health care processes of the unit in great detail.
• Consistently disregards the needs of patients and customers.		• Is patient and customer driven and promotes patient- and customer-focused values throughout his or her unit. – Demonstrates a commitment to the principles of patient and customer satisfaction. – Develops systems to understand patient and customer requirements, strengthen relationships, resolve problems and prevent them from happening again, and obtain information about patient and customer satisfaction and dissatisfaction.		• Is patient and customer driven and actively promotes patient and customer-focused values throughout his or her unit. – Demonstrates a firm commitment to the principles of patient and customer satisfaction. – Develops effective systems to understand patient and customer requirements, strengthen loyalty and patient and customer relationships, resolve problems immediately and prevent them from happening again, and obtain timely information about patient and customer satisfaction and dissatisfaction. – Advocates the needs of patients and customers through the collection and use of information on patient and customer satisfaction, dissatisfaction, and service delivery performance.

Performance Excellence Standards Table

Level 1	Level 2	Level 3	Level 4	Level 5
Performance is unsatisfactory: Individual frequently fails to meet the performance standard for leadership. Is considered a poor leader.	**Better than level 1 and some of level 3.**	**Performance is acceptable: Individual basically meets the performance standard for leadership. Is considered to be a capable leader.**	**All of level 3 and some of level 5.**	**Performance is superior: Individual consistently exceeds the performance standard for leadership. Is considered a role model for leadership.**
• Does not understand and has not taken steps to implement Performance Excellence (may even work against the changes needed).		• Personally uses many Performance Excellence principles and tools for decision making and planning.		• Personally uses nearly all Performance Excellence principles and tools for decision making and planning.
– Intuition tends to dominate decision making, not data or facts. – Organizational goals and actions are not aligned to actions within his or her unit. – May measure and monitor some performance outcomes (such as budget tracking), but most measures are not aligned to organizational goals. – Does not understand and has not taken steps to implement Performance Excellence (may even need work against the changes needed).		– Visibly supports Performance Excellence within the organization. – Usually uses data and facts to drive decisions and ensure that many staff and subordinate managers do the same. – Ensures that key organizational goals are converted to appropriate actions to align most work within his or her organizational unit. – Most goals and actions have defined measures of progress and timelines for achieving desired results.		– Serves as a Performance Excellence champion within the organization and as a resource within the work unit, providing guidance, counsel, and instruction in Performance Excellence tools, processes, and principles. – Is a role model for using data and facts to drive decisions and ensures that staff and subordinate managers do the same. – Ensures that all organizational goals are converted to appropriate actions to align nearly all work within his or her organizational unit. – Each goal and action has defined measures of progress and timelines for achieving desired results.

Performance Excellence Standards Table

Level 1	Level 2	Level 3	Level 4	Level 5
Performance is unsatisfactory: Individual frequently fails to meet the performance standard for leadership. Is considered a poor leader.	**Better than level 1 and some of level 3.**	**Performance is acceptable: Individual basically meets the performance standard for leadership. Is considered to be a capable leader.**	**All of level 3 and some of level 5.**	**Performance is superior: Individual consistently exceeds the performance standard for leadership. Is considered a role model for leadership.**
• Does not effectively promote staff well-being, motivation, and morale.		• Demonstrates some commitment to the principles of staff empowerment, well-being, and satisfaction. Is well regarded by staff for:		• Demonstrates a firm commitment to the principles of staff empowerment, well-being, and satisfaction. Is highly regarded by staff for:
– Tends to micromanage; does not delegate decision-making authority to the lower levels except as directly instructed to do so.		– Involving the workforce in identifying improvement opportunities and developing improvement plans.		– Involving the workforce in setting standards of performance, identifying improvement opportunities, and developing improvement plans.
– Rarely listens to staff or cares what they think.		– Valuing staff input on work-related matters.		– Seeking and valuing staff input on work-related matters.
– Does not consistently promote flexibility and individual initiative.		– Promoting flexibility and individual initiative and ensuring that many subordinate managers do the same.		– Promoting flexibility and individual initiative and ensuring that nearly all subordinate managers do the same.
– Does not consistently encourage and support the personal and professional development of self and staff.		– Encouraging and supporting the personal and professional development and self and staff.		– Encouraging and supporting the personal and professional development of self and staff.
– May send staff to training but does not consistently reinforce the use of new skills on the job.		– Supporting effective training and reinforcing the use of new skills on the job.		– Supporting effective training and reinforcing the use of new skills on the job.
– Has not taken effective steps to ensure compensation and other rewards or recognition are aligned to support health care strategies and actions.		– Ensuring compensation is aligned to support health care strategies and actions.		– Ensuring compensation is aligned to support health care strategies and actions.
– Reward and recognition is not aligned to support organizational goals or the principles of Performance Excellence or patient and customer satisfaction.		– Rewarding and recognizing staff who incorporate the principles of Performance Excellence in their day-to-day work.		– Rewarding and recognizing staff who incorporate the principles of Performance Excellence in their day-to-day work.

Performance Excellence Standards Table

Level 1	Level 2	Level 3	Level 4	Level 5
Performance is unsatisfactory: Individual frequently fails to meet the performance standard for leadership. Is considered a poor leader.	**Better than level 1 and some of level 3.**	**Performance is acceptable: Individual basically meets the performance standard for leadership. Is considered to be a capable leader.**	**All of level 3 and some of level 5.**	**Performance is superior: Individual consistently exceeds the performance standard for leadership. Is considered a role model for leadership.**
• Does not communicate effectively or foster an atmosphere of knowledge sharing among staff and health care units.		• Fosters an atmosphere of open, honest communication and knowledge sharing among staff and health care units throughout the organization.		• Fosters an atmosphere of open, honest communication and knowledge sharing among staff and health care units throughout the organization. – Checks the effectiveness of nearly all communication and makes changes to improve.
• Does not regularly assess or improve work processes, including his or her personal effectiveness as a leader.		Visibly drives continuous improvement of many work processes, including his or her personal effectiveness as a leader.		• Rigorously drives the systematic, continuous improvement of all work processes, including his or her personal effectiveness as a leader. – Develops personal action plan and always incorporates results of 360-degree feedback to continuously improve his/her leadership effectiveness and ensures subordinate managers do the same.
• Does not achieve consistently improving performance outcomes in patient and customer satisfaction; staff well-being, motivation, and satisfaction; operational excellence; and financial (cost/budget) performance.		Achieves consistently improving performance outcomes in patient and customer satisfaction; staff well-being, motivation, and satisfaction; operational excellence; and financial (cost/budget) performance. • The levels of performance outcomes are better than average when compared with organizations providing similar programs or services.		• Achieves consistently improving performance outcomes in patient and customer satisfaction; staff well-being, motivation, and satisfaction; operational excellence; and financial (cost/budget) performance. – The levels of performance outcomes are among the highest in the organization and are also high when compared with organizations providing similar programs or services.

LESSONS LEARNED

Successful leaders will create a customer focus and a context for action at all levels of the organization. Effective leaders will distribute authority and decision making to all levels of the organization. Nearly instantaneous, two-way communication will permit clear strategies, measurable objectives, and priorities to be identified and deployed organizationwide. Problems will be identified and resolved with similar speed. Success in this environment will demand different skills of staff and managers. Unless all managers and staff understand where the organization is going and what must be done to beat the competition, it will be difficult for them to make effective decisions consistent with overall direction and strategy. If staff at all levels are not involved in decision making, organizational effectiveness is reduced—making it more difficult to win in a highly competitive market.

In closing this section, we would like to suggest that the scenario previously described is already happening today among the world's best-performing organizations.

- These organizations have effective leadership at all levels, with a clear strategy focused on maximizing customer value. Middle-level managers support, rather than block, the values and direction of the top leaders.

- They have developed ways to challenge themselves and improve their own processes when doing so promotes patient and customer value and improves operating effectiveness.

- They engage workers fully and promote organizational and personal learning at all levels. They ensure that knowledge is shared within the organization to avoid duplication of effort.

- They have created effective data systems to enhance decision making at all levels.

- They have developed and aligned reward, recognition, compensation, and incentives to support the desired patient and customer-focused behavior among all leaders, managers, and staff.

- They have found ways to design effective work processes and ensure that those processes are improved continuously.

- They closely monitor their performance and the performance of their principal competitors. They use this information to adjust their work and continue to improve.

These organizations are among the best in the world at what they do and they will continue to win, as long as they continue to apply the current principles of Performance Excellence.

AWARD CRITERIA FRAMEWORK

Organizations must position themselves to respond well to the environment within which they compete. They must understand and manage threats and vulnerabilities as well as capitalize on their strengths and opportunities, including the vulnerabilities of competitors. These factors guide strategy development, support operational decisions, and align measures and actions—all of which must be done well for the organization to succeed. Consistent with this overarching purpose, the award Criteria contain the following basic elements: Driver Triad, Work Core, Brain Center, and Health Care Outcomes (Figure 14).

The Driver Triad

The Driver Triad (Figure 15) consists of the categories of Leadership, Strategic Planning, and Patient and Customer and Market Focus. Leaders use these processes to set direction and goals, monitor progress, make resource decisions, and take corrective action when progress does not proceed according to plan. The processes that make up the Driver Triad require leaders to set direction and expectations for the organization to meet customer and market requirements, and fully empower staff (Category 1), provide the vehicle for determining the short- and long-term strategies for success as well as communicating and aligning the organization's work (Category 2), and produce information about critical customer requirements and levels of satisfaction, and strengthen patient and customer relations and loyalty (Category 3).

The Work Core

The Work Core (Figure 16) describes the processes through which the primary work of the organization takes place and consists of Staff Focus (Category 5) and Process Management (Category 6). These Categories recognize that the people of an organization are responsible for doing the work. To achieve peak performance, these people must possess the right skills and must be allowed to work in an environment that promotes initiative and self-direction. The work processes provide the structure for continuous learning and improvement to optimize performance.

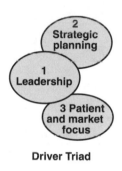

Figure 15 Driver Triad.

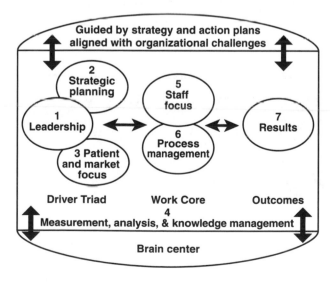

Figure 14 Award Criteria.

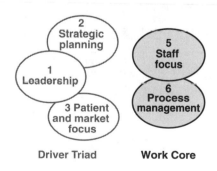

Figure 16 Work Core.

Health Care Results

The processes defined by the Driver Triad, Work Core, and Brain Center produce the Organizational Performance Results (Category 7). Organizational Performance results (Figure 17) reflect the organization's actual performance and serve as the basis for leaders to monitor progress against goals and make adjustments to increase performance. These Organizational Performance include health care results, patient and customer focus, financial and market performance, staff and work system performance, organizational effectiveness and governance and social responsibility.

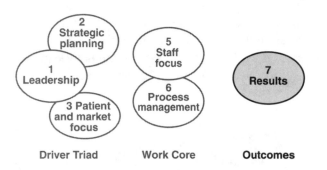

Driver Triad   **Work Core**   **Outcomes**

Figure 17 Results.

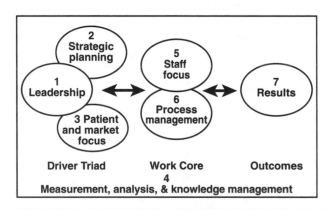

Figure 18 Measurement, analysis, and knowledge management.

Brain Center

The foundation for the entire management system is Measurement, Information, and Analysis (Category 4). Category four processes capture, store, analyze, and retrieve information and data critical to the effective management of the organization and to a fact-based system for improving organization performance and competitiveness. Rapid access and reliable data and information systems are especially critical to enhance effective decision making in an increasingly complex, fast-paced, global competitive environment.

Measurement, Analysis, and Knowledge Management is also called the Brain Center of an effective management system (Figures 18 and 19).

Organizations develop effective strategic plans to help set the direction necessary to achieve future success. Unfortunately, these plans are not always communicated and used to drive actions. The planning process and the resulting strategy are virtually worthless if the organization does not use the plan and strategy to guide decision making at all levels of the organization (Figure 20).

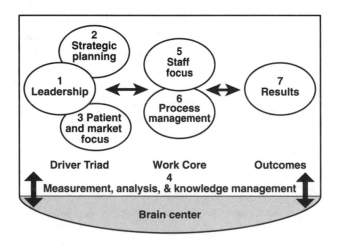

Figure 19 Brain center.

When decisions are not guided by strategy, managers and other staff tend to substitute their own ideas for the correct direction. This frequently causes teams, individuals, and whole health care units to work at cross-purposes, suboptimizing performance and making it more difficult for the organization to achieve desired results.

Taken together, (Figure 21) these processes define the essential ingredients of a complex, integrated management system designed to promote and deliver Performance Excellence. If any part of the system is missing, the performance results suffer. If fully implemented, these processes are sufficient to enable organizations to achieve winning performance.

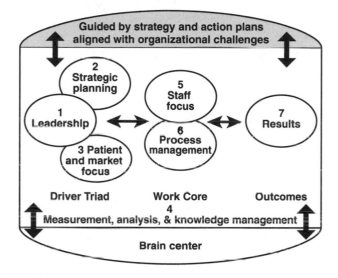

Figure 20

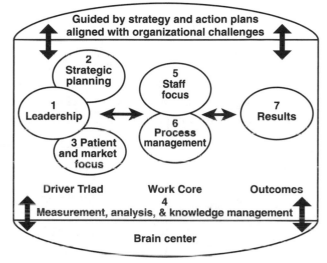

Figure 21 The integrated management system.

Award Criteria Organization

Categories

The seven Criteria categories are subdivided into Items and Areas to Address. Figure 23 demonstrates the organization of Category 1.

Items

There are 19 items, each focusing on a major requirement.

Areas to Address

Items consist of one or more Areas to Address (Areas). Information is submitted by applicants in response to the specific requirements of these Areas. There are 32 Areas to Address.

Subparts

There are 81 subparts in the 2003 Criteria. Areas consist of one or more subparts, where numbers are shown in parentheses. A response should be made to each subpart.

Notes

If a note indicates the process "should" include something, examiners will interpret it as a requirement. If a note indicates that the process "might" include something, examiners will not treat the list as a requirement—only as an example.

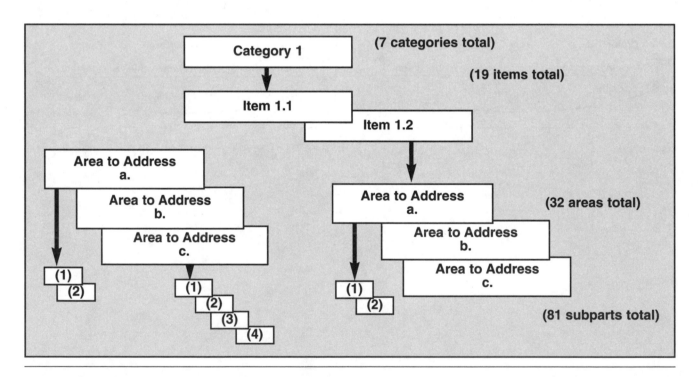

Figure 22 Organization of Category 1.

BALDRIGE CRITERIA CATEGORIES AND POINT VALUES

P	**Preface: Organizational Profile**	**(0 points)**
P.1	Organizational Description	0
P.2	Organizational Challenges	0

Examination Categories/Items	**Maximum Points**
1 Leadership (120 points)	
1.1 Organizational Leadership	70
1.2 Social Responsibility	50
2 Strategic Planning (85 points)	
2.1 Strategy Development	40
2.2 Strategy Deployment	45
3 Focus on Patients, Other Customers, and Markets (85 points)	
3.1 Patient, Other Customer, and Health Care Market Knowledge	40
3.2 Patient and Other Customer Relationships and Satisfaction	45
4 Measurement, Analysis, and Knowledge Management (90 points)	
4.1 Measurement and Analysis of Organizational Performance	45
4.2 Information and Knowledge Management	45
5 Staff Focus (85 points)	
5.1 Work Systems	35
5.2 Staff Learning and Motivation	25
5.3 Staff Well-Being and Satisfaction	25
6 Process Management (85 points)	
6.1 Health Care Processes	50
6.2 Support Processes	35
7 Health Care Results (450 points)	
7.1 Health Care Results	75
7.2 Patient- and Other Customer-Focused Results	75
7.3 Financial and Market Results	75
7.4 Staff and Work System Results	75
7.5 Organizational Effectiveness Results	75
7.6 Governance and Social Responsibility Results	75
Total Points	**1000**

KEY CHARACTERISTICS—2003 PERFORMANCE EXCELLENCE CRITERIA

The Criteria focus on health care results and the processes required to achieve them. Organizational Performance results are a composite of the following:

- Health care results

- Patient and customer-focused results

- Financial and market results

- Staff and work system results

- Organizational effectiveness results, including key internal operational performance measures

- Governance and social responsibility results

The use of this composite of indicators is intended to ensure that strategies are balanced—that they do not inappropriately trade off among important stakeholders, objectives, or short- and longer-term goals.

These results areas cover overall organization performance, including market and financial performance. The results areas also recognize the importance of suppliers and of community and national well-being. The use of a composite of indicators helps to ensure that strategies are balanced—that they do not inappropriately trade off among important stakeholders or objectives or between short- and long-term goals.

The Criteria *do not* prescribe that your organization should or should not have any particular functions, such as departments for quality, planning, or personnel. The Criteria do not prescribe how your organization should be structured or how different units in your organization should be managed. These factors differ among organizations and they are likely to change within an organization over time as needs and strategies evolve. The Criteria are non-prescriptive for the following reasons:

- The focus is on results, not on procedures, tools, or organizational structure. Organizations are encouraged to develop and demonstrate creative, adaptive, and flexible approaches for meeting basic requirements. Non-prescriptive requirements are intended to foster incremental and major ("breakthrough") improvements, as well as basic change.

- The selection of tools, techniques, systems, and organizational structure usually depends on factors, such as health care focus and size, organizational relationships, the organization's stage of development, and staff capabilities and responsibilities.

- A focus on common requirements, rather than on common procedures, fosters better understanding, communication, sharing, and alignment, while supporting innovation and diversity in approaches.

The Criteria support a systems approach to organizationwide goal alignment. The systems approach to goal alignment is embedded in the integrated structure of the Criteria and the results-oriented, cause and effect linkages among the Criteria parts.

The measures in the Criteria tie directly to patient and customer value and to overall performance that relate to key internal and external requirements of the organization. Measures serve both as a communications tool and a basis for deploying performance requirements. Such alignment ensures consistency of purpose while at the same time supporting speed, innovation, and decentralized decision making.

LEARNING CYCLES AND CONTINUOUS IMPROVEMENT

In high-performing organizations, action-oriented learning takes place through feedback between processes and results facilitated by learning or continuous improvement cycles. The learning cycles have four clearly defined and well-established stages (Figure 23).

1. Plan—planning, including design of processes, selection of measures, and deployment of requirements

2. Do—execute plans

3. Study/check—assess progress, taking into account internal and external results

4. Act—revise plans based on assessment findings, learning, new inputs, and new requirements

GOAL-BASED DIAGNOSIS

The Criteria and the Scoring Guidelines are the two elements that combine to make the diagnostic tool, which is part of a developmental assessment. A developmental assessment, unlike a compliance review, seeks to determine how advanced an organization is and then identify the vital few processes that need to be developed to move to the next higher level. The

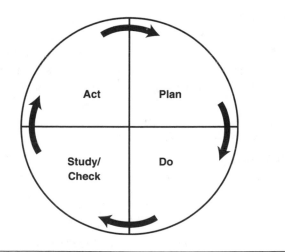

Figure 23 Continuous improvement cycle.

basic systems must be in place before they may be refined and enhanced. In a compliance review, on the other hand, all conditions or requirements must be met or the organization is "out of compliance" and may not be certified or registered. By design, compliance reviews audit against a set of minimum standards. A developmental review, such as that provided through the Baldrige Criteria, identifies continual improvement opportunities to help the organization achieve best-in-class performance—to excel and win.

This diagnostic assessment is a useful management tool that goes beyond most performance reviews and is applicable to a wide range of strategies and management systems.

CHANGES FROM THE 2002 CRITERIA

The Criteria for Performance Excellence continue to evolve, to help health care address a dynamic environment, to focus on strategy-driven performance, to consider the needs of all stakeholders, and to accommodate important changes in health care needs and practices. The increasing importance of a focus on governance and ethics, the need to capitalize on knowledge assets, the need to create value for patients and customers and the health care, and the alignment of all aspects of your performance management system with your results measurements receive greater attention in the 2003 Criteria. In addition, the Criteria emphasize the roles of organizational and personal learning and motivation as key differentiators in high-performing organizations. The Criteria continue to emphasize the central role that patients and customers play in defining and achieving Performance Excellence.

According to the Baldrige Award Office, two underlying concepts framed the overall thought process that led to this year's Criteria changes. The first is the need to have a set of Criteria for "evidence-based management." The second is the need to have a set of Criteria that focuses on the challenges of "running the health care organization" and "changing the health care organization;" to pursue current and future health care success, and to focus on opportunities for innovation.

The increasing importance of a focus on governance and ethics, the need to capitalize on knowledge assets, and the alignment of all aspects of a performance management system with results measurements receive greater attention in the 2003 Criteria. In addition, the Criteria emphasize the roles of organizational and personal learning and motivation as key differentiators in high performing organizations. The Criteria continue to emphasize the central role that patients and customers play in defining and achieving performance excellence.

The number of Items has been increased from 18 to 19 to reflect a reduction of one Item in Category 6 and the creation of two new Items in Category 7, due to the breakout of the former 7.1b (now 7.2) and 7.4b (now 7.6). The number of Areas to Address increased from 29 to 32 to reflect additions in Items 1.1b, 1.2b, 5.1b and c, 5.2b and the elimination of 6.1b and 6.3a.

A more detailed list of changes in the Criteria are summarized as follows:

Preface: Organizational Profile

Item P.1, *Organizational Description*, now requires a description of the organizational governance system and a description of the role of suppliers in key organizational processes. These additions help set the context for the assessment.

Item P.2, *Organizational Challenges*, now requires a list of available sources for comparative data to emphasize the need to develop these sources and to provide a context for selecting sources of comparative data. A Note has been added to Item P.2 to suggest that organizational approaches to process improvement might include six sigma and other performance improvement methodologies.

Category 1: Leadership

Item 1.1, *Organizational Leadership*, has been modified in several ways.

- First, in 1.1a(1) senior leaders must ensure two-way communication with subordinate leaders and other staff, key suppliers, and partners regarding organizational values, directions, and expectations. This two-way communication also provides an opportunity for senior leaders to receive feedback from others about their effectiveness as leaders. It replaces, to some extent, the requirement in previous versions of the Criteria that leaders seek feedback from staff through formal or informal means. Two-way communication should help foster this type of feedback.

- Second, in 1.1a(2) senior leaders must create an organizationwide environment that fosters and requires legal and ethical behavior.

- Third, a new Area to Address 1.1(b) has been added to emphasize the importance of the roles of senior leaders and the governing body to ensure that managers in the organization remain accountable for the organization's actions and performance, and that stakeholder and stockholder interests are protected. In addition, the governance system must ensure fiscal accountability and ensure that internal and external audits are independent (free from manipulation).

- Fourth, 1.1c(3) makes it clear that priorities for improvement and opportunities for innovation—based on organizational performance review findings—must be deployed throughout the organization and to appropriate suppliers and partners. In earlier versions of the Criteria, many applicants and Examiners incorrectly believed that "findings" of performance reviews themselves had to be deployed.

Item 1.2, now *Social Responsibility*, has been modified with a new Area to Address 1.2(b) (which was 1.2a(3) in 2002) to emphasize the requirement for key processes and measures for monitoring and ensuring ethical behavior throughout the organization and with external partners and the governance group.

Category 2: Strategic Planning

Item 2.1, *Strategy Development*, adds several new factors to be considered in the planning process:

- Opportunities the organization may have to redirect resources to higher priority services, or areas

- Changes in the national or global economy

- The impact of ethical issues

In addition, the organization must ensure that strategic objectives not only address short- and longer-term challenges identified in the Organizational Profile (P2) but also balance the needs of all key stakeholders.

Item 2.2, *Strategy Deployment*, has an added focus in 2.2a(1) on sustaining results that were driven by action plans.

Category 3: Patient, Other Customer and Health Care Market Focus

The language in this Category has an enhanced focus on patients and customers, with the addition in 3.2a(1) of specific references to building loyalty and exceeding patient and customer expectations, as well as meeting their absolute requirements.

Category 4: Measurement, Analysis, and Knowledge Management

The title of this category changed to reflect the growing importance of knowledge management, including the sharing of knowledge throughout the organization.

Item 4.1, *Measurement and Analysis of Organizational Performance*, in recognition of the continuously changing measurement and analysis needs of organizations, has an enhanced emphasis on addressing innovation and organizational and health care industry changes. In particular, the following small changes were made:

* 4.1a(1) combines the 2002 requirements of 4.1a(1 and 2) and now requires processes to systematically select, collect (new), align, and integrate data and information for tracking daily operations and organizational performance.

* 4.1a(1) also requires the data and information to be used to support innovation (similar in spirit to the deleted 2002 requirement in 4.1b(3) to use analysis to drive improvements).

* 4.1a(3) now requires the performance measurement system to be sensitive (able to respond) to rapid or unexpected changes from inside or outside the organization.

Item 4.2, now *Information and Knowledge Management* has been restructured.

* Elements of the 2002 requirement in 4.2b(1) pertaining to ensuring software reliability, security, and user-friendliness has been moved to 4.2a(2).

* The 2002 requirement in 4.2b(2) pertaining to keeping hardware and software systems current has been added to 4.2a(3).

* A new Area to Address (4.2b) has been added.

  – Area to address 4.2b(1) looks at the management of organizational knowledge in recognition of the growing importance of the transfer of staff knowledge, the sharing of best practices, and transfer of relevant knowledge from patients and customers, suppliers, and partners.

  – Area to address 4.2b(2) [taken from 2002 Area 4.2a(2)] requires the organization to ensure organizational knowledge (in addition to data and information) to be integral (complete), timely, reliable, secure, accurate, and confidential.

Category 5: Staff Focus

Item 5.1, *Work Systems*, has essentially the requirements as in 2002, but now has three Areas to Address to focus attention on three important aspects:

* 5.1a Organization and Management of Work

* Staff Performance Management

* Recruitment and Career Progression

Item 5.2, now *Staff Learning and Motivation*, has two Areas to Address, with an enhanced emphasis on staff motivation and career development [moved from the 2002 requirement in 5.1a(2)]. Now all key aspects of staff learning and development are located in Item 5.2.

Category 6: Process Management

This category has been restructured to make clear the parallel requirements of effective design, production, and delivery of all core (value creation) and support processes.

Item 6.1, *Health Care Processes*, is a new Item that replaces and combines most of the requirements of

2002 Items 6.1 (Health Care Service Processes) and 6.2 (Business Processes).

- The new Item 6.1 addresses all the critical organizational processes important to health care value for the organization, its patients and customers, and other key stakeholders. These are the processes most important to "running the health care business" and achieving a sustainable competitive advantage.

- All health care processes must demonstrate an effective and efficient design process to ensure patient and customer requirements are met.

- Effective systems must be in place to control and improve the development, and delivery of core (value creation) and health care processes.

Item 6.2, now *Support Processes*, (moved from the 2002 requirements in Item 6.3) requires the organization to identify and describe key processes that support the core health care processes.

- All support processes must demonstrate an effective and efficient design process to ensure patient and customer requirements are met.

- Effective systems must be in place to control and improve the development and delivery of key support processes.

Category 7: Organizational Performance Results

The four Items in the 2002 Category 7 have been spread among 6 Items in 2003. In addition, in 2003 all Items in Category 7 are weighted equally (each is worth 75 points).

Item 7.2, *Health Care Results*, is a stand-alone Results Item in 2003. This new Item was created to provide a greater focus on health care service quality.

Item 7.4, *Staff and Work Systems Results*, for 2003 now requires results to be reported for staff learning and development [7.4a(2)] in addition to the results required in 2002 pertaining to work system performance and effectiveness [7.4a(1)] and staff well-being, satisfaction and motivation [7.4a(3)].

Item 7.5, *Organizational Effectiveness Results* is structured differently from 2002 but requires the same results to be reported.

Item 7.6, *Governance and Social Responsibility Results*, is a stand-alone Item in 2003 that elevates and expands 2002 Area 7.4b (Public Responsibility and Citizenship Results). This new Item was created to provide a greater focus on improving stakeholder trust in organization governance and ensure ethical behavior and legal compliance and requires results for:

- Fiscal accountability [7.6a(1)] (new)

- Ethical behavior and stakeholder trust [7.6a(2)] (new)

- Regulatory, accreditation, assessment, and legal compliance [7.6a(3)], which was part of 7.4b in 2002

- Organizational citizenship [7.6a(4)], which was part of 7.4b in 2002

Other Items in Category 7 were renumbered as the following table indicates.

2003 Item Reference	2002 Item Reference
7.1a(1 and 2)	7.1a(1 and 2)
7.2a	7.1b
7.3a(1 and 2)	7.2a(1 and 2)
7.4a(1, 2, 3), 2 is new	7.3a(1 and 2)
7.5a(1, 2, 3)	7.4a(1 and 2)
7.6a(1, 2, 3, 4), 1 and 2 are new	7.4b

Glossary

New terms have been added to the Glossary:

- Patient and Customer

- Governance

- Key

- Knowledge Assets

- Value Creation

Organizational Profile

The Organizational Profile is a snapshot of your organization, the key influences on how you operate, and the key challenges you face.

Importance of the Organizational Profile

The Organizational Profile is critically important because:

- It is the most appropriate starting point for self-assessment and for writing an application.

- It helps you identify potential gaps in key information and focus on key performance requirements and health care results.

- It is used by the Examiners and Judges in all stages of application review, including the site visit, to understand your organization and what you consider important. It sets the context for the assessment.

- It may be used by itself for an initial self-assessment. If you identify topics for which conflicting, little, or no information is available, it is possible that your assessment need go no further and you can use these topics for action planning.

Page Limit

For Baldrige Award applicants, the Organizational Profile is limited to five pages. These are not counted in the overall 50-page limit for the application. Typing and format instructions for the Organizational Profile are the same as for the application. These instructions are given in the Baldrige Award Application Forms booklet, a copy of which appears on the CD included with this book.

PREFACE: ORGANIZATIONAL PROFILE

The **Organizational Profile** is a snapshot of your organization, the key influences on how you operate, and the key challenges you face.

P.1 ORGANIZATIONAL DESCRIPTION

Describe your organization's environment and your key relationships with patients and other customers, suppliers, and partners.

Within your response, include answers to the following questions:

a. Organizational Environment

(1) What are your organization's main health care services? What are the delivery mechanisms used to provide your health care services to your patients?

(2) What is your organizational culture? What are your stated purpose, vision, mission, and values?

(3) What is your staff profile? What are their education levels? What are your organization's workforce and job diversity, organized bargaining units, use of contract and privileged staff, and special health and safety requirements?

(4) What are your major technologies, equipment, and facilities?

(5) What is the legal and regulatory environment under which your organization operates? What are the applicable occupational health and safety regulations; accreditation, certification, or registration requirements; and environmental and financial regulations relevant to health care service delivery?

b. Organizational Relationships

(1) What is your organizational structure and governance system? What are the reporting relationships among your board of trustees, senior leaders, and your parent organization, as appropriate?

(2) What are your key patient and other customer groups and health care market segments, as appropriate? What are their key requirements and expectations for your health care services? What are the differences in these requirements and expectations among patient and other customer groups and market segments?

(3) What role do suppliers and partners play in your key processes? What are your most important types of suppliers and partners? What are your most important supply chain requirements?

(4) What are your key supplier and partnering relationships and communication mechanisms?

Continued

Notes: *Continued*

N1. Health care service delivery to your patients and other customers [P.1a(1)] might be direct, or through contractors or partners.

N2. Market segments [P.1b(2)] might be based on health care services or features, geography, health care service delivery modes, payors, business volume, population demographics, or other factors that allow your organization to define related market characteristics.

N3. Patient and other customer group and health care market segment requirements [P.1b(2)] might include accessibility, continuity of care, electronic communication, and billing requirements.

N4. Communication mechanisms [P.1b(4)] should be two-way and might be in person, electronic, by telephone, and/or written. For many organizations, these mechanisms might be changing as marketplace requirements change.

P.1 Organizational Description Item Linkages

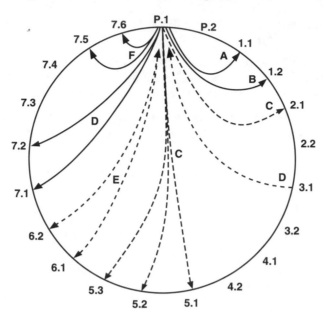

	NATURE OF RELATIONSHIP
A	The organizational structure and governance system described in P.1b(1) sets the context for the review of the management systems for proper governance and ethical behavior [1.1a(2)].
B	The regulatory environment described in P.1a(5) sets the context for the review of the management systems for public responsibility [1.2a(1)].
C	Staff educational levels, diversity, and other characteristics [P.1a(3)] may affect the determination of staff strengths and weaknesses as a part of the strategic planning process [2.1a(2)]. Staff characteristics, such as educational levels, workforce and job diversity, the existence of bargaining units, the use of contract staff, and other special requirements, help set the context for determining the requirements for knowledge and skill sharing across work units, jobs, and locations [5.1a(3)], determining appropriate training needs by staff segment [5.2a(3)] and tailoring benefits, services, and satisfaction assessment methods for staff according to various types of categories [5.3b(1, 2, and 3].
D	The patient and customer and market groups reported in P.1b(2) were determined using the processes described in 3.1a(1 and 2). The information in P.1b(2) helps examiners identify the kind of results, broken out by patient and customer and market segment, that should be reported in Items 7.1 and 7.2.
E	The information in P.1a(1) derives from the delivery processes described in 6.1a and helps set the context for the Examiner review of those processes [6.1a(3)].
F	The legal and regulatory requirements descried in P.1a(5), and the key suppliers and partners listed in P.1b(3) create an expectation that related performance results will be reported in 7.6 and 7.5 respectively.

P.2 ORGANIZATIONAL CHALLENGES

Describe your organization's competitive environment, your key strategic challenges, and your system for performance improvement.

Within your response, include answers to the following questions:

a. Competitive Environment

(1) What is your competitive position? What is your relative size and growth in the health care industry or markets served? What are the numbers and types of competitors and key collaborators for your organization?

(2) What are the principal factors that determine your success relative to your competitors and other organizations delivering similar health care services? What are any key changes taking place that affect your competitive situation or opportunities for collaborating?

(3) What are your key available sources of comparative and competitive data from within the health care industry? What are your key available sources of comparative data for analogous processes outside the health care industry? What limitations, if any, are there in your ability to obtain these data?

b. Strategic Challenges

What are your key health care service, operational, and human resources strategic challenges?

c. Performance Improvement System

(1) What is the overall approach you use to maintain an organizational focus on performance improvement and to guide systematic evaluation and improvement of key processes?

(2) What is your overall approach to organizational learning and sharing your knowledge assets within the organization?

Notes:

N1. Factors [P.2a(2)] might include differentiators such as technology leadership, accessibility, health care and administrative support services offered, cost, and e-services.

N2. Challenges (P.2b) might include cycle times reduced for health care service introduction; mergers and acquisitions; patient and customer loyalty and retention; staff retention; and electronic communication with staff, patients, and other customers.

N3. Performance improvement (P.2c) is an assessment dimension used in the Scoring System to evaluate the maturity of organizational approaches and deployment. This question is intended to help you and the Baldrige Examiners set a context for your approach to performance improvement.

N4. Overall approaches to process improvement [P.2c(1)] might include implementing the use of ISO 9000:2000 standards, six-sigma methodology, Plan-Do-Study-Act (PDSA) improvement cycles, or other process improvement tools.

P.2 Organizational Challenges Item Linkages

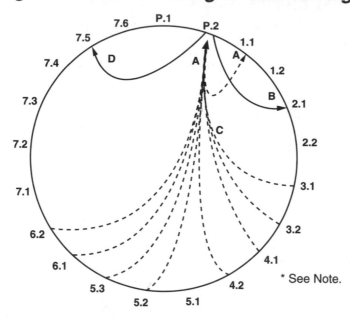

	NATURE OF RELATIONSHIP
A	Leaders [1.1a(2)] are responsible for creating an environment that drives organizational learning, which in turn contributes to the overall focus on performance improvement [P.2c(1)]. The overall approaches to systematic evaluation and improvement, organizational learning, and knowledge sharing identified in P.2c should be consistent with overall *requirements for improvement* specifically required in Items 1.1c(4) leadership effectiveness; 3.1a(3) improving patient and customer requirements definition; 3.2a(4) improving patient and customer relationships and patient and customer access; 3.2b(4) improving processes to determine patient and customer satisfaction; 4.1a supporting innovation and keeping up with rapid or unexpected organizational or external changes; 4.2a(3) keeping data availability (including software and hardware) current, especially in a volatile work environment; 5.2a(6) improving training and education effectiveness; 5.3a(1) improving workforce health, safety, and well-being; 6.1a(6) improving health care processes; and 6.2a(6) improving support services.
B	The competitive environment defined in P.2a should be examined as part of the strategy development process [2.1a(2)]. In addition, the strategic challenges identified in P.2b should be addressed by the strategic objectives in 2.1b(1).
C	Information about competitors, which is needed to create the description for P.2a, uses processes discussed in Items 3.1a(1), 3.2b(3), and 4.1a(2).
D	Progress in achieving strategic challenges, as described in P.2b, should be reported in Item 7.5a(3).

Note: To make the circle diagrams less cluttered, all of the links described in paragraph A will not be repeated on the other diagrams.

1 Leadership—120 Points

*The **Leadership** Category examines how your organization's senior leaders address values, directions, and performance expectations, as well as a focus on patients and customers and other stakeholders, empowerment, innovation, and learning. Also examined are your organization's governance and how your organization addresses its public and community responsibilities.*

The leadership system must promote organizational core values, set high-performance expectations, and promote an organizationwide focus on patients and customers, staff empowerment, learning, and innovation. The Leadership Category looks at how senior leaders guide the organization in setting directions and seeking future opportunities. Senior leaders must communicate clear values and high-performance expectations that address the needs of all stakeholders. The category also looks at the how the organization meets its responsibilities to the public and how it practices good citizenship.

The Category contains two Items:

Organizational Leadership

- Communicating and reinforcing clear values, performance expectations, and a focus on creating value for patients and customers and other stakeholders

- Reinforcing an environment for empowerment and innovation and staff and organizational learning

- Reviewing organizational performance and capabilities, competitiveness, and progress relative to goals, and setting priorities for improvement

- Evaluating and improving the effectiveness of senior leadership and management throughout the organization, including staff input in the process

Social Responsibility

- For regulatory and other legal requirements in areas such as safety, environmental protection, and waste management; anticipating public concerns and addressing risks to the public

- Ensuring ethical health care practices

- For strengthening and supporting key communities

1.1 ORGANIZATIONAL LEADERSHIP (70 PTS.)   Approach/Deployment

Describe how senior leaders guide your organization. Describe your organization's governance system. Describe how senior leaders review organizational performance.

Within your response, include answers to the following questions:

a. Senior Leadership Direction

(1) How do senior leaders set and deploy organizational values, short- and longer-term directions, and performance expectations? How do senior leaders include a focus on creating and balancing value for patients and other customers and stakeholders in their performance expectations? How do senior leaders communicate organizational values, directions, and expectations through your leadership system, to all staff, and to key suppliers and partners? How do senior leaders ensure two-way communication on these topics?

(2) How do senior leaders create an environment for empowerment, innovation, and organizational agility? How do they create an environment for organizational and staff learning? How do they create an environment that fosters legal and ethical behavior?

b. Organizational Governance

How does your organization address the following key factors in your governance system?

- Management accountability for the organization's actions

- Fiscal accountability

- Independence in internal and external audits

- Protection of stockholder and stakeholder interests, as appropriate

c. Organizational Performance Review

(1) How do senior leaders review organizational performance and capabilities? How do they use these reviews to assess organizational success, competitive performance, and progress relative to short- and longer-term goals? How do they use these reviews to assess your organizational ability to address changing health care service needs?

(2) What are the key performance measures regularly reviewed by your senior leaders? What are your key recent performance review findings?

(3) How do senior leaders translate organizational performance review findings into priorities for continuous and breakthrough improvement of key organizational performance results and into opportunities for innovation? How are these priorities and opportunities deployed throughout your organization? When appropriate, how are they deployed to your suppliers and partners to ensure organizational alignment?

(4) How do you evaluate the performance of your senior leaders, including both administrative and health care leaders? How do senior leaders use organizational performance review findings to improve both their own leadership effectiveness and that of your board and leadership system, as appropriate?

Continued

Notes: *Continued*

N1. Senior leaders include the head of the organization and his or her direct reports. In health care organizations with separate administrative/operational and health care provider leadership, "senior leaders" refers to both sets of leaders and the relationships among those leaders.

N2. Organizational directions [1.1a(1)] relate to creating the vision for the organization and to setting the context for strategic objectives and action plans described in Items 2.1 and 2.2.

N3. Senior leaders' organizational performance reviews (1.1c) should be informed by organizational performance analyses described in 4.1b and guided by strategic objectives and action plans described in Items 2.1 and 2.2. Senior leaders' organizational performance reviews also might be informed by internal or external Baldrige assessments.

N4. Leadership performance evaluation [1.1c(4)] might be supported by peer reviews, formal performance management reviews (5.1b), and formal and/or informal staff and other stakeholder feedback and surveys.

N5. Your organizational performance results should be reported in Items 7.1–7.6.

There are three distinctly different aspects to the requirements of Item 1.1. First, 1.1a describes "sending" or outgoing actions of leaders. Through their outward focus they push values, create expectations, and align the work of the organization. Second, 1.1b addresses how the governance or oversight processes ensure fiscal accountability and the protection of stakeholder and stockholder interests. Third, 1.1c requires leaders to receive, rather than send, information. Here they must monitor progress and use this incoming data to determine where resources and priorities must be aligned to ensure appropriate progress is achieved.

The "sending" part of this Item (1.1a) looks at how senior leaders create and sustain values that promote high performance throughout the organization. In promoting high performance, senior leaders set and deploy values, short- and longer-term directions, and performance expectations; and balance the expectations of patients and customers and other stakeholders. Leaders develop and implement systems to ensure values are understood and consistently followed. An organization's failure to achieve high levels of performance can almost always be traced to a failure in leadership.

- To consistently promote high performance, leaders must clearly set direction and make sure

everyone in the organization understands his or her responsibilities. Success requires a strong future orientation and a commitment to improvement, innovation, and the disciplined change that is needed to carry it out. This requires creating an environment for empowerment, learning, innovation, and organizational agility, as well as the means for rapid and effective application of knowledge.

- Leaders also ensure that organizational values actually guide the behavior of leaders and staff throughout the organization or the values are meaningless. To enhance performance excellence the "right" values must be adopted. These values must include a focus on patients and customers and other stakeholders. Since various patient and customer and stakeholder groups often have conflicting interests, leaders must strike a balance that optimizes the interests of all groups. The failure to ensure a patient and customer focus usually causes the organization and its staff to focus internally. The lack of a patient and customer focus forces staff to default to their own ideas of what patients and customers really "need." This increases the risk of becoming arrogant and not caring about the requirements of patients and customers. It also increases the potential for creating and delivering services that no patient or customer wants or values. That, in turn, increases rework, scrap, waste, and added cost/lower value.

- Senior leaders must ensure two-way communication with subordinate leaders and other staff, key suppliers, and partners regarding organizational values, directions, and expectations. This two-way communication also provides an opportunity for senior leaders to receive feedback from others about their effectiveness as leaders. It replaces, to some extent the requirement in previous versions of the Criteria that leaders seek feedback from staff through formal or informal means. Two-way communication should help foster this type of feedback. Accordingly, it is recommended that part of the communication with staff involve formal and informal staff and peer feedback of leader effectiveness, such as using a 360-degree feedback survey or an upward evaluation. This information could be structured to help evaluate the effectiveness of leaders at all levels, as required in Item 1.1c(4).

- Leaders must create an environment for empowerment and agility, as well as the means for rapid and effective application of knowledge.

The new 2003 organizational governance requirement (1.1b) is intended to address the need for a responsible, informed, and accountable governance body that can protect the interests of key stakeholders, including stockholders. It should have independence in review and audit functions. It should also have a performance evaluation function that monitors organizational and CEO performance. The governance structure should ensure that all leaders and supervisors are held accountable for the organization's actions.

The "receiving" part of this Item (1.1c) looks at how senior leaders review organizational performance in a disciplined, fact-based manner, what key performance measures they regularly review, and how review findings are used to drive improvement and innovation. This organizational review should cover all areas of performance, and provide a complete and accurate picture of the "state of health" of the organization. This includes not only how well the organization is currently performing, but also how well it is moving to secure future success.

- Key performance measures should focus on and reflect the key drivers of success leaders regularly review. These measures should relate to the strategic objectives necessary for success.

- Leaders should use these reviews to drive improvement and change. These reviews should provide a reliable means to guide the improvement and change needed to achieve the organization's key objectives, success factors, and measures.

- Leaders must create a consistent process to translate the review findings into an action agenda, sufficiently specific for deployment throughout the organization and to suppliers/partners—people who need to take action to improve.

- In addition, the organization must evaluate the effectiveness of senior leaders, board members, and the entire leadership system. To ensure the evaluation is accurate, staff should provide feedback to the leaders and managers at all levels, which may be accomplished, in part, by the two-way communication required in Item 1.1a(1) and using tools such as 360-degree reviews and upward evaluations.

- Finally, leaders and supervisors at all levels should take action, based on the feedback, to improve their effectiveness. It is critical that leaders, managers, and supervisors at all levels and in all parts of the organization effectively drive and reinforce the principles of Performance Excellence through words and actions. Remember, nearly every failure to achieve and sustain excellence can be traced to a failure on the part of leaders and managers. Jack Welch, former CEO of General Electric, in his last letter to stockholders emphasized the importance of rewarding and nurturing the top 20 percent of staff, and getting rid of the bottom 10 percent. The same is true of health care leaders and managers who do not or will not aggressively and effectively lead the effort to enhance Performance Excellence.

1.1 Organizational Leadership

How senior leaders guide the organization in setting direction and developing and sustaining an effective leadership system throughout the organization

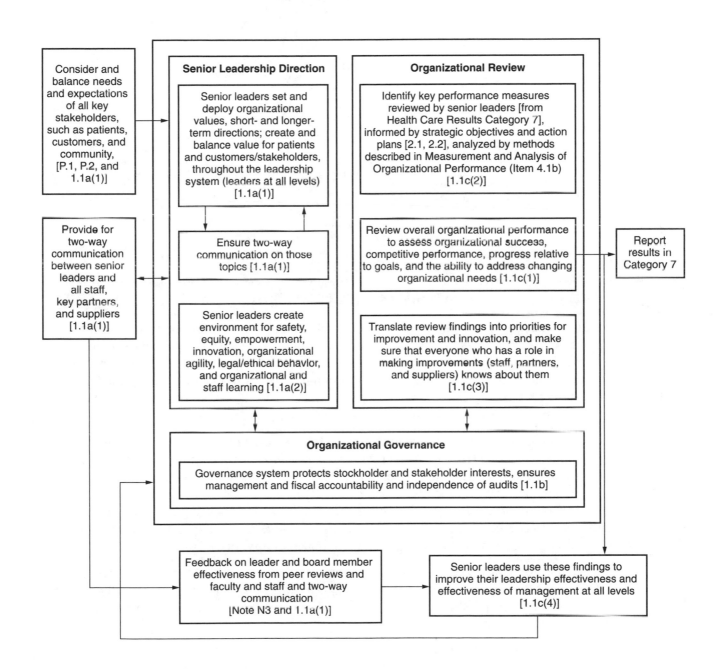

1.1 Leadership Item Linkages

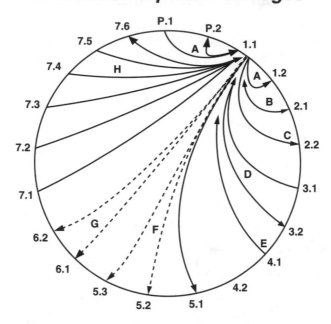

	NATURE OF RELATIONSHIP
A	Leaders [1.1], in support of organizational values, role model and support ethical behavior [1.2b] and public responsibility [1.2a] and practice good citizenship [1.2c]. The organizational structure and governance system described in P.1b(1) sets the context for the review of the management systems for proper governance [1.1b] and ethical behavior [1.1a(2) and 1.2b]. Leaders [1.1a(2)] are responsible for creating an environment that drives organizational learning, which in turn contributes to the overall focus on performance improvement [P.2c].
B	To effectively set organizational direction and expectations, leaders [1.1a(1)] participate in the strategic planning process [2.1]. As part of this effort, leaders [1.1a(1)] ensure that strategic objectives balance the needs of key patients/customers and stakeholders [2.1b(2)]. Leaders also use the time lines for achieving strategic objectives [2.1b(1)] as a basis for defining and monitoring expected progress closely [1.1c(1)], which means the timelines in [2.1b(1)] should define the expected levels of future performance that the leaders use during the performance reviews [1.1c(1)] to determine if the organization is making appropriate progress or not.
C	Leaders [1.1a(1)] ensure that plans are clearly communicated and understood (deployed) at all levels throughout the organization and used to align work [2.2a(1)]. Leaders [1.1a] also approve the overall goals set forth in the plan based, in part, on information about the expected levels of competitor performance [2.2b].
D	Leaders [1.1a(1)] use information from patients and customers about requirements and preferences [3.1a(2)] and satisfaction/dissatisfaction [3.2b] to set direction and create opportunity for the organization. Leaders [1.1] also have a responsibility for creating and driving patient- and customer-focused values to meet patient and customer requirements and expectations throughout the organization [3.2a].

Continued

NATURE OF RELATIONSHIP	*Continued*
E	Leaders [1.1c(1)] use analyses of data [4.1b(1 and 2)] to monitor organizational performance and understand relationships among performance, staff satisfaction, patients and customers, markets, and financial success. These analyses are also used for decision making at all levels to set priorities for action and allocate resources for maximum advantage [1.1c(3)]. They are also responsible for using comparative data [from 4.1a(2)] to set meaningful goals to achieve organizational success.
F	Leaders [1.1a(2)] create an environment for staff empowerment, innovation, and learning throughout the entire organization through the design of work and jobs [5.1a(1)]. They ensure that the compensation and recognition system [5.1b] encourages staff at all levels to achieve performance excellence in areas most critical to the organization. Leaders [1.1a(2)] are also responsible for supporting appropriate skill development of all staff through training and development systems and reinforcing learning on the job [5.2a], as well as creating effective systems to enhance staff satisfaction, well-being, and motivation [5.3b].
G	Leaders [1.1] are responsible for creating an environment that supports high performance, including monitoring processes for value creation [6.1] and support services [6.2] processes. Leaders must ensure that design, delivery, support, and supplier performance processes are aligned and consistently evaluated and refined.
H	Senior leaders [1.1c] use performance results data [from Category 7] for many activities, including monitoring organizational performance [1.1c(1)]; deploying priority improvement areas to focus work and ensure alignment [1.1c(3)]; strategic planning [2.1a]; setting goals and priorities [2.1b(1)]; reinforcing or rewarding staff performance [5.1b]; and for improving their effectiveness and the effectiveness of leaders at all levels [1.1c(4)]. In addition, key results of leadership behavior, such as results of ethical behavior [1.1a(2)] and fiscal accountability [1.1b], are reported in Governance and Social Responsibilities Results [7.6a(1 and 2)].

	IF YOU DON'T DO WHAT THE CRITERIA REQUIRE...
Item Reference	**Possible Adverse Consequences**
1.1a(1)	If senior leaders fail to make performance expectations clear (especially defining them in measurable terms), it may create uncertainty among managers and staff throughout the organization about what they must accomplish and the direction they must follow. This may cause managers to substitute their own ideas, objectives, and directions, which may not be in alignment with those of top leadership. The lack of alignment may also contribute to redundancy and wasted resources. As a consequence, some parts of the organization may work at cross-purposes with other parts of the organization.
1.1a(1)	If senior leaders do not create an environment that focuses on creating value for patients and customers and other stakeholders, staff and managers within the organization may become internally focused and risk negatively impacting the patient and customer focus on which the organization was built. An internal focus may contribute to a climate where staff are not primarily interested in listening to patient and customer requirements or concerns. This may produce a high level of organizational arrogance where staff believe they know what the patients and customers want better than the patient and customer. This type of behavior can antagonize patients and customers and produce high levels of patient and customer dissatisfaction. In a related area, if senior leaders do not create an environment that focuses on balancing value for patients and customers and other stakeholders—especially when different patient and customer groups have competing interests—it may erode patient and customer confidence and eventually cause a loss of patients and customers. For example, patients want inexpensive, pain-free, quick, health care services while the board and stockholders want profits and revenues to increase. Excessive focus on one group over the other makes it difficult to maximize value and keep both patients and stockholders loyal.
1.1a(2)	If senior leaders do not create an environment that promotes staff empowerment, they risk not leveraging the power of a formidable asset—their people. As a consequence, leaders may be effectively sending a message that staff do not have the skills or ability to make decisions on their own—that micromanagement is the preferred approach within the organization. This kind of environment tends to migrate decision making to higher and higher levels in the organization, creating excessive delay and working against organizational agility. Unnecessary levels of review and approval may also tend to minimize innovation and creativity throughout the organization. Taken together, these problems are likely to add cost but not value—making it increasingly difficult to be successful in a highly competitive industry.

Continued

	IF YOU DON'T DO WHAT THE CRITERIA REQUIRE... *Continued*
Item Reference	**Possible Adverse Consequences**
1.1b	The adverse consequences of unconcerned or incompetent organizational governance can be sudden and spectacular. One need only consider the impact of the Severe Acute Respiratory Syndrome (SARS) on the public and particularly on health care workers. With increased public scrutiny, organizations that do not have visible and effective processes in place to ensure management accountability and protection of all stakeholder and staff interests may not be able to maintain public trust and confidence. Their market share and consumer confidence may remain flat. Intrusive government oversight may increase, which diverts leadership attention and organizational resources away from value-adding outcomes needed to beat competitors, enhance services, and satisfy patients and customers and other stakeholders.
1.1c(1)	If senior leaders do not have a systematic, fact-based process in place that enables them to review organizational performance and assess progress toward goals, it may send a message throughout the organization that performance outcomes are really not that important. If results are not important to top leaders, they may not be considered important to lower levels within the organization and staff at all levels may not contribute optimum effort to achieve these (unimportant) results.
1.1c(2)	If key performance measures that are used to review organizational performance have not been defined or are not consistent with organizational strategic priorities [Item 2.1b(1)] and related actions [Item 2.2a(1)], people in the organization may not be focusing their work in areas essential to organizational success, further suboptimizing organizational performance and value to the patient and customer. The wrong performance measures may prevent senior leaders from monitoring the things that are most critical to organizational success and making appropriate adjustments when needed.
1.1c(3)	Even if senior leaders have an effective process to review organizational performance [Item 1.1c(1)], but do not effectively use these review findings to identify priorities for improvement and areas that should be targets of innovation, they may not be providing appropriate focus and alignment throughout the organization and to affected suppliers and partners. This may make it difficult for staff, managers, partners, and suppliers to make the changes needed to correct problems or comply with the new priorities for improvement, contributing to wasted resources and performance failures. The long-standing failure to identify priorities for improvement or targets of innovation may contribute to the perception that the status quo is acceptable and continuous improvement is not important. This may further contribute to organizational stagnation and may make it difficult to keep pace with competitors and increasing patient and customer requirements.

IF YOU DON'T DO WHAT THE CRITERIA REQUIRE...	Continued

Item Reference	Possible Adverse Consequences
1.1c(4)	Even new staff can tell the difference between an effective leader and an incompetent one. Unfortunately, an incompetent leader is frequently blind to this fact. *(Where do you think Scott Adams gets his material for the "Dilbert" cartoon?)* The combination of organizational performance outcomes and staff (subordinate) feedback can provide critical information to help leaders throughout the leadership system identify personal strengths and opportunities for improvement. Without this information leaders may not be able to focus effectively on areas where improvement would be essential not only to personal growth and development, but to better organizational results. Leaders that do not have accurate feedback about their strengths and weaknesses may not be able to keep pace with changing health care needs and directions as they are challenged to work smarter by patients and customers, competitors, and the demands of stockholders and other stakeholders. They may not be able to lead their organization to winning levels of Performance Excellence.

1.1 ORGANIZATIONAL LEADERSHIP—SAMPLE EFFECTIVE PRACTICES

Perhaps most critical is that senior leaders demonstrate absolute, unwavering commitment to performance excellence—even aligning reward and recognition to provide incentives and disincentives. The best senior leaders do not tolerate a lack of aggressive commitment and urgent action from subordinate managers at any level. They send a clear message to staff that the effort is serious.

A. Senior Leadership Direction

- All senior leaders are personally involved in performance improvement.

- Senior leaders spend a significant portion of their time on performance improvement activities.

- Senior leaders carry out many visible activities (for example, goal setting, planning, and recognition and reward of performance and process improvement).

- Senior leaders regularly communicate Performance Excellence values to staff and managers and ensure that all demonstrate those values in their work.

- Senior leaders participate on performance improvement teams and use performance excellence tools and practices.

- Senior leaders mentor managers and ensure that promotion criteria reflect organizational values, especially patient and customer satisfaction.

- Senior leaders study and learn about the improvement practices of other organizations.

- Senior leaders clearly and consistently articulate values (patient and customer focus, patient and customer satisfaction, role model leadership, continuous improvement, staff involvement, and performance optimization) throughout the organization.

- Senior leaders ensure that organizational values are used to provide direction to all staff in the organization to help achieve the mission, vision, and performance goals.

- Senior leaders use effective and innovative approaches to reach out to all staff to spread the organization's values and align its work to support organizational goals.

- Senior leaders effectively surface problems and encourage staff risk-taking.

- Roles and responsibilities of managers are clearly defined, understood by them, and used to evaluate and improve their performance.

- Managers serve as role models (walk the talk) in leading systematic performance improvement.

- Job definitions with quality indices are clearly delineated for each level of the organization, objectively measured, and presented in a logical and organized structure.

- Many different communication strategies are used to reinforce organizational values. Leaders at all levels make two-way communication easy through personal methods, such as voice mail, e-mail, town hall meetings, and face-to-face meetings. They also use anonymous methods such as 360-degree surveys to ensure feedback is honest and complete.

- Leader behavior (not merely words) clearly communicates what is expected of the organization and its staff.

- Systems and procedures are deployed that encourage cooperation and a cross-functional approach to management, team activities, and problem solving.

- Leaders monitor staff acceptance and adoption of vision and values using annual surveys, staff focus groups, and e-mail questions.

- A systematic process is in place for evaluating and improving the integration or alignment of Performance Excellence values throughout the organization.

B. Organizational Governance

- Independence of the board of directors is ensured by requiring that a substantial percentage of directors come from outside the organization.

- Fiscal accountability is assured by a variety of processes including independent audits and separation of consultants from auditing functions. Audit and consulting services are not provided by the same or affiliated companies.

- Stockholders (if appropriate) approve the election slates for the board of directors and even place names on the slate.

- Board term limits ensure rotating membership to ensure a fresh and objective voice is present on the board.

- Board audit committees contain at least one financial expert who is independent of the company.

- The full board of directors reviews financial statements quarterly after the CEO and CFO certifies accuracy.

- Directors with competing interests, such as key suppliers or interlocking directors, are eliminated or influence is minimized.

- Dissent, debate, and open criticism are encouraged among board members.

- CEOs promote candor and meaningful discussion at board meetings by sharing relevant information with directors before meetings to permit careful analysis before the deliberation begins.

- Board members formally assess their peers in writing and ask poorly performing members to resign.

- A climate of trust and candor exists among board members. No secret group wields power to make back-room decisions.

C. Organizational Performance Review

- Reviews against measurable performance standards are held frequently.

- Actions are taken to assist units that are not meeting goals or performing to plan.

- Senior leaders systematically and routinely check the effectiveness of their leadership activities (for example, seeking feedback at least annually from staff and peers using an upward or 360-degree evaluation), and taking steps to improve.

- Leaders at all levels determine how well they carried out their activities (what went right or wrong and how they could be done better).

- There is evidence of adopting changes to improve leader effectiveness.

- Patients and customers, performance, and financial data drive priorities for organizational improvement and innovation.

- Senior leaders base their health care decisions on reliable data and facts pertaining to patients and customers, operational processes, and staff performance and satisfaction.

- Senior leaders hold regular meetings to review performance data and communicate problems, successes, and effective approaches to improve work.

- Senior leaders conduct monthly reviews of organizational performance. This requires that subordinates conduct biweekly reviews, and workers and work teams provide daily performance updates. Corrective actions are developed to improve performance that deviates from planned performance.

- A culture of continuous improvement has been developed. The number of benchmarking visits by health care and other organizations is a strong indicator of the strength of an organizational culture.

- In alignment with their mission, the organization has adopted a culture of non-violence, avoiding any use of language that could be perceived to imply violence.

- Senior leadership has established a set of "Organization Requirements for Suppliers" that is balanced by a set of "Supplier Requirements for the Organization." A similar set of balanced requirements has been established with Physician Partners. This sets a standard of balanced obligations between the organization and suppliers and the organization and its physician partners.

- To ensure effective communication of important leadership messages across the multi-state organization, a consistent package of materials is sent to each location. This package includes video, brochures, and Personal Commitment cards.

- Decision-making authority is deployed through the organization through the Mutual Accountability process. This has had a significant impact on staff satisfaction and turnover.

- Senior leaders conduct monthly reviews of organizational performance. This requires that subordinates conduct biweekly reviews, and staff and work teams provide daily performance updates. Corrective actions are developed to improve performance that deviates from planned performance.

1.2 SOCIAL RESPONSIBILITY (50 PTS.)   **Approach/Deployment**
Describe how your organization addresses its responsibilities to the public, ensures ethical behavior, practices good citizenship, and contributes to the health of its community.

Within your response, include answers to the following questions:

a. **Responsibilities to the Public**

   (1) How do you address the impacts on society of your health care services and operations? What are your key processes, measures, and goals for achieving and surpassing regulatory, legal, and accreditation requirements, as appropriate? What are your key processes, measures, and goals for addressing risks associated with your management of health care services and other organizational operations?

   (2) How do you anticipate public concerns with current and future services and operations? How do you prepare for these concerns in a proactive manner?

b. **Ethical Behavior**

   How do you ensure ethical behavior in all stakeholder transactions and interactions? What are your key processes and measures or indicators for monitoring ethical behavior throughout your organization, with key partners and collaborators, and in your governance structure?

c. **Support of Key Communities and Community Health**

   How does your organization actively support and strengthen your key communities? How do you identify key communities and determine areas of emphasis for organizational involvement and support? What are your key communities? How do your senior leaders and your staff contribute to improving these communities and to building community health?

Continued

Notes: *Continued*

N1. Societal responsibilities in areas critical to your organization also should be addressed in Strategy Development (Item 2.1) and in Process Management (Category 6). Key results, such as results of regulatory and legal compliance (including malpractice) and accreditation, should be reported as Governance and Social Responsibility Results (in Item 7.6).

N2. Public concerns [1.2a(2)] might include patient safety; cost; equitable and timely access to providers; emergence of new health care threats; and the handling of medical waste.

N3. Ethical behavior (1.2b) includes business, professional, health care practice, and patient rights issues. It also includes public accountability and disclosure of information about your organization health care performance.

N4. Measures or indicators of ethical behavior (1.2b) might include the percentage of independent board members, measures of relationships with stockholder and nonstockholder constituencies, and results of ethics reviews and audits.

N5. Actions to build community health (1.2c) are population-based services supporting the general health of your community. Such services might include health education programs, immunization programs, unique health services provided at a financial loss, population-screening programs (e.g., hypertension), safety program sponsorship, and indigent care. You should address these results of community health services in item 7.6.

N6. In addition to actions to build community health, areas of community support appropriate for inclusion in 1.2c might include your efforts to strengthen local community services and education; the environment; and practices of trade, business, or professional associations.

N7. The health and safety of staff are not addressed in Item 1.2; you should address these staff factors in Item 5.3. The Strategic Planning Category examines how your organization develops strategic objectives and action plans. Also examined are how your chosen strategic objectives and action plans are deployed and how progress is measured.

This Item [1.2] looks at how the organization fulfills its public responsibilities and encourages, supports, and practices good citizenship.

The first part of this Item [1.2a] looks at how the organization addresses current and future impacts on society in a proactive manner. The impacts and practices are expected to cover all relevant and important areas—products, services, and operations.

- An integral part of performance management and improvement is proactively addressing legal and regulatory requirements and risk factors. Addressing these areas requires establishing appropriate measures and/or indicators that senior leaders track in their overall performance review. The organization should be sensitive to issues of public concern, whether or not these issues are currently embodied in law. The failure to address these areas can expose the organization to future problems when it least expects them. Problems can range from a sudden decline in public confidence to extensive and costly litigation. In this regard, it is important to anticipate potential problems the public may have with both current and future health care services. Sometimes a well-intended service could create adverse public consequences.

Good public responsibility implies going beyond minimum compliance with laws and regulations. Top-performing health care organizations frequently serve as role models of responsibility and provide leadership in areas key to health care success. For example, a hospital that must dispose of hazardous waste materials might go beyond the requirements of the environmental protection regulations and develop innovative and award-winning systems to protect the environment and reduce pollution. This has a double benefit. Not only do they develop good relations with regulators (and occasionally receive the "benefit-of-the-doubt"), but when regulators increase requirements, the high-performing organizations are already in compliance, usually way ahead of competitors who only met minimum requirements.

- Good citizenship opportunities are available to organizations of all sizes. These opportunities include encouraging and supporting staff community service.

- Ensuring that ethical health care practices are followed by all staff lessens the organization's risk of adverse public reaction as well as criminal prosecution. Programs to ensure ethical health care practices typically seek to prevent activities that might be perceived as criminal or near criminal. Examples of unethical health care practices might include falsifying records or quality-control data, accepting lavish gifts from a contractor, or seeking kickbacks.

The second part of this Item [1.2b] looks at how the organization, its senior leaders, and its staff ensure ethical health care practices are followed in all stakeholder transactions and interactions. Standards of ethical behavior should be defined (preferably in measurable terms) and everyone in the organization should understand and follow the standards. The organization must systematically monitor ethical behavior throughout the organization and with key suppliers, partners, and within the governance structure. Failing to follow the standards of ethical behavior should have prompt and serious consequences for every governing board member, leader, manager, staff, supplier, and partner.

The third part of this Item [1.2c] looks at how the organization, its senior leaders, and its staff identify, support, and strengthen key communities as part of good citizenship practices.

- Good citizenship practices typically vary according to the size, complexity, and location of the organization. Larger organizations are generally expected to have a more comprehensive approach to citizenship than small organizations.

- Examples of organizational community involvement include: influencing the adoption of higher standards in education by communicating health care employability requirements to schools and school boards; partnering with other businesses and health care providers to improve health in the local community by providing education and volunteer services to address public health issues; and partnering to influence trade and health care associations to engage in beneficial, cooperative activities such as sharing best practices to improve overall U.S.-global health and the environment.

- In addition to activities directly carried out by the organization, opportunities to practice good citizenship include staff community service that is encouraged and supported by the organization. Frequently, the organization's leaders actively participate on community boards and actively support their work. Usually, organizations—like people—support causes and issues that they value. Top-performing organizations are not content to simply donate money, people, and services to these causes without examining the impact of this support. They look carefully at the impact their support or involvement will have and how this aligns with their mission and goals.

1.2 Social Responsibility

How the organization addresses public responsibilities, ensures ethical behavior, practices good citizenship, and contributes to community health

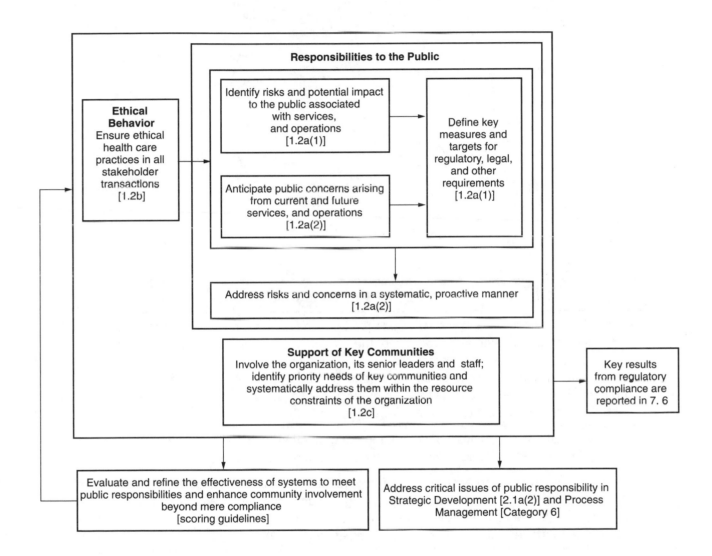

1.2 Social Responsibility Item Linkages

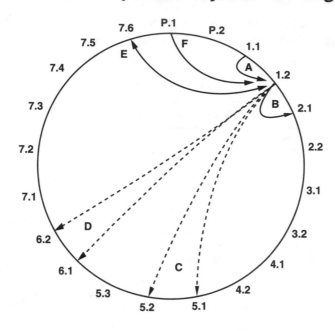

NATURE OF RELATIONSHIP	
A	Leaders, in support of organizational values [1.1a(1)], have a responsibility for setting policies and ensuring that practices and products of the organization and its staff do not adversely impact society or violate ethical standards, regulations, or law [1.2a and b]. They are also responsible to be personally involved and to ensure that the organization and its staff strengthen key communities in areas such as local community services, education, health, the environment, and health care, professional, and trade associations [1.2c].
B	Public health and safety concerns, environmental protection, and waste management issues [1.2a] are important factors to consider in strategy development [2.1a(2)].
C	Training [5.2] is provided to ensure all staff understand organization ethical health care practices [1.2b] as well as the importance of strengthening key communities [1.2c]. In addition, recruitment and hiring and the design of work systems should capitalize on the ideas, culture, and thinking of key communities and their impact on the organization [5.1c(2)].
D	Leaders at all levels have responsibility for ensuring that work practices of the organization [6.1 and 6.2] are consistent with the organization's standards of ethics and public responsibility [1.2a and b].
E	Key results, such as results of regulatory and legal compliance [1.2a], anticipate public concerns [1.2a(2)], ethical behavior [1.2b], and support to key communities [1.2c], and are reported in Governance and Social Responsibilities Results [7.6a(2 and 3)]. In addition, these results are monitored to determine if process changes are needed. (Results in areas of staff safety and well-being are reported in 7.4, based on processes described in Item 5.3, Staff Well-Being and Satisfaction, and are not a part of the requirements in 1.2.)
F	The regulatory environment described in P.1a(5) sets the context for the review of the management systems for public responsibility citizenship [1.2a(1)].

IF YOU DON'T DO WHAT THE CRITERIA REQUIRE...	
Item Reference	**Possible Adverse Consequences**
1.2a(1)	Organizations that fail to consider the impact of their service and operations on the public may be seriously impaired in the future if it is determined that these services cause harm. In the short term, organizations that fail to comply with regulatory and legal requirements may find themselves facing costly sanctions or be prohibited from conducting health care. The failure to consider risks associated with services and operations may contribute to costly corrective action or litigation.
1.2a(2)	Organizations that fail to anticipate and consider potential concerns that the public may have with current and future services and operations may be faced with costly redesign or redirection. When an organization appears to treat the public and the community within which it works with impunity and disregards their concerns, it becomes extremely difficult to recover trust and confidence. When the organization finds it needs public support to carry out its work or expand its operations, it may find it difficult to secure that support from the public.
1.2b	Organizations that do not ensure ethical health care practices in all transactions and interactions with stakeholders (public, patients and customers, stockholders, staff, suppliers, and so on) run the risk of violating the public trust. Accordingly, these organizations may face serious adverse consequences when their misdeeds are discovered. (One only needs to consider the difference between Enron and Tylenol. Both companies faced disasters that threatened their existence. Tylenol responded ethically and is still thriving.) Moreover, if the unethical practices of leaders are considered an acceptable health care standard in the organization and repeated by others, it can contribute to numerous unpredictable problems that divert human and financial resources to correct.
1.2c	Organizations that fail to act as good corporate citizens and support the local community may find it difficult to get support in return, especially for projects or initiatives that require local approval. For example, local communities typically provide the bulk of support for services as well as new workers. Organizations that fail to support local education, or trade and professional associations may find themselves faced with a shortage of skilled workers in key areas and important services they need to conduct health care.

1.2 SOCIAL RESPONSIBILITY— SAMPLE EFFECTIVE PRACTICES

A. Responsibilities to the Public

- The organization's principal health care activities include systems to analyze, anticipate, and minimize public hazards or risk.

- Indicators for risk areas are identified and monitored.

- Improvement strategies are used consistently, target performance levels are set, and progress is reviewed regularly and tied to recognition and reward.

- The organization considers the impact that its operations and services might have on society and considers those impacts in planning.

- The effectiveness of systems to meet or exceed regulatory or legal requirements is systematically evaluated and improved.

B. Ethical Behavior

- A formal system to train all staff about ethical health care requirements is in place.

- A process is in place to test the understanding of ethical principles for all people who must follow the principles. This may include staff, governing board members, suppliers, and partners.

- An audit process is in place to communicate and ensure ethical requirements and practices are deployed to all levels of the organization and to key partners, suppliers, and members of the board of directors (governance group).

- The effectiveness of systems to meet or exceed ethical requirements is systematically evaluated and improved.

C. Support of Key Communities

- Senior leaders and staff at various levels in the organization are involved in professional organizations, committees, task forces, or other community activities.

- Organizational resources are allocated to support involvement in community activities outside the organization. The effectiveness of these allocations is examined to determine if expectations are met and resources are used wisely.

- Staff participate in local, state, or national quality award programs and receive recognition from the organization.

- Staff participate in a variety of professional and health care improvement associations.

- The effectiveness of processes to support and strengthen key communities is systematically measured, evaluated, and improved.

- A process has been developed to ensure compliance with Medicare and Medicaid fraud and abuse requirements and regulations.

- A social responsibility process addresses societal responsibility, including regulatory, legal, and ethical compliance. This process also takes the organization beyond "mere compliance" in addressing key areas that support the vision, mission, and values.

- A corporate risk department ensures a safe environment for patients, employees, and visitors.

- Recognizing the threat posed by terrorist attacks after September 11, 2001, a systemwide team has been set up to ensure appropriate and timely response to biological or chemical exposure.

- In support of the organization's vision and mission, care is provided to anyone, regardless of their ability to pay. Policy requires 25 percent of prior year operating profit to be set aside for charity care.

2 Strategic Planning—85 Points

*The **Strategic Planning** Category examines how your organization develops strategic objectives and action plans. Also examined are how your chosen strategic objectives and action plans are deployed and how progress is measured.*

The Strategic Planning Category looks at the organization's process for strategic and action planning, and deployment of plans to make sure everyone is working to achieve those plans. Patient- and customer-driven quality and operational performance excellence are key strategic issues that need to be integral parts of the organization's overall planning.

- Patient- and customer-driven quality is a strategic view of quality. The focus is on the drivers of patient and customer satisfaction, patient and customer retention, new markets, and market share—key factors in competitiveness, profitability, and health care success.

- Operational performance improvement contributes to short- and longer-term productivity growth and cost/price competitiveness. Building operational capability—including speed, responsiveness, and flexibility—represents an investment in strengthening the organization's competitive position now and into the future.

Over the years, much debate and discussion have taken place around planning. Professors in our colleges and universities spend a great deal of time trying to differentiate strategic planning, long-term planning, short-term planning, tactical planning, operational planning, quality planning, health care planning, and staff planning, to name a few. However, a much simpler view might serve us better. For our purposes, the following captures the essence of planning:

- Strategic planning is simply an effort to identify the things we must do to be successful in the future.

- Once we have determined what we must do to be successful (the plan), we must take steps to execute that plan (the actions).

Accordingly, the key role of strategic planning is to provide a basis for aligning the organization's work processes with its strategic directions, thereby ensuring people and processes in different parts of the organization are not working at cross-purposes. To the extent that alignment does not occur, the organization's effectiveness and competitiveness is reduced.

The Strategic Planning Category looks at how the organization:

- Understands the key patient and customer, market, and operational requirements as input to setting strategic directions. This helps to ensure that ongoing process improvements are aligned with the organization's strategic directions.

- Optimizes the use of resources and ensures bridging between short- and longer-term requirements that may entail capital expenditures, supplier development, new staff recruitment strategies, reengineering key processes, and other factors affecting health care success.

- Ensures that deployment will be effective—that there are mechanisms to transmit requirements and achieve alignment on three basic levels: (1) the organization/executive level; (2) the key process level; and (3) the work-unit/individual-job level.

The requirements for the Strategic Planning Category are intended to encourage strategic thinking and acting—to develop a basis for achieving and maintaining a competitive position. These requirements do not demand formalized plans, planning systems, departments, or specific planning cycles. They also do not imply that all improvements could or should be planned in advance. They do, however, require plans and the alignment of actions to those plans at all levels of the organization. An effective improvement system combines improvements of many types and degrees of involvement. An effective system to improve performance and competitive advantage requires fact-based strategic guidance, particularly when improvement alternatives compete for limited resources. In most cases, priority setting depends heavily upon a cost rationale. However, an organization might also have to deal with critical requirements, such as public responsibilities, that are not driven by cost considerations alone.

Strategic planning consists of the planning process, the identification of goals and actions necessary to achieve success, and the deployment of those actions to align the work of the organization.

Strategy Development

- Patients and Customers: market requirements and evolving expectations and opportunities

- Competitive environment and capabilities relative to competitors: industry and market

- Technologies and other innovations that might affect products and services and future health care operations

- Internal strengths and weaknesses, including staff capabilities and needs, resource availability and operational capabilities and needs

- Financial, societal, ethical, regulatory, and other potential risks that may affect health care success risks

- Opportunities to redirect resources to higher priority services or health care areas

- Changes in economic/health conditions (local, national, or global) that might affect health care

- Unique organizational factors, such as supplier and supply chain, capabilities and needs

- Develop clear strategic objectives with timetables that help leaders determine where the organization should be at given points in time so they can effectively monitor progress

Strategy Deployment

- Translate strategy into action plans and related staff plans.

- Align and deploy action plan requirements, performance measures, and resources throughout the organization to ensure changes or improvements are sustained.

- Define measures for tracking progress on action plans and ensure actions are aligned throughout the organization.

- Project expected performance results, including assumptions of competitor performance increases.

2.1 STRATEGY DEVELOPMENT (40 PTS.)

Describe how your organization establishes its strategic objectives, including how it enhances its performance relative to other organizations providing similar health care services, overall performance as a health care provider, and future success.

Within your response, include answers to the following questions:

a. Strategy Development Process

(1) What is your overall strategic planning process? What are the key steps? Who are the key participants? What are your short- and longer-term planning time horizons? How are these time horizons set? How does your strategic planning process address these time horizons?

(2) How do you ensure that strategic planning addresses the key factors listed below? How do you collect and analyze relevant data and information to address these factors as they relate to your strategic planning:

- Your patient, other customer, and health care market needs, expectations, and opportunities

- Your competitive environment, and/or your collaborative environment to conserve community resources and your capabilities relative to competitors

- Technological and other key innovations or changes that might affect your health care services and how you operate

- Your strengths and weaknesses, including staff and other resources

- Your opportunities to redirect resources to higher priority health care services or areas

- Financial, societal and ethical, regulatory, and other potential risks

- Changes in the local, regional, or national economic environment

- Factors unique to your organization, including partner and supply chain needs, strengths, and weaknesses

b. Strategic Objectives

(1) What are your key strategic objectives and your timetable for accomplishing them? What are your most important goals for these strategic objectives?

(2) How do your strategic objectives address the challenges identified in response to p.2 in your organizational profile? How do you ensure that your strategic objectives balance short- and longer-term challenges and opportunities? How do you ensure that your strategic objectives balance the needs of patients and other key customers and stakeholders?

Continued

Notes: *Continued*

N1. "Strategy development" refers to your organization's approach (formal or informal) to preparing for the future. Strategy development might utilize various types of forecasts, projections, options, scenarios, and/or other approaches to envisioning the future for purposes of decision making and resource allocation

N2. "Strategy" should be interpreted broadly. Strategy might be built around or lead to any or all of the following: new health care services and/or delivery processes and markets; revenue growth via various approaches, including acquisitions; and new partnerships and alliances. Strategy might be directed toward becoming a center for clinical and service excellence, a preferred provider, a research leader, or an integrated service provider.

N3. Strategies to address key challenges [2.1b(2)] might include access and locations; rapid response; customization; rapid innovation; ISO 9000:2000 registration; Web-based provider, patient, and other customer relationship management; and health care.

N4. Item 2.1 addresses your overall organizational strategy, which might include changes in health care services and programs. However, the Item does not address service and program design; you should address these factors in Item 6.1, as appropriate.

This Item [2.1] looks at how the organization sets strategic directions and develops strategic objectives, with the aim of strengthening overall performance and competitiveness.

The first part of this Item [2.1a(1)] asks the organization to describe its strategic planning process and identify the key participants, key steps, and planning time horizons. This helps examiners understand the steps and data used in the planning process. It is usually a good idea to provide a flowchart of the planning process. This helps examiners understand how the planning process works without wasting valuable space in the application.

Organizations must consider the key factors that affect its future success. These factors cover external and internal influences on the organization. Each factor must be addressed and outlined to show how relevant data and information are gathered and analyzed. Although the organization is not limited to the number of factors it considers important in planning, the eight factors identified in Item 2.1a(2) must be addressed unless a valid rationale can be offered as to why the factor is not appropriate. Together, these eight factors will cover the most important variables for any organization's future success.

- The planning process should examine all the key influences, risks, challenges, and other requirements that might affect the organization's future

opportunities and directions—taking as long-term a view as possible. This approach is intended to provide a thorough and realistic context for the development of a patient-, customer- and market-focused strategy to guide ongoing decision making, resource allocation, and overall management.

- This planning process should cover all types of health care services and sites, competitive situations, strategic issues, planning approaches, and plans. The requirement calls for a future-oriented basis for action, but does not specifically require formalized planning, planning departments, planning cycles, or a specified way of visualizing the future. If the organization is seeking to create an entirely new health care service or program, it is necessary to set and to test the objectives that define and guide critical actions and performance.

- This Item also focuses on identifying the factors and actions the organization must take to achieve a leadership position in a competitive market. This usually requires ongoing revenue growth and improvements in operational effectiveness. Achieving and sustaining a leadership position in a competitive market requires a view of the future that includes not only the markets or segments in which the organization competes, but also how it competes. How it competes presents many options and requires understanding of the organization's and competitors' strengths and weaknesses. No specific time horizon for planning is required by the Criteria; the thrust of this Item is finding ways to create and ensure sustained competitive leadership.

In order to maintain competitive leadership, an increasingly important part of strategic planning requires processes to project the competitive environment accurately. Such projections help detect and reduce competitive threats, shorten reaction time, and identify opportunities. Depending on the size and type of health care, maturity of markets, pace of change, and competitive parameters (such as price or innovation rate), organizations might use a variety of modeling, scenario, or other techniques and judgments to project the competitive environment.

The second part of this Item [2.1b] asks for a summary of the organization's key strategic objectives and the timetable for accomplishing them. It also asks how these objectives address the challenges outlined in the Organizational Profile.

- The purpose of the timetable is to provide a basis for projecting the path that improvement is likely to take. This allows the leaders who monitor progress to determine when performance is deviating from plan and when adjustments should be made to get back on track. Consider Figure 24. The performance goal four years into the future is to achieve a level of performance of 100. Currently the organization is at 20. At the end of year one, the organization achieved a performance level of 40, represented by the circle symbol. It appears that that level of performance is on track toward the goal of 100. However, the path from the current state to the future state is rarely a straight line. Unless the expected trajectory is known (or at least estimated), it is not possible to evaluate the progress accurately. Without timetables or trajectories, leaders are forced to default to use best guess or intuition as a basis for comparing actual, measurable progress against expected progress.

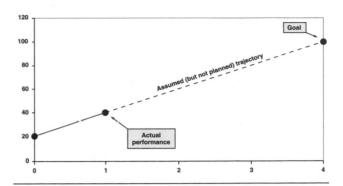

Figure 24 Assumed trajectory.

In Figure 25, the planned trajectory is represented by the triangle symbols. When compared with the current level of performance (the circle symbol), it is clear that there is a performance shortfall of approximately 30.

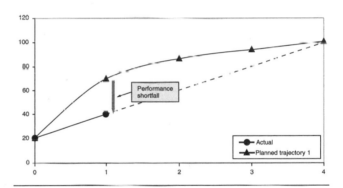

Figure 25 Planned trajectory no. 1.

In Figure 26, the planned trajectory is represented by the square symbols. When compared with the current level of performance (the circle symbol), it is clear that the performance is ahead of schedule.

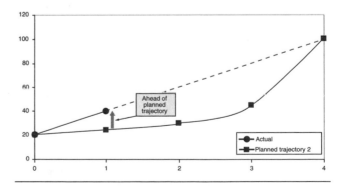

Figure 26 Planned trajectory no. 2.

There are several possible decisions that leaders could make based on this information. It might mean that the original estimates/goals were low and should be reset. It might also mean that the process did not need all of the resources it had available. These resources may be better used in areas where performance is not ahead of schedule.

In any case, without knowing the expected path toward a goal, it requires leaders to guess whether the level of progress is appropriate or not.

- Finally, the last part of this Item requires the organization to evaluate the options it considered in the strategic planning process to ensure it responded fully to the six factors identified in Item 2.1a(2) that were most important to health care success. This last step helps the organization "close the loop" to make sure that the factors influencing organization success were adequately analyzed and support key strategic objectives

2.1 Strategy Development

How the organization establishes strategic objectives, including how it enhances its competitive position, overall performance, and future success

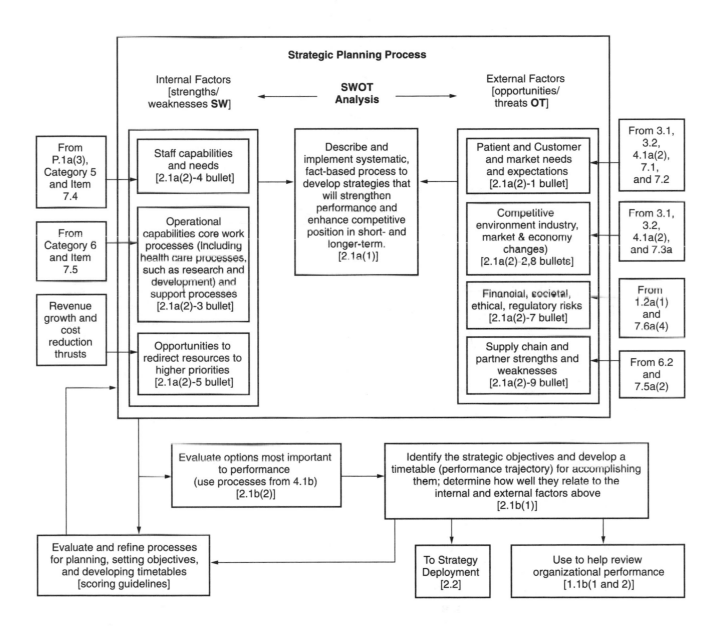

2.1 Strategy Development Item Linkages

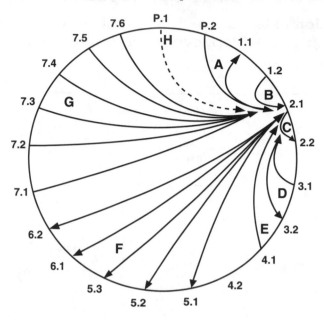

NATURE OF RELATIONSHIP	
A	The planning process [2.1] includes senior leaders—as part of their responsibilities for setting direction, expectations, and ensuring a strong focus on patients and customers and staff empowerment [1.1a], and the protection of stakeholder interests [1.1b]. In addition, the timelines or expected performance trajectories [2.1b(1)] provide a basis for leaders to determine if progress is on track or not when they monitor progress [1.1c(1)]. The competitive environment [partly defined in P.2a] is also examined as part of the strategy development process [2.1a(2)]. In addition, before the planning cycle is complete, leaders must ensure that the strategic objectives [2.1b(2)] address the challenges identified in the Organizational Profile [P.2b].
B	Public health, environmental, waste management, and related concerns [1.2a], as well as the need to promote ethical behavior in all transactions [1.2b], are considered, as appropriate, in the strategy development process [2.1a(2)].
C	The planning process [2.1a] produces a set of strategic objectives [2.1b(1)] that must be converted into action plans that are deployed to the workforce [2.2a].
D	The planning process [2.1] includes information on current and potential patient and customer requirements and preferences, and the projected competitive environment [3.1], as well as intelligence obtained from patient- and customer-contact people (complaints and comments) [3.2a] and patient and customer satisfaction data [3.2b].
E	Key organizational and competitive comparison data [4.1a(2)] and analytical data, including various forecasts and projections [4.1b], are used for planning [2.1a(2)] and setting objectives [2.1b].

Continued

	NATURE OF RELATIONSHIP	*Continued*
F	Information on staff capabilities [Category 5] and work process capabilities [Category 6] is considered in the strategic planning process as part of the determination of internal strengths and weaknesses and to help determine if resources should be redirected to higher priority products, services, or areas [2.1a(2)]. Staff educational levels, diversity, and other characteristics [P.1a(3)] may affect the determination of staff strengths and weaknesses as a part of the strategic planning process [2.1a(2)]. *To avoid cluttering diagrams in Categories 5 and 6, these linkage arrows will not be repeated there.*	
G	Patient- and customer-focused [7.2], health care [7.1], financial and market [7.3], staff [7.4], organization effectiveness [7.5], and governance and social responsibility [7.6] results are used in the planning process [2.1a(2)] to set strategic objectives [2.1b(1)]. In addition, results in 7.5a(3) must specifically report on progress toward achieving the strategic objectives and are used in subsequent planning.	
H	Staff educational levels, diversity, and other characteristics [P.1a(3)] relate to staff strengths and weaknesses, and are considered during the strategic planning process [2.1a(2)].	

	IF YOU DON'T DO WHAT THE CRITERIA REQUIRE...
Item Reference	**Possible Adverse Consequences**
2.1a(1)	Without clearly defined short- and longer-term planning horizons, it may be difficult to properly align the analysis and collection of market and health care industry forecast data to support effective planning. The shorter the planning horizon, the easier it is to be accurate in forecasting. However, the planning horizon must be at least as long as the time it takes the organization to design, develop, and deliver new services required by patients and customers and markets. For example, if the design-delivery cycle is seven years, then to be effective an organization must be able to forecast or anticipate patient/customer and market requirements seven years out—which may be difficult to do accurately. Shorter planning cycles may facilitate more accurate patient/customer and market requirements.
2.1a(2)	The failure to address the eight key factors (patient/customer and market needs; competitive environment; technological and other key innovations or changes that might affect operations; internal strengths and weaknesses; opportunities to redirect resources to higher priority areas or services; external risks such as financial, societal, ethical, and regulatory; changes in the economy; and partner and supply chain strengths and weaknesses) usually results in a flawed strategic plan—a plan that has overlooked an element critical to future success. For example, an organization may fail to achieve strategic objectives if it assumed (incorrectly) that a key supplier would be able to deliver critical components at a certain time. Likewise, a strategic plan that does not adequately account for the arrival of competitive offerings or new technologies in the marketplace can be faced with major challenges. (Consider the impact of new, longer lasting filling materials coupled with successful prevention of dental decay on modern dentistry.) Failing to consider or incorrectly forecast these eight elements may result in a strategic plan that cannot be achieved.
2.1b(1)	Knowing whether the strategy is unfolding as expected is critical to the successful performance of the organization and the leadership. The failure to develop a timetable with clearly defined targets for accomplishing strategic objectives makes it extremely difficult for leaders to monitor organizational performance effectively [as required by Item 1.1c(1)]. Without defined milestones, leaders must guess whether the rate of progress is appropriate or not. Without clear timelines or trajectories for growth, leaders frequently assume the path between current state and desired state (goals) is linear. Data indicate that the actual path is almost never linear; so the assumptions of linearity that leaders make in the absence of clear timelines and trajectories are usually incorrect.
2.1b(2)	Strategy development is an ongoing, dynamic process. It is often a difficult process that takes a considerable amount of time to complete initially and then requires continual attention to address a rapidly changing marketplace. However, if leaders fail to ensure that planning has fully addressed organizational changes and ensure that the strategic objectives effectively balance the needs of all key stakeholders, the plan may be ineffective and the time it took to develop the plan may be wasted.

2.1 STRATEGY DEVELOPMENT— SAMPLE EFFECTIVE PRACTICES

A. Strategy Development Process

- Health Care goals, strategies, and issues are addressed and reported in measurable terms. Strategic objectives consider future requirements needed to achieve organizational leadership after considering the performance levels that other organizations are likely to achieve in the same planning time frame. Key changes in services or patients and customers/markets consider Web-based or e-commerce or e-learning initiatives integrated within or separate from current health care.

- The planning and objective-setting process encourages input (but not necessarily decision making) from a variety of people at all levels throughout the organization.

- Data on patient and customer requirements, key markets, benchmarks, supplier and partner, staff, and organizational capabilities (internal and external factors) are used to develop health care plans.

- Plans and the planning process itself are evaluated each cycle for accuracy and completeness—more often if needed to keep pace with changing health care requirements.

- Opportunities for improvement in the planning process are identified systematically and carried out each planning cycle.

- Refinements in the process of planning, plan deployment, and receiving input from work units have been made. Improvements in plan cycle time, plan resources, and planning accuracy are documented.

B. Strategic Objectives

- Strategic objectives are identified and a timetable (or planned growth trajectory) for accomplishing the objectives are set. The timelines match the senior leaders' review cycle. For example, if leaders review progress against goals quarterly, the timelines identify the expected level of performance by quarters.

- Options to obtain best performance for the strategic objectives are systematically evaluated against the internal and external factors used in the strategy development process.

- The process of setting timelines or trajectories, and the accuracy of the projections, are analyzed and refined.

- Best practices from other providers, competitors, or outside benchmarks are identified and used to provide better estimates of trajectories.

- The strategic planning process incorporates setting direction, strategy development, human resources, and financial planning.

- A minimum data set of information from internal and external sources is required from each entity within the organization as input into the strategic planning process.

- Suppliers and payors are included in the strategic planning process when their efforts will impact the success of the organization in reaching a goal.

2.2 STRATEGY DEPLOYMENT (45 PTS.)

Describe how your organization converts its strategic objectives into action plans. Summarize your organizations action plans and related key performance measures or indicators. Project your organization's future performance on these key performance measures or indicators.

Within your response, include answers to the following questions:

a. Action Plan Development and Deployment

(1) How do you develop and deploy action plans to achieve your key strategic objectives? How do you allocate resources to ensure accomplishment of your action plans? How do you ensure that the key changes resulting from action plans can be sustained?

(2) What are your key short- and longer-term action plans? What are the key changes, if any, in your health care services and programs, your customers and markets (including patient populations), and how you will operate?

(3) What are your key staffing plans that derive from your short- and longer-term strategic objectives and action plans?

(4) What are your key performance measures or indicators for tracking progress on your action plans? How do you ensure that your overall action plan measurement system reinforces organizational alignment? How do you ensure that the measurement system covers all key deployment areas and stakeholders?

b. Performance Projection

For the key performance measures or indicators identified in 2.2a(4), what are your performance projections for both your short- and longer-term planning time horizons? How does your projected performance compare with competitors' projected performance or other organizations providing similar health care services? How does it compare with key benchmarks, goals, and past performance, as appropriate service quality? Responses to Item 2.1 should focus on your specific challenges—those most important to your organizational success and to strengthening your organization's overall performance as a health care provider.

Notes:

N1. Strategy and action plan development and deployment are closely linked to other Items in the Criteria. Examples of key linkages are:

- Item 1.1 for how your senior leaders set and communicate directions
- Category 3 for gathering patient, other customer, and health care market knowledge as input to your strategy and action plans and for deploying action plans
- Category 4 for measurement, analysis, and knowledge management to support your key information needs to support your development of strategy, to provide an effective basis for your performance measurements, and to track progress relative to your strategic objectives and action plans
- Category 5 for your work system needs; staff education, training, and development needs; and related human resource factors resulting from action plans
- Category 6 for process requirements resulting from your action plans
- Item 7.5 for specific accomplishments relative to your organizational strategy and action plans.

N2. Measures and indicators of projected performance (2.2b) might include changes resulting from new ventures; acquisitions or mergers; health care market entry and shifts; and significant anticipated innovations in health care service delivery and technology.

The first part of this Item [2.2a] looks at how the organization translates its strategic objectives (which were identified in item 2.1b) into action plans to accomplish the objectives and to enable assessment of progress relative to action plans. Overall, the intent of this item is to ensure that strategies are deployed at all levels throughout the organization to align work for goal achievement.

The first part of this Item [2.2a] calls for information on how action plans are developed and deployed. This includes spelling out key performance requirements and measures, as well as allocating resources and aligning work throughout the organization. Leaders must develop action plans that address the key strategic objectives (which were developed using the processes in Item 2.1). Organizations must summarize key short- and longer-term action plans. Particular attention is given to services, patients and customers/markets, how the organization operates, and key staff plans that will enable accomplishment of strategic objectives and action plans.

The organization should provide the key measures/indicators used in tracking progress relative to the action plans. The organization should also use these measures or indicators to achieve organizational alignment and coverage of all key work units and patients, customers, and other stakeholders.

Consistently accomplishing action plans and making necessary course corrections or adjustments requires resources and performance measures, as well as the alignment of work unit and supplier/partner plans. Alignment and consistency are intended to provide a basis for setting and communicating priorities for ongoing improvement activities—part of the daily work of all units. Also required are the key measures and/or indicators used in tracking progress relative to the action plans, how they are communicated, and how strategic objectives, action plans, and performance are aligned. Action plans include staff plans that support the overall strategy.

Without effective alignment, routine work and acts of improvement can be random and serve to suboptimize organizational performance. In Figure 27, the arrows represent the well-intended work carried out by staff of organizations who lack a clear set of expectations and direction. Each person, each manager, and each work unit works diligently to achieve goals they believe are important. Each is pulling hard—but not

necessarily in ways that ensure Performance Excellence. This encourages the creation of "fiefdoms" or "silos" within organizations.

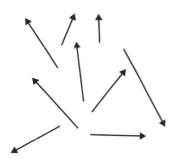

Figure 27 Nonaligned work.

With a clear, well-communicated strategic plan, it is easier to know when daily work is out of alignment. The large arrow in Figure 28 represents the strategic plan pointing the direction the organization must take to be successful and achieve its mission and vision. The strategic plan and accompanying measures make it possible to analyze work and health care practices to know when they are not aligned and to help staff, including leaders, to know when adjustments are required.

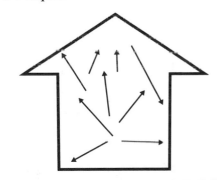

Figure 28 Strategic direction.

A well-deployed and understood strategic plan helps everyone in the organization distinguish between random acts of improvement and aligned improvement. Random acts of improvement give a false sense of accomplishment and rarely produce optimum benefits for the organization. For example, a decision to improve a health care process that is not aligned with the strategic plan (as the small bold arrow in Figure 29 represents) usually results in a wasteful expenditure of time, money, and staff—improvement without benefiting patients and customers or enhancing operating effectiveness.

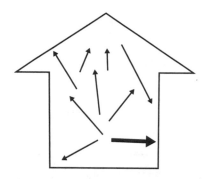

Figure 29 Random improvement.

On the other hand, by working systematically to strengthen processes that are aligned with the strategic plan, the organization moves closer to achieving success, as Figure 30 indicates.

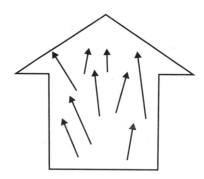

Figure 30 Moving toward alignment.

Ultimately, all processes and procedures of an organization should be aligned to maximize the achievement of strategic plans, as Figure 31 demonstrates.

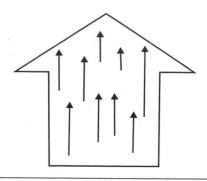

Figure 31 Systematic alignment.

Critical action plan resource requirements include staff plans that support the overall strategy. Examples of possible staff plan elements are:

- Redesign of work organization and/or jobs to increase staff empowerment and decision making

- Initiatives to promote greater labor-management and clinical-administrative cooperation, such as union and other types of partnerships

- Initiatives to foster knowledge sharing and organizational learning

- Modification of compensation and recognition systems to recognize team, organizational, patient and customer, or other performance attributes

- Education and training initiatives, such as developmental programs for future leaders, partnerships with universities to help ensure the availability of future staff, and/or establishment of technology-based training capabilities

Finally, the second part of this Item [2.2b] asks the organization to provide a projection of key performance measures and/or indicators, including key performance targets and/or goals for both short- and longer-term planning time horizons. This projected performance is the basis for comparing past performance and performance relative to competitors and benchmarks, as appropriate.

- Projections and comparisons in this Area are intended to help the organization's leaders improve their ability to understand and track dynamic, competitive performance factors. Through this tracking process, they should be better prepared to take into account its rate of improvement and change relative to competitors and relative to their own targets or stretch goals. Such tracking serves as a key diagnostic management tool.

- In addition to improvement relative to past performance and to competitors, projected performance also might include changes resulting from new health care ventures, entry into new markets, e-commerce initiatives, service innovations, or other strategic thrusts. Without this comparison information, it is possible to set goals that, even if attained, may not result in competitive advantage. More than one high-performing organization has been surprised by a

competitor that set and achieved more aggressive goals. Consider the following example represented by Figure 32. Imagine that you are ahead of your competition and committed to a 10 percent increase in market share over your base year. After eight years you are twice as profitable. To your surprise, you find that your competitor has increased 20 percent each year. You have achieved your goal, but your competitor has beaten you, making slightly more. After 10 years, the competitor has a significant lead. It is not good enough to achieve your goals unless your goals place you in a competitive position.

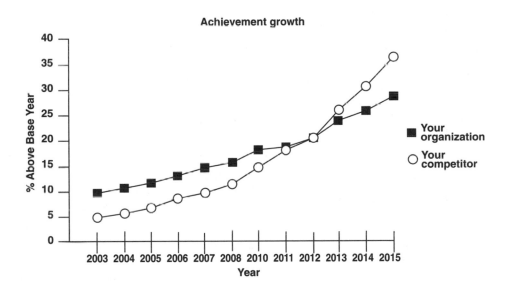

Figure 32 Projecting competitor's future performance.

2.2 Strategy Deployment

Summary of strategy, action plans, and related key performance measures and indicators and performance projections; how they are developed, communicated, and deployed

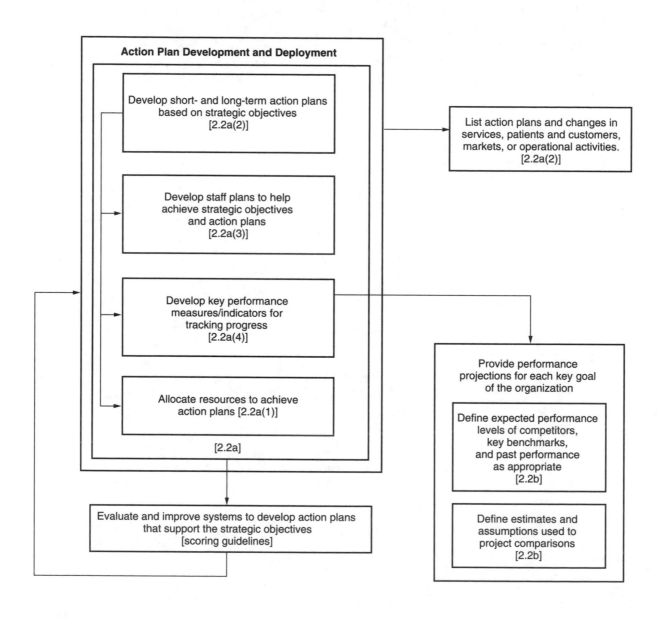

2.2 Strategy Deployment Item Linkages

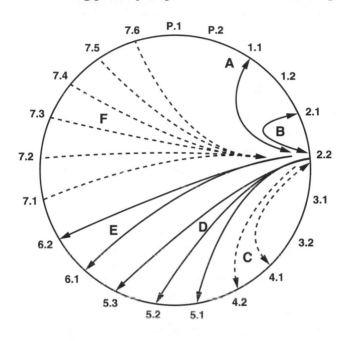

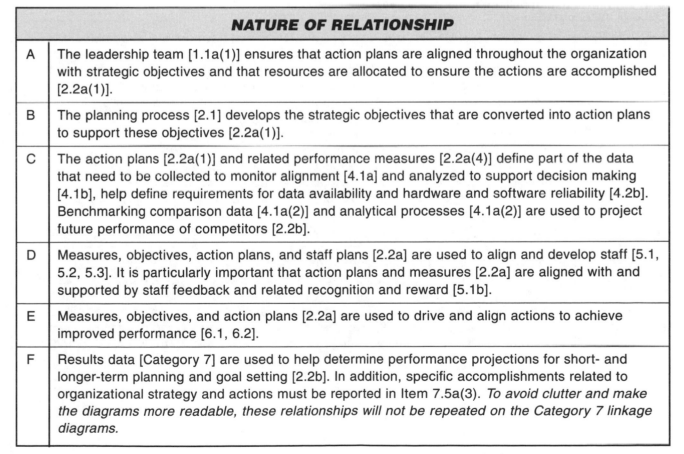

	NATURE OF RELATIONSHIP
A	The leadership team [1.1a(1)] ensures that action plans are aligned throughout the organization with strategic objectives and that resources are allocated to ensure the actions are accomplished [2.2a(1)].
B	The planning process [2.1] develops the strategic objectives that are converted into action plans to support these objectives [2.2a(1)].
C	The action plans [2.2a(1)] and related performance measures [2.2a(4)] define part of the data that need to be collected to monitor alignment [4.1a] and analyzed to support decision making [4.1b], help define requirements for data availability and hardware and software reliability [4.2b]. Benchmarking comparison data [4.1a(2)] and analytical processes [4.1a(2)] are used to project future performance of competitors [2.2b].
D	Measures, objectives, action plans, and staff plans [2.2a] are used to align and develop staff [5.1, 5.2, 5.3]. It is particularly important that action plans and measures [2.2a] are aligned with and supported by staff feedback and related recognition and reward [5.1b].
E	Measures, objectives, and action plans [2.2a] are used to drive and align actions to achieve improved performance [6.1, 6.2].
F	Results data [Category 7] are used to help determine performance projections for short- and longer-term planning and goal setting [2.2b]. In addition, specific accomplishments related to organizational strategy and actions must be reported in Item 7.5a(3). *To avoid clutter and make the diagrams more readable, these relationships will not be repeated on the Category 7 linkage diagrams.*

	IF YOU DON'T DO WHAT THE CRITERIA REQUIRE...
Item Reference	**Possible Adverse Consequences**
2.2a(1)	The failure to develop action plans to carry out strategic objectives and employ them at all levels of the organization usually means that work may not be aligned to achieve the strategy. Instead, there is a tendency for managers and other staff to focus their work on things they believe are important. This can result in significant resources being spent on activities that do not contribute to the objectives the organization's leaders have determined are critical for its future success. In addition, the failure to allocate resources appropriately to accomplish action plans frequently means that some plans are not accomplished because of insufficient resources, while other plans are accomplished inefficiently because of too many resources. In both cases, the value to the patient and customer and the organization is suboptimized.
2.2a(2)	The inability to articulate and communicate key short- and longer-term action plans usually means those plans do not exist, or they are only expressed as vague generalities. Unclear plans make it more difficult to help staff at all levels of the organization understand what work they must do to help the organization achieve future success. Again, without clear direction from the top, staff will still work hard but their work may be unfocused as they follow their own ideas for appropriate action—everyone is not pulling in the same direction.
2.2a(3)	By definition, "plans" describe activities or actions that have not yet taken place. Many times, in order to achieve plans, staff must possess skills, knowledge, or abilities that they do not currently possess. Without appropriate plans to develop, acquire, or motivate the staff necessary to carry out desired actions, the organization may not be able to achieve its strategic objectives. Its staff may not have the knowledge, skills, or abilities to carry out the actions required for success in the future.
2.2a(4)	Without appropriate measures or indicators, it is difficult for leaders, managers, and staff throughout the organization to determine if they are making appropriate progress. It is also more difficult to communicate expectations accurately. Unclear expectations increase the likelihood that staff will not understand what they are required to do to achieve strategic objectives. Consider the adage, "What gets measured gets done." Without appropriate measures it is difficult to focus everyone on doing the right things.
2.2b	In the best-performing organizations, strategic goals are designed to enable the organization to win in highly competitive situations. If an organization desires to achieve a leadership position, it must understand where the competition is likely to be in the future before it sets its goals. Unless the organization's leaders understand the likely future performance levels of key competitors (in the same planning horizon), they may set an aggressive goal, achieve that goal, and still lose—finding themselves behind the competition.

2.2 STRATEGY DEPLOYMENT— SAMPLE EFFECTIVE PRACTICES

A. Action Plan Development and Deployment

- Plans are in place to optimize operational performance and improve patient and customer focus using tools such as reengineering, streamlining work processes, and reducing cycle time.

- Actions have been defined in measurable terms, which align with strategic objectives and enable the organization to sustain established leadership positions for major products and services for key patients and customers or markets.

- Strategies to achieve key organizational results (operational performance requirements) are defined.

- Planned performance and productivity levels are defined in measurable terms for key features of products and services.

- Planned actions are challenging, realistic, achievable, and understood by staff throughout the organization. Each staff understands his or her role in achieving strategic and operational goals and objectives.

- Resources are available and committed to achieve the plans (no unfunded mandates). Capital projects are funded according to health care improvement plans.

- Plans are absolutely used to guide operational performance improvements. Plans drive budget and action, not the other way around.

- Incremental (short-term) strategies to achieve long-term plans are defined in measurable terms and timelines are in place to help monitor progress.

- Health Care plans, short- and long-term goals, and performance measures are understood and used to drive actions throughout the organization.

- Each individual in the organization, at all levels, understands how his or her work contributes to achieving organizational goals and plans.

- Plans are followed to ensure that resources are deployed and redeployed as needed to support goals.

- Human resource plans support strategic plans and goals. Plans show how the workforce will be developed to enable the organization to achieve its strategic goals.

- Key issues of training and development, hiring, retention, staff participation, involvement, empowerment, and recognition and reward are addressed as a part of the staff plan. Appropriate measures and targets for each are defined.

- Innovative strategies may involve one or more of the following:

  - Redesign of work to increase staff responsibility

  - Improved labor-management relations (that is, prior to contract negotiations, train both sides in effective negotiation skills so that people focus on the merits of issues, not on positions. A goal, for example, is to improve relations and shorten negotiation time by 50 percent.)

  - Forming partnerships with education institutions to develop staff and ensure a supply of well-prepared future staff

  - Developing gain-sharing or equity-building compensation systems for all staff to increase motivation and productivity

  - Broadening staff responsibilities; creating self-directed or high-performance work teams

- Key performance measures (for example, staff satisfaction or work climate surveys) have been identified to gather data to manage progress. (Note: Improvement results associated with these measures should be reported in 7.4.)

- The effectiveness of staff planning and alignment with strategic plans is evaluated systematically.

- Data are used to evaluate and improve performance and participation for all types of staff (for example, absenteeism, turnover, grievances, accidents, recognition and reward, and training participation).

- Routine, two-way communication about performance of staff occurs.

- The process to develop action plans to support strategic objectives is systematically evaluated.

B. Performance Projection

- Projections of two- to five-year changes in performance levels are developed and used to collect data (measure) and track progress.

- Data from competitors, key benchmarks, and/or past performance form a valid basis for comparison. The organization has valid strategies and goals in place to meet or exceed the planned levels of performance for these competitors and benchmarks.

- Plans include expected future levels of competitor or comparison performance and are used to set and validate the organization's own plans and goals.

- Future plans and projections of performance consider new acquisition, optimum but secure growth, reducing costs through operational excellence processes, and research and development of innovations internally or among competitors. The accuracy of these projections is mapped and analyzed. Techniques to improve accuracy are developed and implemented.

- To ensure alignment of strategic plan to individual activity, a "personal commitment" card is distributed to all employees. This card includes the mission, vision, values, the characteristics of exceptional health care services, spaces for departmental and individual goals and measures, and a place for employee and manager signatures.

- Strategy is deployed through chartering of projects that support the vision and mission. Allocation of capital is determined by priority of these projects in helping to accomplish the vision and mission.

- A variety of tools are used to ensure staff recognition of the alignment of departmental goals to the organization's mission. These include posters, video presentations, mutual accountability, and personal commitment cards.

- Human resource needs are incorporated into each strategic goal and project in order to ensure appropriate resource availability.

3 Focus on Patients, Other Customers, and Markets–85 Points

The **Patient, Other Customer and Market Focus** Category examines how your organization determines requirements, expectations, and preferences of patients and customers and markets. Also examined is how your organization builds relationships with patients and customers and determines the key factors that lead to patient and customer acquisition, satisfaction, loyalty, and retention, and to health care expansion.

This Category addresses how the organization seeks to understand the voices of patients and customers, and of the marketplace. It stresses relationships as an important part of an overall listening, learning, and performance excellence strategy. Patient and customer satisfaction and dissatisfaction results provide vital information for understanding patients and customers, and the marketplace. In many cases, such results and trends provide the most meaningful information, not only on patients' and customers' views, but also on their marketplace behaviors—repeat health care services when needed and positive referrals.

Patient, Other Customer, and Market Focus contains two Items that focus on understanding patient and customer and market requirements, and building relationships and determining satisfaction.

Patient, Other Customer, and Market Knowledge

- Determining market or patient and customer segments

- Determining patient and customer information validity

- Determining important health care service features

- Using complaint information and data from potential and former patients and customers

Patient and Other Customer Relationships and Satisfaction

- Make patient and customer contact and feedback easy and useful

- Handle complaints effectively and responsively

- Ensure complaint data are used to eliminate causes of complaints

- Build patient and customer relationships and loyalty

- Systematically determine patient and customer satisfaction and the satisfaction of competitor's patients and customers

3.1 PATIENT, OTHER CUSTOMER, AND HEALTH CARE MARKET KNOWLEDGE (40 PTS.)

Approach/Deployment

Describe how your organization determines requirements, expectations, and preferences of patients, other customers, and markets to ensure the continuing relevance of your health care services and to develop new health care service opportunities.

Within your response, include answers to the following questions:

a. Patient/Customer and Health Care Market Knowledge

(1) How do you determine or target patients, other customers, customer groups, and health care market segments? How do you include customers of competitors and other potential customers and markets in this determination?

(2) How do you listen and learn to determine key patient/customer requirements and expectations (including health care service features) and their relative importance to patients'/customers' health care purchasing decisions? How do determination methods vary for different patients/customers or customer groups? How do you use relevant information from current and former patients/customers, including marketing information, patient/customer loyalty and retention data, win/loss analysis, and complaints? How do you use this information for purposes of health care service planning, marketing, process improvements, and other business development?

(3) How do you keep your listening and learning methods current with health care service needs and directions?

Notes:

N1. Patients, as a key customer group, are frequently identified separately in the Criteria. Other customer groups could include patients' families, the community, insurers and other third-party payors, employers, health care providers, patient advocacy groups, Departments of Health, and students. Generic references to customers include patients.

N2. Your responses to this Item should include patients, other customer groups, and market segments identified in P.1b(2).

N3. "Health care service features" [3.1a(2)] refers to all the important characteristics of your health care services that patients and other customers receive. This includes all customers' overall interactions with you and their service experiences. The focus should be on features that affect customer health care-related preference and loyalty and the customers' view of clinical and service quality—for example, those features that differentiate your organization's services from other providers offering similar services. Beyond specific health care provision, those features might include factors such as extended hours, family support services, cost, assistance with billing/paperwork processes, and transportation assistance. Key health care service features and purchasing decisions [3.1a(2)] might take into account how transactions occur and factors such as confidentiality and security.

N4. The determination of health care service features and their relative importance [3.1a(2)] should take into account the potentially differing expectations of patients and other customers.

N5. Listening and learning [3.1a(2)] might include gathering and integrating surveys, focus group findings, Web-based data, and other data and information that bear upon health care purchasing decisions. Keeping your listening and learning methods current with health care service needs and directions [3.1a(3)] also might include use of newer technology, such as Web-based data gathering.

This Item [3.1] looks at the organization's key processes for gaining knowledge about its current and future patients and customers and markets, in order to offer relevant products and services, understand emerging patient and customer requirements and expectations, and keep pace with changing markets and marketplaces. Processes required by Item 3.1 permit the organization to gather intelligence about its patients and customers and competition. It is a critical starting place for determining direction and strategic planning.

This information is intended to support marketing, health care development, and planning. In a rapidly changing competitive environment, many factors may affect patient and customer preference and loyalty, and the interface with patients and customers in the marketplace, making it necessary to listen and learn on a continuous basis. To be effective, such listening and learning strategies need to have a close connection with the organization's overall health care strategy. For example, if the organization customizes its products and services, the listening and learning strategy needs to be backed by a capable information system—one that rapidly accumulates information about patients and customers and makes this information available where needed throughout the organization or elsewhere within the overall value chain.

The organization must have a process for determining or segmenting key patient and customer groups and markets. To ensure that a complete and accurate picture of patient and customer requirements and concerns is obtained, organizations should consider the requirements of potential patients and customers, including competitors' patients and customers. (Note: a potential patient and customer is a patient and customer the organization wants but is currently being served by a competitor.)

The organization should show how these determinations include relevant information from current and former patients and customers. In addition, the organization should tailor its listening and learning techniques to different patient and customer groups and market segments. A relationship or listening strategy might work with some patients and customers, but not with others.

Information sought should be sensitive to specific health care service requirements and their relative importance or value to different patient and customer groups. This determination should be supported by use of information and data, such as complaints and gains and losses of patients and customers.

In addition to defining patient and customer requirements, organizations must determine key requirements and drivers of purchase decisions and key product/service features. In other words, the organization must be able to prioritize key patient and customer requirements and drivers of health care consumer decisions. These priorities are likely to be different for different patient and customer groups and market segments. Knowledge of patient and customer groups and market segments allows the organization to tailor listening and learning strategies and marketplace offerings, to support marketing strategies, and to develop new health care.

In a rapidly changing competitive environment, many factors may affect patient and customer preference and loyalty. This makes it necessary to listen and learn on a continuous basis. To be effective as an organization, listening and learning need to be closely linked with the overall health care strategy and strategy planning process.

E-commerce is changing the competitive arena rapidly. This may significantly affect the relationships with patients and customers and the effectiveness of listening and learning strategies. It may also force the organization to redefine patient and customer groups and market segments.

A variety of listening and learning strategies are commonly used by top-performing organizations. Increasingly, companies interact with patients and customers via multiple modes. Some examples of listening and learning strategies include:

- Close integration with key patients and customers

- Rapid innovation and field trials of products and services to better link research and development (R&D) and design to the market

- Close tracking of technological, competitive, and other factors that may bear upon patient and customer requirements, expectations, preferences, or alternatives

- Defining the patients' and customers' value chains and how they are likely to change

- Focus groups with key patients and customers

- Use of critical incidents, such as complaints, to understand key service attributes from the point of view of patients and customers and patient- and customer-contact staff

- Interviewing lost patients and customers to determine the factors they use in their health care buying decisions

- Survey/feedback information, including information collected on the Internet

- Won/lost analysis relative to competitors

Finally, the organization must have a system in place to improve its patient and customer listening and learning strategies to keep current with changing health care needs and directions. If the organization competes in a rapidly changing environment, it may need to evaluate and improve its patient and customer listening and learning strategies more frequently. The organization should be able to demonstrate that it has made appropriate improvements to ensure its techniques for understanding patient and customer requirements and priorities keeps pace with changing health care needs.

3.1 Patient, Other Customer, and Health Care Market Knowledge

How the organization determines requirements, expectations, and preferences of target or potential patients, other customers and markets to anticipate their needs and to develop health care opportunities

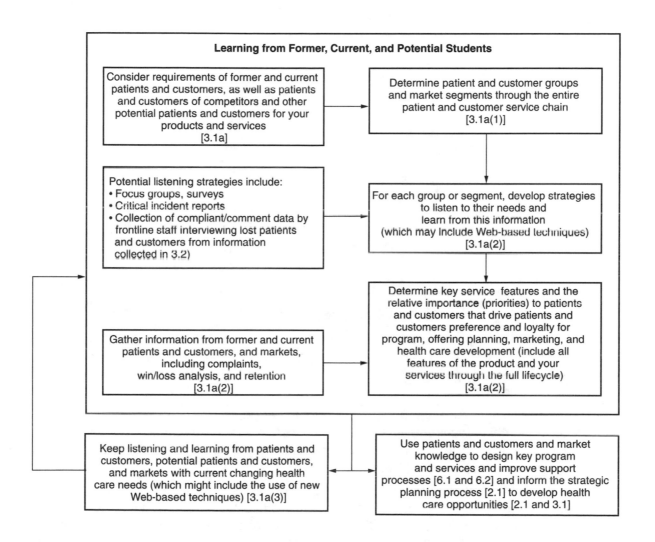

3.1 Patient, Other Customer, and Health Care Market Knowledge Item Linkages

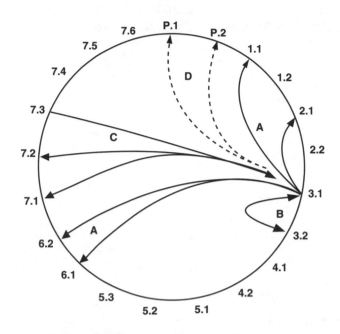

	NATURE OF RELATIONSHIP
A	Patient and customer input and related information about current and future patient and customer and market requirements and preferences [3.1a(2)] is used for strategic planning [2.1a], to design key health services and revise work processes [6.1a(2, 3, and 4)] and to help leaders set directions for the organization [1.1a(1)].
B	Patient and customer complaints [3.2a(3)] are used to help assess current patient and customer expectations and refine requirements [3.1a(2)]. Information about patient and customer requirement priorities [3.1a(2)] is used to build instruments and better target questions to assess patient and customer satisfaction [3.2b(1)].
C	Patient and customer satisfaction, complaint, and health care service data and trends [7.2a(2) and 7.1a] and market data [7.3a(2)] are used to help validate patient and customer expectations and refine requirements [3.1a(2)]. In addition, processes to gather intelligence about patient and customer requirements [3.1] are used to define and report patient and customer satisfaction and health care service quality results [7.2 and 7.1].
D	The products and services reported in P.1b(2) were determined using the processes described in 3.1a(2). The information in P.1b(2) helps examiners identify the kind of results, broken out by patient and customer and market segment, which should be reported in Items 7.1 and 7.2.

	IF YOU DON'T DO WHAT THE CRITERIA REQUIRE...
Item Reference	**Possible Adverse Consequences**
3.1a(1)	The failure to classify or group patients and customers or markets into meaningful segments may make it difficult to identify and differentiate key requirements that may be critical to one group but not another. For example, frequent or high service volume patients and customers may have different expectations than infrequent or low-volume patients and customers. Unless these differences are understood it may be difficult for the organization to customize information collection techniques as well as programs and services according to the needs and expectations of different groups of patients and customers.
3.1a(2)	Different techniques may be needed to understand the requirements of different groups of patients and customers. The failure to listen and learn about the key patient and customer requirements for health care services, especially those features that are most important to patient and customer buying decisions, may make it difficult to design and develop those key services that are most likely to satisfy patients and customers and increase market share. In addition to gathering feedback directly from current and former patients and customers, complaint and lost patient and customer data may provide additional insights to unmet requirements and present opportunities. If an organization does not know why it lost or gained patients and customers, it makes it more difficult to deliver the right services to keep patients and customers.
3.1a(3)	The failure to systematically evaluate the processes used to listen and learn about patient and customer requirements may make it difficult to identify specific areas needing change. For example, it does not do much good to create a survey to identify patient and customer requirements if the questions asked on the survey are not the right questions. Incorrect information generated by this survey may cause the organization to design and deliver the wrong products or services. Furthermore, it does not do much good to use a written survey tool when face-to-face interviews may be a better way to acquire accurate and actionable information. The failure to evaluate the effectiveness of the approaches used to identify and prioritize patient and customer requirements may make it difficult to keep up with changing patient and customer and market needs and gather critical information necessary for strategic planning [Item 2.1a(2)], as well as the design and development of new health care services [Item 6.1a(3)].

3.1 PATIENT, OTHER CUSTOMER AND HEALTH CARE MARKET KNOWLEDGE—SAMPLE EFFECTIVE PRACTICES

A. Patient, Other Customer, and Market Knowledge

- Various systematic methods are used to gather data and identify current requirements and expectations of patients and customers (for example, surveys, focus groups, and the use of Web-based systems).

- Key service features are defined. Service features refer to all important characteristics and to the performance of health care services that patients and customers experience or perceive throughout. Factors that bear on patient and customer preference and loyalty—for example, those features that enhance or differentiate services from competing offerings—are defined in measurable terms.

- Patient and customer requirements are identified or grouped by patient and customer segments. These segments are consistently used for planning, data analysis, service design, and delivery devices, and for reporting and monitoring progress.

- Patient and customer data such as complaints and gains or losses of patients and customers are used to support the identification or validation of key patient and customer requirements.

- Fact-based, systematic methods are used to identify the future requirements and expectations of patients and customers. These are tested for accuracy, and estimation techniques are improved.

- Patients and customers of competitors are considered and processes are in place to gather expectation data from potential patients and customers.

- Effective listening and learning strategies include:

  – Close monitoring of technological, competitive, societal, environmental, economic, and demographic factors that may bear on patient and customer requirements, expectations, preferences, or alternatives

  – Focus groups with demanding or key patients and customers

  – Training of frontline staff in patient and customer listening

  – Use of critical incidents in service performance or quality to understand key service attributes from the point of view of patients and customers and frontline staff

  – Interviewing lost patients and customers

  – Won/lost analysis relative to competitors

  – Analysis of major factors affecting key patients and customers

- Tools such as forced- or paired-choice analysis are used (where patients and customers select between options A and B, A and C, B and C, and so forth). Using this technique, organizations quickly prioritize requirements and focus on delivering those that make the greatest impact on satisfaction, repeat health care service, and loyalty.

- Methods to listen and learn from patients and customers are evaluated and improved through several cycles. Examples of factors that are evaluated include:

  – The adequacy and timeliness of patient- and customer-related information

  – Improvement of survey design

  – Approaches for getting reliable and timely information—surveys, focus groups, patient- and customer-contact personnel

  – Improved aggregation and analysis of information

- Best practices for gathering patient and customer requirements and forecasting are identified and used to make improvements.

- A variety of methods are used to gather information about competitor's customers. Focus groups of competitor's customers, telephone surveys, physician interviews, and literature searches are a few of the methods employed.

- Patients are segmented primarily by location of care, such as inpatient, emergency department, and home care. They are further segmented by health care need and individual patient requirements.

3.2 PATIENT AND OTHER CUSTOMER RELATIONSHIPS AND SATISFACTION (45 PTS.)

Describe how your organization builds relationships to acquire, satisfy, and retain patients and other customers; to increase loyalty; and to develop new health care service opportunities. Describe also how your organization determines patient and other customer satisfaction.

Within your response, include answers to the following questions:

a. Patient/Customer Relationship Building

(1) How do you build relationships to acquire patients and other customers, to meet and exceed their expectations, to increase loyalty and secure their future interactions with your organization, and to gain positive referrals?

(2) What are your key access mechanisms for patients and other customers to seek information, obtain services, and make complaints? How do you determine key contact requirements for each mode of patient and other customer access? How do you ensure that these contact requirements are deployed to all people and processes involved in the customer response chain?

(3) What is your complaint management process? How do you ensure that complaints are resolved effectively and promptly? How are complaints aggregated and analyzed for use in improvement throughout your organization and by your partners?

(4) How do you keep your approaches to building relationships and providing patient/customer access current with health care service needs and directions?

b. Patient/Customer Satisfaction Determination

(1) How do you determine patient and other customer satisfaction and dissatisfaction? How do these determination methods differ among patient/customer groups? How do you ensure that your measurements capture actionable information for use in exceeding your patients' and other customers' expectations, securing their future interactions with your organization, and gaining positive referrals? How do you use patient and other customer satisfaction and dissatisfaction information for improvement?

(2) How do you follow up with patients and other customers on health care services and transaction quality to receive prompt and actionable feedback?

(3) How do you obtain and use information on patients' and other customers' satisfaction relative to satisfaction with your competitors, other organizations providing similar health care services, and/or benchmarks?

(4) How do you keep your approaches to determining satisfaction current with health care service needs and directions?

Continued

Notes: *Continued*

N1. Customer relationships (3.2a) might include the development of partnerships or alliances with customers.

N2. Determining patient and other customer satisfaction and dissatisfaction (3.2b) might include use of any or all of the following: surveys, formal and informal feedback, customer account histories, complaints, win/loss analysis, and information on timeliness of service delivery. Information might be gathered on the Internet, through personal contact or a third party, or by mail.

N3. Patient and other customer satisfaction measurements might include both a numerical rating scale and descriptors for each unit in the scale. Actionable satisfaction measurements provide useful information about specific service features, delivery, relationships, and transactions that bear upon the customers' future actions—choice of health care provider and positive referral.

N4. Your patient and other customer satisfaction and dissatisfaction results should be reported in Item 7.2.

Item 3.2 describes processes that examine the impact of health care services on patient and customer relationships and satisfaction. In particular, this Item looks at the organization's processes for building patient and customer relationships and determining patient and customer satisfaction, with the aim of acquiring new patients and customers, retaining existing patients and customers, and developing new opportunities. Relationships provide an important means for organizations to understand and manage patient and customer expectations and to develop new health care services. Also, patient- and customer-contact employees may provide vital information to build partnerships and other longer-term relationships with patients and customers.

Overall, Item 3.2 emphasizes the importance of obtaining actionable information, such as feedback and complaints from patients and customers. To be actionable, the information gathered should meet two conditions:

- Patient and customer responses should be tied directly to key service and health care processes, so that opportunities for improvement are clear.

- Patient and customer responses should be translated into cost/revenue implications to support the setting of improvement and change priorities.

The first part of this Item [3.2a(1)] looks at the organization's processes for providing easy access for patients and customers and potential patients and customers to seek information or assistance and/or to comment and complain.

- This access makes it easy to get timely information from patients and customers about issues that are of real concern to them. Timely information, in turn, is transmitted to the appropriate place in the organization to drive improvements or new levels of health care service.

- Information from patients and customers should be actionable. To be actionable, organizations should be able to tie the information to key health care processes, and be able to determine cost/revenue implications for improvement priority setting.

Organizations must also determine key patient- and customer-contact requirements and how these vary for different modes of access, and make sure all employees who are involved in responding to patients and customers understand these requirements. As part of this response, the organization is asked to describe key access mechanisms for patients and customers to seek information, conduct health care-related business, and make complaints. Also important is how patient- and customer-contact requirements are deployed along the entire response chain.

- Patient- and customer-contact requirements essentially refer to patient and customer expectations for service after contact with the organization has been made. Typically, the organization translates patient- and customer-contact requirements into patient and customer service standards. Patient- and customer-contact requirements should be set in measurable terms to permit effective monitoring and performance review.

- A good example of a measurable patient- and customer-contact requirement might be the patient and customer expectation that a malfunctioning computer information site would be back online within 24 hours of the request for service. Another example might be the patient and customer requirement that a knowledgeable and polite human being is available within 10 minutes to resolve a problem with software. In both cases, a clear requirement and a measurable standard were identified.

- A bad example of a patient and customer service standard might be, "We get back to the patient and customer as soon as we can." With this example, no standard of performance is defined. Some patient- and customer-contact representatives might get back to a patient and customer within a matter of minutes. Others might take hours or days. The failure to define precisely the contact requirement makes it difficult to allocate appropriate resources to meet that requirement consistently.

- These patient and customer service standards must be deployed to all staff who are in contact with patients and customers. Such deployment needs to take account of all key points in the response chain—all units or individuals in the organization that make effective interactions possible. These standards then become one source of information to evaluate the organization's performance in meeting patient- and customer-contact requirements.

Organizations should capture, aggregate, analyze, and learn from the complaint information and comments they receive. A prompt and effective response and solutions to patient and customer needs and desires are a source of satisfaction and loyalty. Effective complaint management requires the prompt and courteous resolution of complaints. This leads to recovery of patient and customer confidence. Patient and customer loyalty and confidence is enhanced when problems are resolved by the first person the patient and customer contacts. In fact, prompt resolution of problems helps to ensure higher levels of loyalty than if the patient and customer never had a problem in first place. Even if the organization ultimately resolves a problem, the likelihood of maintaining a loyal patient and customer is reduced by 10 percent when a customer is referred to another place or person in the organization.[1]

The organization must also have a mechanism for learning from complaints and ensuring that design/delivery process staff receive information needed to eliminate the causes of complaints. Effective elimination of the causes of complaints involves aggregation of complaint information from all sources for evaluation and use in overall organizational improvement—both design and delivery stages (see Items 6.1 and 6.2).

Complaint aggregation, analysis, and root-cause determination should lead to effective elimination of the causes of complaints and to priority setting for process and service improvements. Successful outcomes require effective deployment of information throughout the organization.

For long-term success, organizations should build strong relationships with patients and customers since health care development and service innovation increasingly depend on maintaining close relationships with patients and customers.

- Organizations should keep approaches to all aspects of patient and customer relationships current with changing health care needs and directions, since approaches to and bases for relationships may change quickly.

- Organizations should also develop an effective process to determine the levels of satisfaction and dissatisfaction for the different patient and customer groups, including capturing actionable information that reflects patients' and customers' future health care and/or positive referral intentions. Satisfied patients and customers are a requirement for loyalty, repeat health care service, and positive referrals.

The second part of this Item [3.2b] looks at how the organization determines patient and customer satisfaction and dissatisfaction.

The organization must gather information on patient and customer satisfaction and dissatisfaction, including any important differences in approaches for different patient and customer groups or market segments. This highlights the importance of the measurement scale in determining those factors that best reflect patients' and customers' market behaviors—future business, new health care service, and positive referral. The organization must keep its approaches to determining patient and customer satisfaction current with changing health care needs and directions. Changing health care needs and directions might include new modes of patient and customer access, such as the Internet. In such cases, key contact requirements might include online security for patients and customers, and access to personal assistance.

The organization should systematically follow-up with patients and customers regarding services and recent transactions to receive feedback that is prompt and actionable. Prompt feedback enables problems to be identified quickly to help prevent them from recurring.

The organization should determine the satisfaction levels of the patients and customers of competitors in

---

1. From the article, "Basic Facts on Customer Complaint Behavior and the Impact of Service on Bottom Line," by John Goodman. First published in *Competitive Advantage* (June 1999): pp. 1-5. The article can be read at www.e-satisfy.com/pfd/basicfacts.pdf.

order to identify threats and opportunities to improve future performance. Such information might be derived from the organization's own comparative studies or from independent studies. The factors that lead to patient and customer preference are of critical importance in understanding factors that drive markets and potentially affect longer-term competitiveness and are particularly helpful during strategic planning.

The patient and customer satisfaction data gathered from the complaint management process in Item 3.2a ensure timely resolution of problems and can help recover or build patient and customer loyalty. Data from the complaint processes in Item 3.2a are collected at the patient and customer's convenience.

However, data collected by survey or similar means, as required by Item 3.2b, produce information at the convenience of the organization. Patients and customers complain when they have a problem. They do not tend to hold their complaint until the organization finds it convenient to ask them.

Although the complaint-type patient and customer feedback (from Item 3.2a) is timely, it is often difficult to develop reliable trend data. The processes in Item 3.2b make it easier to track satisfaction over time. Both techniques are required to fully understand the dynamics that build loyalty, retention, and positive referral. To be effective, both techniques should be used to drive improvement actions.

3.2 Patient and Other Customer Relationships and Satisfaction

How patient and customer satisfaction is determined, relationships strengthened, and services enhanced to support patient and customer- and market-related planning

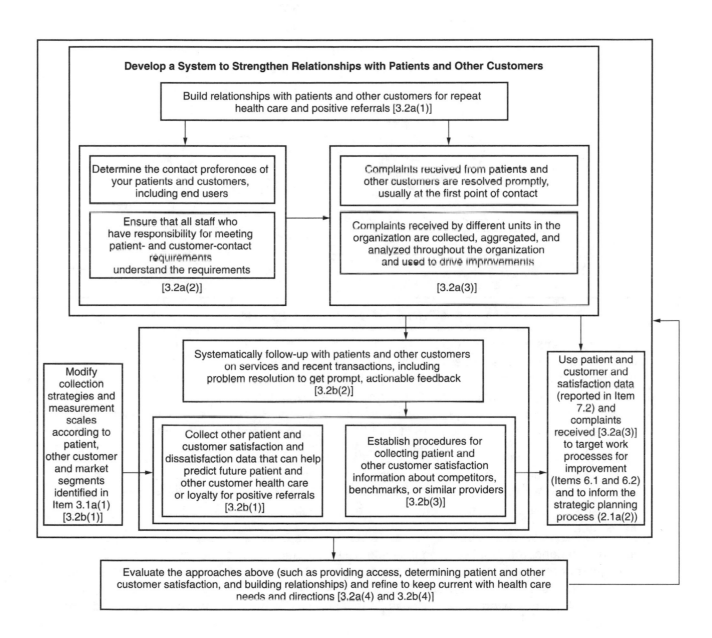

Develop a System to Strengthen Relationships with Patients and Other Customers

Build relationships with patients and other customers for repeat health care and positive referrals [3.2a(1)]

Determine the contact preferences of your patients and customers, including end users

Ensure that all staff who have responsibility for meeting patient- and customer-contact requirements understand the requirements

[3.2a(2)]

Complaints received from patients and other customers are resolved promptly, usually at the first point of contact

Complaints received by different units in the organization are collected, aggregated, and analyzed throughout the organization and used to drive improvements

[3.2a(3)]

Systematically follow-up with patients and other customers on services and recent transactions, including problem resolution to get prompt, actionable feedback [3.2b(2)]

Modify collection strategies and measurement scales according to patient, other customer and market segments identified in Item 3.1a(1) [3.2b(1)]

Collect other patient and customer satisfaction and dissatisfaction data that can help predict future patient and other customer health care or loyalty for positive referrals [3.2b(1)]

Establish procedures for collecting patient and other customer satisfaction information about competitors, benchmarks, or similar providers [3.2b(3)]

Use patient and customer and satisfaction data (reported in Item 7.2) and complaints received [3.2a(3)] to target work processes for improvement (Items 6.1 and 6.2) and to inform the strategic planning process (2.1a(2))

Evaluate the approaches above (such as providing access, determining patient and other customer satisfaction, and building relationships) and refine to keep current with health care needs and directions [3.2a(4) and 3.2b(4)]

3.2 Patient and Other Customer Relationships and Satisfaction Item Linkages

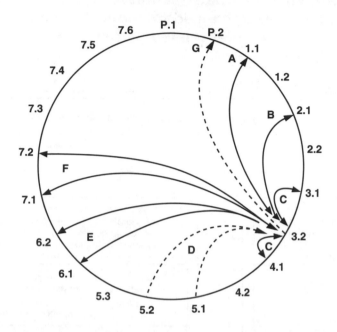

NATURE OF RELATIONSHIP	
A	The climate establishing patient- and customer-focused priorities and patient- and customer-contact requirements (service standards) for patient and customer service personnel [3.2a(2)] is driven by top leadership [1.1a(1)]. They receive useful information from those patients and customers to improve management decision making. Patient and customer relationships/complaint data [3.2a(3)] and satisfaction data [3.2b(1)] are typically used by senior leaders to review performance [1.1c (1 and 2)] and set priorities for action [1.1c(3)].
B	Information about patient and customer satisfaction [3.2b(1)] and complaints [3.2a(3)] collected by patient- and customer-contact employees is used in the planning process [2.1a(2)]. In addition, strategic objectives [2.1b(1)] influence patient and customer relationship management [3.2a] and patient and customer satisfaction determination processes [3.2b] by identifying key focus areas.
C	Information concerning patient and customer requirements and expectations [3.1a] and benchmark data [4.1a(2)] are used to help identify, set, and deploy patient and customer contact requirements (service standards) [3.2a(2)]. Patient and customer complaint data [3.2a(3)] are analyzed [4.1b] and used to help assess patient and customer requirements and expectations [3.1a(2)].
D	Training [5.2] and feedback, reward, and recognition tied to patient and customer satisfaction [5.1b] should enhance the ability of patient- and customer-contact staff [3.2a(2)] to understand requirements and develop the skills to resolve complaints and satisfy patients and customers [3.2a(3)].

Continued

	NATURE OF RELATIONSHIP	*Continued*
E	Information collected through patient and customer relations staff [3.2a(2 and 3)] is used to enhance design of health care services and to improve health care and support processes [6.1 and 6.2].	
F	Information and complaints from patient and customer relations processes [3.2a(3)] can help in the design of patient and customer satisfaction measures [3.2b(1)] and produce data on patient and customer satisfaction [7.2] and related health care service results [7.1]. In addition, patient and customer satisfaction results [7.21a] are used to set patient and customer contact requirements (service standards) [3.2a(2)]. Efforts of improved accessibility and responsiveness in compliant management [3.2a(3 and 4)] should result in improved complaint response time, effective compliant resolution, and a higher percentage of complaints resolved on first contact. These results should be reported in 7.1 and/or 7.2.	
G	Processes in Item 3.2b(3) produce information about the satisfaction of competitors' patients and customers, which is needed to create the description for P.2a(1 and 2).	

	IF YOU DON'T DO WHAT THE CRITERIA REQUIRE...
Item Reference	**Possible Adverse Consequences**
3.2a(1)	The failure to build lasting relationships and loyalty with patients and customers makes it easier for patients and customers to "jump ship" when problems arise. Loyal patients and customers are twice as likely to use services than those who are simply satisfied. Without a disciplined approach for building relationships and cultivating loyalty, the benefits of loyal patients and customers become a hit-or-miss opportunity for the organization. For example, in many manufacturing companies today, service is a key differentiator. This is similar for health care organizations. Programs and services that were once considered specialty items, such as wellness centers and courses and birthing classes, are now common commodities. Therefore, service can become the factor that differentiates organizations and cultivates loyal patients and customers. Furthermore, since it is more costly to acquire a new patient and customer than to keep an existing patient and customer, organizations can avoid unnecessary expenses by building relationships and strengthening the loyalty of current patients and customers. Loyal patients and customers are far more likely to provide positive referrals than a dissatisfied or even minimally satisfied patient and customer.
3.2a(2)	Patient and customer contact requirements (sometimes called patient and customer service standards) help define the patients' and customers' expectations for service after initiating a contact, question, or complaint. For example, a large health care organization surveyed its patients and customers and determined that they expected to have a nurse clinician help solve their problems after outpatient surgery within ten minutes of making the initial contact. By knowing the patient and customer contact requirements and the hour-to-hour call volume, the organization was able to put enough nurse clinicians in place to ensure the average response time was nine minutes or less. The failure to understand and meet patient and customer contact requirements and make it easy for patients and customers to contact the organization makes it more difficult to build loyalty and learn quickly about patient and customer problems.
3.2a(3)	Once the organization learns about a patient and customer problem, the speed and efficiency with which it resolves that problem contributes a great deal to patient and customer loyalty and willingness to make positive referrals. The failure to resolve a problem to patient and customer's satisfaction at the first point of contact almost cuts in half the likelihood of maintaining a loyal patient and customer. In addition, the failure to collect, aggregate, analyze, and use complaint data to drive improvements throughout the organization (and as appropriate to key suppliers or partners) increases the likelihood that the problem will recur again and again. Failing to prevent the problem from recurring directly adds cost but no value to the services delivered to patients and customers. Rework associated with repeating problems is a pure waste of resources and can be a significant source of patient and customer dissatisfaction.

Continued

	IF YOU DON'T DO WHAT THE CRITERIA REQUIRE... *Continued*
Item Reference	**Possible Adverse Consequences**
3.2a(4)	The failure to evaluate systematically the processes used to build relationships, resolve complaints, and prevent them from recurring may make it difficult to identify specific areas needing change. Making it easy for patients and customers to complain but not resolving those complaints effectively and promptly may create even higher levels of dissatisfaction. Ignorance about the effectiveness of patient and customer access and complaint resolution processes may blind the organization to a problem of its own creation, especially in a highly competitive arena where patient and customer and market requirements can change quickly. Without an ongoing system to evaluate and improve processes to build relationships and satisfy patients and customers, current processes may not be able to keep up with changing health care or market demands.
3.2b(1)	The failure to accurately determine patient and customer satisfaction and dissatisfaction may make it difficult for the organization to make timely adjustments in the services it offers. Furthermore, if the data collection processes do not help the organization understand what drives patient and customer behavior, the organization may not know until it is too late (the patient and customer goes elsewhere) that they have a serious problem. The failure to predict patient and customer behavior and the likelihood for positive referral also makes it difficult to forecast demand, which may create supply chain difficulties, such as excessive delays in scheduling and other services. In addition, the failure to take into account differences in patient and customer or market segments and adjust the techniques for collecting patient and customer satisfaction and dissatisfaction data appropriately may cause the organization to collect inaccurate or unreliable information, which threatens the accuracy of the organization's decision making and planning.
3.2b(2)	The longer an organization waits to gather patient- and customer- satisfaction data, the more time it takes to identify and correct a problem. Organizations that fail to follow up with patients and customers whenever a transaction occurs and learn about problems promptly increase the likelihood that other patients and customers will experience the same problem because it will not have been identified or corrected. Similarly, organizations that fail to follow up with patients and customers may be unaware of elements that drive satisfaction and loyalty that could be spread to other parts of the organization or to other health care services.
3.2b(3)	By failing to obtain information on the satisfaction of the competitors' patients and customers, the organization may not learn what it must do differently to satisfy and acquire (win over) the patients and customers of its competitors.

IF YOU DON'T DO WHAT THE CRITERIA REQUIRE... *Continued*	
Item Reference	**Possible Adverse Consequences**
3.2b(4)	Organizations that do not evaluate the effectiveness of their techniques to determine patient and customer satisfaction and dissatisfaction run the risk of making bad decisions based on misleading or even useless information. It does not do much good to gather patient and customer satisfaction data unless the organization asks the right questions. Failing to ask the right questions rarely produces accurate, actionable information to support effective decision making. Moreover, the failure to evaluate the effectiveness of the approaches used to assess patient and customer satisfaction may make it difficult to keep up with changing patient and customer and market needs, and gather critical information necessary for strategic planning and the development of new or improved services.

3.2 PATIENT AND OTHER CUSTOMER RELATIONSHIPS AND SATISFACTION—SAMPLE EFFECTIVE PRACTICES

A. Patient and Customer Relationships

- Several methods are used to ensure ease of patient and customer contact, 24 hours a day if necessary (for example, toll-free numbers, patient information hot lines, pagers for contact staff, Web sites, e-mail, surveys, interviews, focus groups, electronic bulletin boards).

- Patient- and customer-contact staff are empowered to make decisions to address patient and customer concerns.

- Adequate staff members are available to maintain effective patient and customer contact, within the time limits expected by patients and customers.

- Measurable performance expectations are set for staff whose job brings them in regular contact with patients and customers. The performance of employees against these expectations is tracked.

- A system exists to ensure that patient and customer complaints are resolved promptly and effectively by the first point of contact. This often means training patient- and customer-contact staff and giving them authority for resolving a broad range of problems.

- Complaint data are tracked, analyzed, and used to initiate prompt corrective action to prevent the problem from recurring.

- Training and development plans exist for patient- and customer-contact staff. These processes have been measured and refined.

- Measurable patient- and customer-contact requirements (service standards) have been derived from patient and customer expectations (for example, accuracy, timeliness, courtesy, efficiency, thoroughness, and completeness).

- Requirements for building relationships are identified and may include factors such as clinical knowledge, staff responsiveness, and various patient and customer contact methods.

- A systematic approach is in place to evaluate and improve service levels, patient- and customer-focused decision making, and patient and customer relationships

B. Patient and Customer Satisfaction Determination

- Several patient- and customer- satisfaction indicators are used (for example, repeat health care measures, praise letters, and direct measures using survey questions and interviews).

- Comprehensive satisfaction and dissatisfaction data are collected and segmented or grouped to enable the organization to predict patient and customer behavior (likelihood of remaining a patient and customer).

- Patient and customer satisfaction and dissatisfaction measurements include both a numerical rating scale and descriptors assigned to each unit in the scale. An effective (actionable) patient and customer satisfaction and dissatisfaction measurement system provides the organization with reliable information about patient and customer ratings of specific service features and the relationship between these ratings and the patient and customer's likely market behavior.

- Patient and customer dissatisfaction indicators include complaints, claims, repeat services, litigation, performance rating downgrades, and incomplete orders.

- Satisfaction data are collected from former patients and customers.

- Competitors' patient and customer satisfaction is determined using external or internal studies. This information is used to refine services and program features.

- Procedures are in place and evaluated to ensure that patient and customer contact is initiated to follow-up on recent transactions to build relationships. Data from these contacts are used.

- The process of collecting complete, timely, and accurate patient and customer satisfaction and dissatisfaction data is regularly evaluated and improved. Patient and customer preferences, by patient and customer segment, are considered when designing procedures to determine satisfaction levels. Some prefer surveys while others prefer face-to-face interactions or focus groups. Several improvement cycles are evident.

- A variety of listening and learning tools are used. Recognizing the differing needs within their various operating groups, the listening and learning tools are applied at the local level.

- Senior leaders perform daily rounds, similar to physician rounds but with the purpose of receiving prompt and actionable feedback from patients and their families. This feedback is followed up promptly with a report to the patient and their family.

- Patient-satisfaction information is statistically validated and correlated with other results to understand the relationship of satisfaction to organization results.

- Scripting is used to ensure standard communication with patients and their families.

4 Measurement, Analysis, and Knowledge Management—90 Points

*The **Measurement, Analysis, and Knowledge Management** Category examines how your organization selects, gathers, analyzes, manages, and improves its data, information, and knowledge assets.*

The Measurement, Analysis, and Knowledge Management Category is the main point within the Criteria for all key information about effectively measuring and analyzing performance and managing organizational knowledge to drive improvement and organizational competitiveness.

This category is like the "motherboard" on a personal computer. All information flows into and out of it. In the simplest terms, Category 4 is the "brain center" for the alignment of the organization's operations and its strategic objectives. Moreover, since information and analysis might themselves be a source of competitive advantage and productivity growth, the category also may have strategic value and its capabilities should be considered as part of the strategic planning process.

Information and analysis evaluates the selection, management, and effectiveness of the use of information and data to support processes, action plans, and the performance management system. Systems to analyze, review, capture, store, retrieve, and distribute data to support decision making are also evaluated.

Measurement and Analysis of Organizational Performance

- This Item looks at the mechanical processes associated with data collection, information, and measures (including comparative data) for planning, decision making, improving performance, and supporting action plans and operations.

- The Item also looks at the analytical processes used to make sense out of the data. It also looks at how these analyses are deployed throughout the organization and used to support organization-level review, decision making, and planning

Information and Knowledge Management

- This Item looks at how the organization ensures that needed data and information are accessible to staff, suppliers and partners, and patients and customers as needed and appropriate to support decision making. This Item also seeks to ensure that hardware and software are reliable and user-friendly throughout the organization. In many organizations, people with minimal computer skills must be able to access and use data to support decision making.

- The data system must provide for and ensure data integrity, reliability, accuracy, timeliness, security, and confidentiality.

4.1 MEASUREMENT AND ANALYSIS OF ORGANIZATIONAL PERFORMANCE (45 PTS.)

Approach/Deployment

Describe how your organization measures, analyzes, aligns, and improves performance data and information as a health care provider at all levels and in all parts of your organization.

Within your response, include answers to the following questions:

a. Performance Measurement

(1) How do you select, collect, align, and integrate data and information for tracking daily operations and for tracking overall organizational performance? How do you use these data and information to support organizational decision making and innovation as a health care provider?

(2) How do you select and ensure the effective use of key comparative data and information to support operational and strategic decision making and innovation?

(3) How do you keep your performance measurement system current with health care service needs and directions? How do you ensure that your performance measurement system is sensitive to rapid or unexpected organizational or external changes?

b. Performance Analysis

(1) What analyses do you perform to support your senior leaders' organizational performance review? What analyses do you perform to support your organization's strategic planning?

(2) How do you communicate the results of organizational-level analyses to work group and functional-level operations to enable effective support for their decision making?

Notes:

N1. Performance measurement is used in fact-based decision making for setting and aligning organizational directions and resource use at the work unit, key process, departmental, and whole organization levels.

N2. Comparative data and information sources [4.1a(2)] are obtained by benchmarking and by seeking competitive comparisons. "Benchmarking" refers to identifying processes and results that represent best practices and performance for similar activities, inside or outside the health care industry. Competitive comparisons relate your organization's performance to that of competitors and other organizations providing similar health care services. Comparative data might include data from similar organizations and health care industry benchmarks. Such data might be derived from surveys, published and public studies, participation in indicator programs, or other sources. These data may be drawn from local or national sources.

N3. Analysis includes examining trends; organizational, health care industry, and technology projections; and comparisons, cause-effect relationships, and correlations intended to support your performance reviews, help determine root causes, and help set priorities for resource use. Accordingly, analysis draws upon all types of data: patient- and other customer-related, health care outcomes, financial and market, operational, and competitive/comparative.

N4. The results of organizational performance analysis should contribute to your senior leaders' organizational performance review in 1.1c and organizational strategic planning in Category 2.

N5. Your organizational performance results should be reported in Items 7.1–7.6.

Item 4.1, the Measurement and Analysis of Organizational Performance, looks at the selection, collection, alignment, integration, management, analysis, and use of data and information in support of organizational decision making, planning, and performance improvement. The processes and systems required by this item:

- Provide a key foundation for consistently good decision making

- Serve as a central collection and analysis point in the management system to guide the organization's process management toward the achievement of key health care results and strategic objectives

The first part of this Item, Performance Measurement [4.1a], requires the organization to select and use measures to better track daily operations and enhance decision making accuracy. It should select and integrate measures for monitoring overall organizational performance.

Data alignment and integration are key concepts for successful implementation of the performance measurement system. They are viewed in terms of extent and effectiveness of use to meet performance assessment needs. Alignment and integration include how measures are aligned throughout the organization, how they are integrated to yield organizationwide measures, and how performance measurement requirements are deployed by senior leaders to track work group and process level performance on key measures targeted for organizationwide significance and/or improvement. Comparative data should be selected and used to help drive performance improvement.

Performance data and information are especially important in health care networks, alliances, and supply chains. Once determining the data and information requirements, the organization should determine data and information requirements of the strategic planning and goal-setting process.

The organization should show how competitive comparisons and benchmarking data are selected and used to help drive performance improvement.

The use of competitive and comparative information is important to all organizations. The major premises for using competitive and comparative information are: (1) the organization needs to know where it stands relative to competitors and best practices; (2) comparative and benchmarking information often provides the impetus for significant ("breakthrough") improvement or change; and (3) preparation for comparing performance information frequently leads to a better understanding of the processes and their performance. Benchmarking information also may support health care analysis and decisions relating to core competencies, alliances, and outsourcing.

Effective selection and use of competitive comparisons and benchmarking information require: (1) determination of needs and priorities; (2) criteria for seeking appropriate sources for comparisons—from within and outside the organization's industry and markets; and (3) use of data and information to set stretch targets and to promote major, nonincremental improvements in areas most critical to the organization's competitive strategy.

The last part of Item 4.1a examines how the organization's performance measurement system keeps current with changing health care needs. This involves ongoing evaluation and demonstrated refinement.

The second part of this Item, Performance Analysis [4.1b], examines how the organization analyzes data to support decision making. Isolated facts and data do not usually provide an effective basis for setting organizational priorities and effective decision making. Accordingly, close alignment is needed between analysis and organizational performance review and between analysis and organizational planning. This ensures that analysis is relevant to decision making and that decision making is based on relevant data and information.

Effective decision making usually requires leaders to understand cause-effect connections among and between processes and health care/performance results. Process actions and their results may have many resource implications. High-performing organizations find it necessary to have support systems that provide an effective analytical basis for decisions because resources for improvement are limited and cause-effect connections are often unclear. In addition, organizations must have the ability to perform effective analyses to support senior leaders' assessment of overall organizational performance and strategic planning. Moreover, the results of organizational-level analysis must be effectively communicated by leaders to support decision making throughout the organization and ensure those decisions are aligned with health care results, strategic objectives, and action plans.

Accordingly, systematic processes must be in place for analyzing all types of data and to determine overall organizational health, including key health care results, action plans, and strategic objectives. In addition, organizations must evaluate the effectiveness of its analytical processes and make improvements based on the evaluation.

Facts, rather than intuition, are used to support most decision making at all levels based on the analyses conducted to make sense out of the data collected. Analyses that organizations typically conduct to gain an understanding of performance and needed actions vary widely depending on the type of organization, size, competitive environment, and other factors. These analyses help the organization's leaders understand the following:

- How service improvement correlates with key patient and customer indicators, such as patient and customer satisfaction, patient and customer retention, and market share

- Cost/revenue implications of patient- and customer-related problems and effective problem resolution

- Interpretation of market share changes in terms of patient and customer gains and losses and changes in patient and customer satisfaction

- The impact of improvements in key operational performance areas such as productivity, cycle time, waste reduction, and new program introduction

- Relationships between staff/organizational learning and value added per staff

- Financial benefits derived from improvements in staff safety, absenteeism, and turnover

- Benefits and costs associated with education and training, including Internet-based, or e-learning opportunities

- Benefits and costs associated with improved organizational knowledge management and sharing

- The extent to which identifying and meeting staff requirements correlate with staff retention, motivation, and productivity

- Cost/revenue implications of staff-related problems and effective problem resolution

- Individual or aggregate measures of productivity and quality relative to competitors

- Cost trends relative to competitors.

- Relationships among service quality, operational performance indicators, and overall financial performance trends as reflected in indicators such as operating costs, revenues, asset utilization, and value added per staff

- Allocation of resources among alternative improvement projects based on cost/benefit implications or environmental/community impact

- Net earnings derived from quality, operational, and staff performance improvements

- Comparisons among health care units showing how quality and operational performance improvement affect financial performance

- Contributions of improvement activities to cash flow, working capital use, and shareholder value

- Profit impacts of patient and customer retention

- Cost/revenue implications of new market entry, or expansion

- Cost/revenue, patient and customer, and productivity implications of engaging in and/or expanding e-commerce/e-health care and use of the Internet and intranets

- Market share versus profits if applicable

- Trends in economic, market, and shareholder indicators of value

The availability of electronic data and information of many kinds (for example, financial, operational, patient- and customer-related, accreditation/regulatory) and from many sources (for example, internal, third-party, and public sources; the Internet; Internet tracking software) permits extensive analysis and correlations. Effectively utilizing and prioritizing this wealth of information are important to the success of top-performing organizations.

4.1 Measurement and Analysis of Organizational Performance

How the organization measures, aligns, improves, analyzes, and uses information and data to support decision making for key processes and to improve performance at all levels and parts of the organization

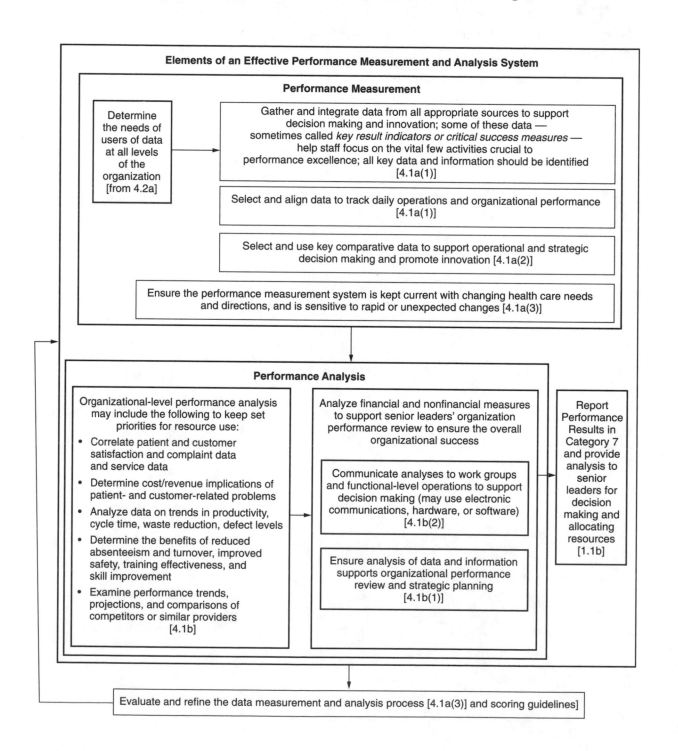

Elements of an Effective Performance Measurement and Analysis System

Performance Measurement

Determine the needs of users of data at all levels of the organization [from 4.2a]

Gather and integrate data from all appropriate sources to support decision making and innovation; some of these data — sometimes called *key result indicators or critical success measures* — help staff focus on the vital few activities crucial to performance excellence; all key data and information should be identified [4.1a(1)]

Select and align data to track daily operations and organizational performance [4.1a(1)]

Select and use key comparative data to support operational and strategic decision making and promote innovation [4.1a(2)]

Ensure the performance measurement system is kept current with changing health care needs and directions, and is sensitive to rapid or unexpected changes [4.1a(3)]

Performance Analysis

Organizational-level performance analysis may include the following to keep set priorities for resource use:

• Correlate patient and customer satisfaction and complaint data and service data

• Determine cost/revenue implications of patient- and customer-related problems

• Analyze data on trends in productivity, cycle time, waste reduction, defect levels

• Determine the benefits of reduced absenteeism and turnover, improved safety, training effectiveness, and skill improvement

• Examine performance trends, projections, and comparisons of competitors or similar providers [4.1b]

Analyze financial and nonfinancial measures to support senior leaders' organization performance review to ensure the overall organizational success

Communicate analyses to work groups and functional-level operations to support decision making (may use electronic communications, hardware, or software) [4.1b(2)]

Ensure analysis of data and information supports organizational performance review and strategic planning [4.1b(1)]

Report Performance Results in Category 7 and provide analysis to senior leaders for decision making and allocating resources [1.1b]

Evaluate and refine the data measurement and analysis process [4.1a(3)] and scoring guidelines

4.1 Measurement and Analysis of Organizational Performance Item Linkages

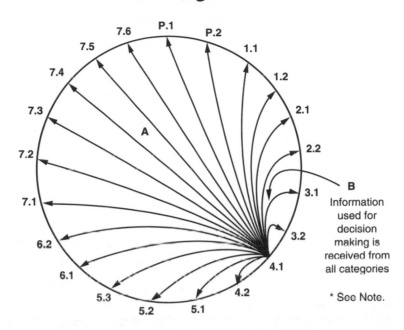

NATURE OF RELATIONSHIP	
A	Data and information are collected and analyzed [4.1] and made available [4.2] for developing the Organizational Profile [P.1 and P.2], planning [2.1a(2)], setting strategic objectives [2.1b(1)], benchmarking priority setting [4.1], day-to-day leadership decisions [1.1], setting public responsibility standards (regulatory, legal, ethical) for community involvement [1.2], reporting performance results [7.1, 7.2, 7.3, 7.4, 7.5, and 7.6], improving work processes [6.1 and 6.2] and staff systems [5.1, 5.2, and 5.3], determining patient and customer requirements [3.1], managing patient and customer complaints and building patient and customer relations [3.2a, and determining patient and customer satisfaction [3.2b].
B	Data and information used to support analysis, decision making, and continuous improvement [4.1] are received from all processes. Information from patient and customer satisfaction data [7.2] are analyzed [4.1b] and used to help determine ways to assess patient and customer requirements [3.1a(2)], to determine appropriate standards or required levels of patient and customer service [3.2a(2)], and to design instruments to assess patient and customer satisfaction [3.2b(1)]. Data and information are received from the following areas and analyzed to support decisions: staff capabilities, including work system efficiency, initiative, and self-direction [5.1a(1)]; training and development needs [5.2a(3)] and effectiveness [5.2a(4)]; and safety, retention, absenteeism, organizational effectiveness, and well-being and satisfaction [5.3]. Data are aggregated and analyzed [4.1] to improve health care processes [6.1] and support processes [6.2] that will reduce cycle time, waste, and defect levels. Performance data from all parts of the organization are integrated and analyzed [4.1] to assess performance in key areas such as patient- and customer-related performance [7.2], health care results [7.1], operational performance [7.5], financial and market performance [7.3], and staff performance [7.4], and regulatory and legal compliance [7.6] relative to competitors or similar providers in all areas.

*Note: The information collected and used for decision making links with all other Items, all of the linkage arrows will not be repeated on the other item maps. Only the most relevant will be repeated.

IF YOU DON'T DO WHAT THE CRITERIA REQUIRE...	
Item Reference	**Possible Adverse Consequences**
4.1a(1)	The failure to systematically gather appropriate data and information from throughout the organization to support the daily operational and organizational decision making can create an environment where decisions are typically based on intuition, gut feel, or guesswork. Furthermore, information gathered in this way may ignore some of the linkages critical to sustaining high performance in an organization. Decisions based on intuition or guesswork tend to be highly variable, which introduce error. Furthermore, in an environment where decisions are based on intuition, it is usually the boss's intuition that drives the decision—which can lead to the disengagement of the people in the organization. Decisions made in this manner erode the organization's efforts to promote staff empowerment and innovation [Item 1.1a(2)]. Finally, the failure to integrate data and information may make it difficult to monitor overall organizational performance. Disjointed, nonintegrated data are difficult to consolidate and report in a manageable, easy to understand "dashboard" to support effective decision making.
4.1a(1)	Data and information provide a basis for decision making at all levels of the organization: top leaders use the data to make decisions about the direction of the organization and staff use data to make decisions about operational matters. Unless measures are selected and aligned to provide the right information, at the right time, in the right format, the decisions of the leaders and the staff are likely to be suboptimized. Moreover, although the failure to gather appropriate data tends to reduce decision making quality, spending resources to gather data and information that do not support decision making throughout the organization (useless data) typically adds unnecessary cost. It is difficult to collect the right data and information if the organization has failed to determine what data are needed to support decision making at all levels. In addition, the failure to collect appropriate information makes it more difficult to monitor performance against goals [Item 1.1c(1)], effectively communicate expectations throughout the organization [Item 1.1a(1)], and deploy actions needed to carry out strategy [Item 2.2a].
4.1a(2)	The failure to collect and effectively use the right comparative data makes it difficult for the organization to learn and take appropriate action. Learning from the best helps provoke an understanding of what systems and processes may be required to make quantum leaps in performance as well as the levels that must be reached to achieve a leadership position projected during the planning process [Item 2.2b]. For example, comparisons showing that the organization's projected performance outpaces the industrial *average* will have little meaning if the *best* competitor's rate of improvement is greater. Furthermore, if an organization collects comparative data from world-class benchmarks, but does not effectively use comparative data for planning [Item 2.1a(2)], identifying areas needing breakthrough performance, or setting improvement priorities [Item 1.1c(2)], then it is simply wasting resources. If an organization does not collect comparative performance outcome data, it is not able to determine if its own rate of progress is sufficient to keep ahead of the competition or evaluate the strength of its own performance results [required by Category 7].

Continued

IF YOU DON'T DO WHAT THE CRITERIA REQUIRE...	*Continued*

Item Reference	Possible Adverse Consequences
4.1a(3)	Organizations that fail to improve the speed and accuracy of decision making typically do not perform well in a competitive environment. Without a process to evaluate the information system and how well it responds to the needs of health care, organizations may not know they are collecting insufficient or incorrect data and information. In addition, organizations may not know if the data effectively support daily operations and organizational decision making. They may not know if the resources spent to collect benchmarking and comparison data are producing appropriate benefits.
4.1b(1)	The lack of a system to analyze and make sense out of raw data may make it difficult for senior leaders to understand cause-and-effect relationships, root causes of problems, and the impact of various processes on performance outcomes. This may make it more difficult for leaders to identify specific areas within the organization where improvement is required. It also makes it more difficult for leaders to effectively set priorities. Consider the following examples: (a) without a cost-benefit analysis, it is more difficult to determine whether project A or project B should receive support because it is difficult to know which project is likely to be of greater benefit to the organization; (b) calculating Cpk (the capability of a process) helps leaders understand the extent to which their key processes are in control of need adjustment (the raw run data cannot support this kind of decision making); and (c) failing to understand root causes makes it more difficult to prevent problems from recurring, which adds cost but not value.
4.1b(1)	Strategy identifies the things an organization must do to be successful in the future. Many actions must be taken in an organization to ensure strategic objectives are achieved. Data analysis helps leaders understand critical relationships between actions and outcomes to effectively allocate resources and achieve desired results. The failure to examine and understand the relationship between performance outcomes, action plans, and strategic objectives may cause senior leaders to make inappropriate decisions about the allocation of limited resources. This means that the organization may not realize the maximum benefit from the expenditure of those resources. For example, failing to understand the correlation between health care service quality improvement and improved patient and customer satisfaction and retention may cause the leader to divert resources to less important activities.
4.1b(2)	Staff and managers at all levels of the organization need useful information to support decision making. The failure to ensure that people at every level understand the impact that their work has on overall organizational performance makes it more difficult for them to identify and understand why they need to perform at certain agreed levels and why change may need to occur. Without this information, staff and managers throughout the organization must rely on intuition or incomplete data to support decision making—typically reducing the accuracy of those decisions and, in some cases, suboptimizing the overall performance of the organization.

4.1 MEASUREMENT AND ANALYSIS OF ORGANIZATIONAL PERFORMANCE—SAMPLE EFFECTIVE PRACTICES

A. Performance Measurement

- Above all, data and information are favored as a decision making support tool, rather than a quick and easy reliance on intuition or "gut feel."

- Data collected at the individual staff level are consistent across the organization to permit consolidation and organizationwide performance monitoring.

- The cost of quality (including rework, delay, waste, scrap, errors) and other financial concerns are measured for internal operations and processes.

- Data are maintained on staff-related issues of satisfaction, morale, safety, education, and training, use of teams, and recognition and reward.

- A systematic process exists for data review and improvement, standardization, and easy staff access to data. Training on the use of data systems is provided as needed.

- Data used for management decisions focus on critical success factors and are integrated with work processes for the planning, design, and delivery of products and services.

- A systematic process is in place for identifying and prioritizing comparative information and benchmark targets.

- Research has been conducted to identify best-in-class organizations, which may be competitors or noncompetitors. Critical health care processes or functions are the subject of benchmarking. Activities, such as those that support the organization's goals and objectives, action plans, and opportunities for improvement and innovation, are the subject of benchmarking. Benchmarking also covers key services, patient and customer satisfiers, suppliers, staff, and support operations.

- The organization reaches beyond its own health care business to conduct comparative studies.

- Benchmark or comparison data are used to improve the understanding of work processes and to discover the best levels of performance that have been achieved. Based on this knowledge, the organization sets goals or targets to stretch performance as well as drive innovations.

- A systematic process is in place to improve the use of benchmark or comparison data in the understanding of all work processes.

B. Performance Analysis

- Systematic processes are in place for analyzing all types of data and to determine overall organizational health, including key health care results, action plans, and strategic objectives. Part of the process is a method to evaluate the effectiveness of the analysis process and improve upon it.

- Facts, rather than intuition, are used to support most decision making at all levels based on the analyses conducted to make sense out of the data collected.

- The analysis process itself is analyzed to make the results more timely and useful for decision making for quality improvement at all levels.

- Analysis processes and tools, and the value of analyses to decision making, are systematically evaluated and improved.

- Analysis is linked to work groups to facilitate decision making (sometimes daily) throughout the organization.

- Analysis techniques enable meaningful interpretation of the cost and performance impact of organization processes. This analysis helps people at all levels of the organization make necessary trade-offs, set priorities, and reallocate resources to maximize overall organization performance.

- Common information-gathering platforms are used across the organization to ensure comparative data across the various entities. Forty-nine various Departmental Indicators roll up to Entity Indicators, which then roll up to System Indicators.

- Quality indicators focus on four areas: clinical quality, patient safety, employee safety, and patient satisfaction.

- Patient and family satisfaction in a children's hospital was increased after a benchmarking trip to learn about Disney approaches to satisfying children.

- System level indicators are correlated inpatient loyalty. This information is used as a basis for planning and project prioritization.

4.2 INFORMATION AND KNOWLEDGE MANAGEMENT (45 PTS.)

Approach/Deployment

Describe how your organization ensures the quality and availability of needed data and information for staff, suppliers and partners, and patients and other customers. Describe how your organization builds and manages its knowledge assets.

Within your response, include answers to the following questions:

a. Data and Information Availability

(1) How do you make needed data and information available? How do you make them accessible to staff, suppliers and partners, and patients and other customers, as appropriate?

(2) How do you ensure that hardware and software are reliable, secure, and user friendly?

(3) How do you keep your data and information availability mechanisms, including your software and hardware systems, current with health care service needs and directions?

b. Organizational Knowledge

(1) How do you manage organizational knowledge to accomplish?

- The collection and transfer of staff knowledge

- The transfer of relevant knowledge from patients and other customers, suppliers, and partners

- The identification and sharing of best practices

(2) How do you ensure the following properties of your data, information, and organizational knowledge:

- Integrity

- Timeliness

- Reliability

- Security

- Accuracy

- Confidentiality

Notes:

N1. Data and information availability (4.2a) are of growing importance as the internet, electronic communication and information transfer, and e-business are used increasingly for provider, provider-to-patient/customer, and business-to-business interactions and as intranets become more important as a major source of organizationwide communications.

N2. Data and information access [4.2a(1)] might be via electronic and other means.

The first part of this Item, Data and Information Availability [4.2a], examines how the organization ensures the availability of high-quality, timely data and information for all key users—staff, suppliers/partners, and patients and customers. Top-performing organizations make data and information available and accessible to all appropriate users. The organization's hardware systems and software must be reliable and user friendly, facilitating full access and encouraging routine use.

As the sources of data and information and the number of users within the organization grow dramatically, systems to manage information technology often require significant resources. Top-performing organizations consider the management of information technology as a strategic imperative. The expanding use of electronic information within organizational operations, more comprehensive knowledge networks, new data from the Internet, and increasing health care-to-health care and health care-to-consumer communications challenges make it absolutely critical that the organization develops systems to ensure data reliability and availability in a user-friendly format.

Data and information are especially important in health care networks, alliances, and supply chains. Information management systems should facilitate the use of data and information and should recognize the need for rapid data validation and reliability assurance, given the increasing use of electronic data transfer.

The second part of this Item, Organizational Knowledge [4.2b], focuses on the need to transfer knowledge: from staff, patients and customers, suppliers, and partners for the benefit of the organization. It also includes the sharing of practices that might benefit the organization and key partners.

Required data and information should meet user needs, including integrity (completeness—tells the whole story), reliability (consistency), accuracy (correctness), timeliness (available when needed), and appropriate levels of security and confidentiality (free from tampering and inappropriate release).

Organizations must ensure data and information reliability since reliability is critical to good decision making, successful monitoring of operations, and successful data integration for assessing overall performance.

Processes should be in place to protect against external threats, including attacks from hackers, viral infections, power surges, and other storm-related damage.

Processes should be in place to protect against system failure which may damage critical data. This may require redundant systems as well as effective backup and storage of data.

Finally, as with the other items required for performance excellence, the organization must systematically evaluate and improve data availability mechanisms, software, and hardware to keep them current with changing health care needs and directions.

4.2 Information and Knowledge Management

How the organization ensures the quality and availability of data and information for staff, suppliers and partners, and patients and customers

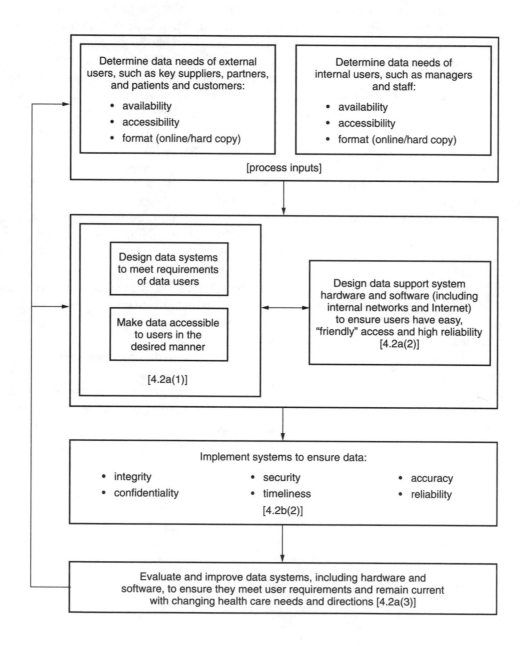

Determine data needs of external users, such as key suppliers, partners, and patients and customers:

- availability
- accessibility
- format (online/hard copy)

Determine data needs of internal users, such as managers and staff:

- availability
- accessibility
- format (online/hard copy)

[process inputs]

Design data systems to meet requirements of data users

Make data accessible to users in the desired manner

[4.2a(1)]

Design data support system hardware and software (including internal networks and Internet) to ensure users have easy, "friendly" access and high reliability [4.2a(2)]

Implement systems to ensure data:

- integrity
- confidentiality
- security
- timeliness
- accuracy
- reliability

[4.2b(2)]

Evaluate and improve data systems, including hardware and software, to ensure they meet user requirements and remain current with changing health care needs and directions [4.2a(3)]

4.2 Information and Knowledge Management
Item Linkages

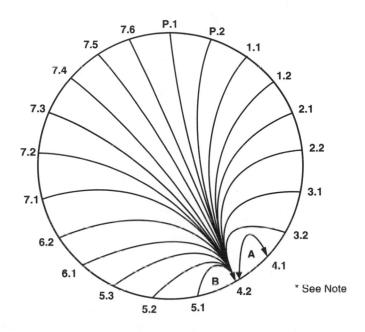

NATURE OF RELATIONSHIP	
A	Information and Knowledge Management [4.2] enables the data flow within the organization and indirectly interacts with all other items (similar to the relationships identified and reported in the Item 4.1 diagram). The simplest way to show these relationships is to tie this Item [4.2] with the Measurement and Analysis of Organizational Performance Item [4.1].
B	In order to ensure that hardware and software systems are reliable and user-friendly [4.2a(2)], information from the following types of system users is gathered: leaders [Category 1]; planners [Category 2]; patient and customer relationships and contact staff [Category 3]; information specialists [Category 4]; staff managers, and staff [Category 5]; operations workers and managers [Category 6]; and people who monitor and interpret results [Category 7] for use in decision making.

*Note: Because the information collected and used for decision making links with all other Items, all of the linkage arrows will not be repeated on the other item maps. Only the most relevant will be repeated.

	IF YOU DON'T DO WHAT THE CRITERIA REQUIRE...
Item Reference	**Possible Adverse Consequences**
4.2a(1)	Getting the right information to the right people at the right time and in the right format enables effective decision making. Just as different types of staff in an organization need different data to support decision making, they may need to access information in different ways. Similarly, patients and customers and suppliers may need access to information to facilitate ordering and delivery of required products and services. The failure to provide appropriate access to data may make it more difficult for staff to make timely decisions about work, for patients and customers to place orders for products and services, or lead to disruptions in the supply chain. Providing inappropriate access for individuals inside or outside the organization may compromise data confidentiality and security or even violate certain privacy statutes.
4.2a(2)	The breadth, depth, and speed of decision making continue to increase as artificial intelligence plays a larger and larger role in our lives. Hardware and software are at the heart of this phenomenon. More people than ever before are being asked to interact with computers. In the best-performing organizations, staff frequently use computers to access data and use them to develop relevant analyses that enable better decisions about their work. People with very little computer literacy must now enter and retrieve data from these systems. A user interface that may be easily understood by information management technicians may be incomprehensible to a line worker, patient and customer, or supplier. The failure to make these systems reliable and easy to use (user-friendly) makes it difficult, if not impossible, for some people to use them effectively. This may create significant problems for organizations, particularly those venturing into areas where e-commerce plays a larger and larger role. Consider, for example, a clinic that wants to expand and promote distance invoicing and payment via the Internet or through home-to-bank modem connections. If the software is not reliable and very user-friendly, many patients and customers may be unwilling or unable to take advantage of these services. This may limit the organization's agility to achieve strategic and/or market share goals that should have been considered during the strategy development process [Item 2.1a(2)].
4.2a(3)	n a rapidly changing world, access to information and the use of that information to provide insight and help decision making can provide a strategic advantage. Rapid data availability is becoming more and more critical for health care success, especially in e-health care situations. As product and delivery cycle times grow shorter, the need for rapid access to information grows greater. Without evaluating the suitability of data and information systems, and making refinements based on this evaluation, the organization leaves itself open to falling behind and not being able to respond rapidly to changing health care needs and directions.

Continued

	IF YOU DON'T DO WHAT THE CRITERIA REQUIRE... *Continued*
Item Reference	**Possible Adverse Consequences**
4.1b(1)	Knowledge is of little or no use unless the people who need it, have it. Knowledge sequestered in one corner of an organization cannot benefit the entire organization unless it is transferred to other staff in other units. The same is true for knowledge held by key patients and customers, suppliers, and partners. Knowledge withheld is knowledge (and resources) wasted.
4.2b(2)	Decisions that are based on data and information may be compromised if the data are inaccurate or unreliable. For example, when a data entry error is made and goes unnoticed (sometimes referred to as "garbage in, garbage out"), it could drive decisions to deliver the wrong product at the wrong time to the wrong patient and customer. At the very least this is likely to cause the product to be returned and restocked, adding cost, but not value. The lack of timely information may cause decisions to be delayed inappropriately. Consider, for example, an organization that conducts a staff (or patient and customer) satisfaction survey but does not analyze or make the data available for eight months. This not only sends a message to the organization that staff (or patient and customer) concerns are unimportant, it also makes it difficult to identify real problems that may be contributing to patient and customer dissatisfaction, low worker morale, and poor productivity.
4.2b(2)	Concerns about security, data loss, sophisticated hackers, and increased patient and customer requirements for better access and availability places steadily increasing demands on hardware and software systems. The failure to keep these systems current may expose them to internal or external threats. For example, the failure to update virus protections frequently and maintain up-to-date, effective firewalls can expose the computer system (and the organization) to catastrophic and costly losses. (Please note that this Item does not require improvements in software and hardware simply for the sake of buying new gadgets. Improvements should help support changing health care needs and directions—as a means to an end, not the end itself. This is another example where a cost-benefit data analysis [Item 4.1b(2)] may be crucial to making good decisions about maintaining appropriate software and hardware systems.)

4.2 INFORMATION AND KNOWLEDGE MANAGEMENT— SAMPLE EFFECTIVE PRACTICES

A. Data and Information Availability

- Users of data help determine what data systems are developed and how data are accessed.

- Every person has access to the data they need to make decisions about their work, from top leaders to individual staff or staff teams.

- The performance measurement system is systematically evaluated and refined. Improvements have been made to reduce cycle time for data collection and to increase data access, reliability, and use.

- Data are protected against misuse from external sources through encryption and randomly changing user passwords.

- Procedures required to interface with the hardware and software were designed to meet the needs and capabilities of all computer users, to ensure they are not excluded.

- Disciplined, automatic file backup occurs. Backup data are stored in a secure, external facility.

- Hardware and software systems have been protected against external threats from hackers, viral threats, water, and electrical damage. Protection systems are updated as appropriate (for example, viral updates are made several times daily).

- Data systems are benchmarked against best-in-class systems and continually refined.

B. Organizational Knowledge

- All key work processes are documented and stored in a searchable and accessible data base and used to share improvements and avoid rework associated with re-inventing effective processes.

- A data and knowledge exchange is in place to receive useful knowledge and information from patients and customers, suppliers, partners and other key stakeholders. The system is automated for easy update end access. Face-to-face and/or electronic meetings are held regularly to share information.

- A "sunset" review is conducted to determine what data no longer need to be collected and can be dropped.

- A data reliability (consistency) team routinely and randomly checks data. Systems are in place to minimize or prevent human error in data entry and analysis.

- Three categories are used to classify information systems: Required (standardized across the system), Standard (standard systems integrated at entities as appropriate), and Non-Standard (non-standard systems integrated at entities as appropriate).

- An infrastructure is in place that allows physician partners to access data and information from any location using a variety of methods: PDA, PCs, pagers, and Fax.

- The Information Management department has moved their focus from reporting to "improvement assistance" focus.

- Staff are recognized and rewarded for sharing knowledge through the Information Anywhere database.

5 Staff Focus—85 Points

*The **Staff Focus** Category examines how your organization's work systems and staff learning and motivation enable staff to develop and utilize their full potential in alignment with your organization's overall objectives and action plans. Also examined are your organization's efforts to build and maintain a work environment and staff support climate conducive to performance excellence and to personal and organizational growth.*

Staff Focus addresses key human resource practices —those directed toward creating a high-performance workplace and toward developing staff to enable them and the organization to adapt to change. The Category covers staff development and management requirements in an integrated manner, aligned with the organization's strategic directions. Included in the focus on human resources is a focus on the work environment and the staff support climate.

To ensure the basic alignment of human resource management with overall strategy, the Criteria also include human resource planning as part of organizational planning in the Strategic Planning Category. Staff Focus also evaluates how the organization enables staff to develop and use their full potential.

Work Systems

- Design, organize, and manage work and jobs to optimize staff performance and potential

- Performance feedback to staff and recognition and reward practices support objectives for patient and other customer satisfaction, high performance objectives, and staff and organization learning goals

- Identify skills and capabilities needed by potential (future) staff, and then recruit, hire and effectively retain them

Staff Learning and Motivation

- Deliver, evaluate, and reinforce appropriate training to achieve action plans and address organization needs including building knowledge, skills, and abilities to improve staff development and performance

- Enhance staff motivation and career progression

Staff Well-Being and Satisfaction

- Improve staff safety, well-being, development, and satisfaction and maintain a work environment free from distractions to high performance

- Systematically evaluate staff well-being, satisfaction, and motivation, and identify improvement priorities that promote key health care results

5.1 WORK SYSTEMS (35 pts.)   Approach/Deployment

Describe how your organization's work and jobs enable all staff and the organization to achieve high performance. Describe how compensation, career progression, and related work-force practices enable staff and the organization to achieve high performance.

Within your response, include answers to the following questions:

a. Organization and Management of Work

(1) How do you organize and manage work and jobs to promote cooperation, initiative, empowerment, innovation, and your organizational culture? How do you organize and manage work and jobs to achieve the agility to keep current with health care service needs?

(2) How do your work systems capitalize on the diverse ideas, cultures, and thinking of your staff and the communities with which you interact (your staff recruitment and your patient/customer communities)?

(3) How do you achieve effective communication and skill sharing across health care professions, departments and work units, jobs, and locations?

b. Staff Performance Management System

How does your staff performance management system, including feedback to staff, support high-performance work? How does your staff performance management system support a patient/customer and health care service focus? How do your compensation, recognition, and related reward and incentive practices reinforce high-performance work and a patient and other customer and health care service focus?

c. Recruitment and Career Progression

(1) How do you identify characteristics and skills needed by potential staff?

(2) How do you recruit, hire, and retain new staff? How do you ensure the staff members represent the diverse ideas, cultures, and thinking of your staff recruitment community?

(3) How do you accomplish effective succession planning for leadership and management positions, including senior administrative and health care leadership, as appropriate? How do you manage effective career progression for all staff throughout the organization? Education and training delivery [5.2a(4)] might occur inside or outside your organization and involve on-the-job, classroom, computer-based, distance learning, and other types of delivery (formal or informal).

Continued

Notes: *Continued*

N1. "Staff " refers to all people who contribute to the delivery of your organization's services, including paid staff (e.g., permanent, temporary, and part-time personnel, as well as any contract employee supervised by your organization), independent practitioners (e.g., physicians, physician assistants, nurse practitioners, acupuncturists, and nutritionists not paid by the organization), volunteers, and health profession students (e.g., medical, nursing, and ancillary). Staff includes team leaders, supervisors, and managers at all levels. Contract employees supervised by a contractor should be addressed in Category 6.

N2. "Your organization's work" refers to how your staff are organized or organize themselves in formal and informal, temporary, or longer-term units. This might include work teams, process teams, project teams, patient/ customers action teams, problem-solving teams, centers of excellence, functional units, remote (e.g., at-home) workers, cross-functional teams, and departments—self-managed or managed by supervisors. "Jobs" refers to responsibilities, authorities, and tasks of individuals. In some work systems, a team might share jobs.

N3. "Recruitment" refers to how potential staff are hired and brought into the organization. This includes paid staff, privileged staff, and volunteers.

N4. Compensation and recognition (5.1b) include promotions and bonuses that might be based upon performance, skills acquired, and other factors. Recognition includes monetary and non-monetary, formal and informal, and individual and group mechanisms. Recognition systems for volunteers and independent practitioners who contribute to the work of the organization should be included, as appropriate.

This Item [5.1] looks at the organization's systems for work and jobs, compensation, career progression, staff performance management, motivation, recognition, communication, and hiring, with the aim of enabling and encouraging all staff to contribute effectively and to the best of their ability. These systems are intended to foster high performance, to result in individual and organizational learning, and to enable adaptation to change.

Work and jobs should be designed in such a way as to allow staff to exercise optimum discretion and decision making, resulting in higher involvement and better performance. *In order to exercise effective decision making, staff need access to appropriate data and analyses concerning their work.* (This links to the information and knowledge management systems required in Category 4.)

Unless staff have access to data to support effective decision making and understand how to analyze and interpret data, their decisions, by default, revert to intuition—which is highly variable. Managers are less likely to permit staff to substitute their intuition for that of managers. Therefore, staff decision mak-

ing is likely to be limited, even if managers were inclined to release decisions to subordinates. Accordingly, systems to promote staff empowerment and agility should ensure staff have the authority to make decisions about their work, as well as data and analysis systems to support effective and consistently good decisions.

Work and job factors important to consider include simplification of job classifications (less specialization and work isolation), which can be addressed by cross training, job rotation, use of teams (including self-directed teams), and changes in work layout and location. Another important factor to combat worker isolation is to foster communication across functions and work units, maintain a focus on patient and other customer requirements, and create an environment of knowledge sharing and respect.

High-performance work is also enhanced by systems that promote staff flexibility, innovation, knowledge and skill sharing, alignment with organizational objectives, patient and other customer focus, and rapid response to changing health care needs and requirements of the marketplace. Work should support the achievement of organizational objectives. Creativity and innovation from all staff should be specifically required, measured, and recognized. Suggestion boxes are not enough. The number of innovative ideas actually *implemented* per person is s better indicator of innovation and idea quality than the number if ideas *proposed*.

Hierarchical, command-and-control management styles work directly against fast response and high-performance capability. Agility reflects the speed with which staff and the organization does its work, including rapid response to changing needs and requirements. Work that is bogged down with bureaucratic inefficiencies cannot be agile. Unnecessary layers of management approval typically add delay and cost, but not value.

Developing and sustaining high-performance work systems requires ongoing education and training, and information systems (see Category 4) that ensure adequate information availability. To help staff realize their full potential, many organizations use individual development plans prepared with the input of staff and designed to address his/her career and learning objectives.

The best organizations put in place a staff performance management system that provides measurable feedback to staff, supports high-performance objectives, and supports a patient and other customer and health care focus. Furthermore, staff compensation, recognition, and reward is aligned to support these health care objectives. In addition, to make sure all staff understand their responsibilities, systems exist to promote effective communication and cooperation, at all levels of the organization.

Once the organization determines its key strategic objectives, it should review compensation, reward, and recognition systems to ensure they support those objectives. The failure to do this creates an environment where staff are focused on one set of activities (based on their compensation plan), but the organization has determined that another set of activities (the action plans to achieve the strategic objectives) is necessary for success.

Compensation and recognition systems must be matched to support the work necessary for health care success. Consistent with this, compensation and recognition might be tied to demonstrated skills and to peer evaluations. Compensation and recognition approaches also might include profit sharing, rewarding exemplary team or unit performance, and links to patient and other customer satisfaction and loyalty measures or other health care objectives.

The organization must perform effective succession planning for senior leadership and managers at all levels of the organization. The rate of new knowledge acquisition is accelerating throughout the world. Significantly more new knowledge is causing change to occur faster than ever before in history. To manage effectively in this climate of rapid change, organizations must prepare its future leaders and managers. The best organizations do not wait for vacancy to occur before it thinks about the requirements and skills needed. Succession planning enables organizations to identify future skill needs against current skill gaps, enabling them to recruit and develop the necessary human resources.

Finally, organizations must profile, recruit, and hire staff who will meet skill requirements required to position the organization for future success. Obviously, the right workforce is a key driver of high performance. As the pool of skilled talent continues to shrink, it becomes more important than ever for organizations to specifically define the capabilities and skills needed by potential staff of all types and create a work environment to attract them. Accordingly, it is critical to take into account characteristics of diverse populations to make sure appropriate support systems exist that make it possible to attract skilled workers.

5.1 Work Systems

How the organization's work and job design, compensation, career progression, and related workforce practices enable and encourage all staff to contribute effectively to achieving high performance

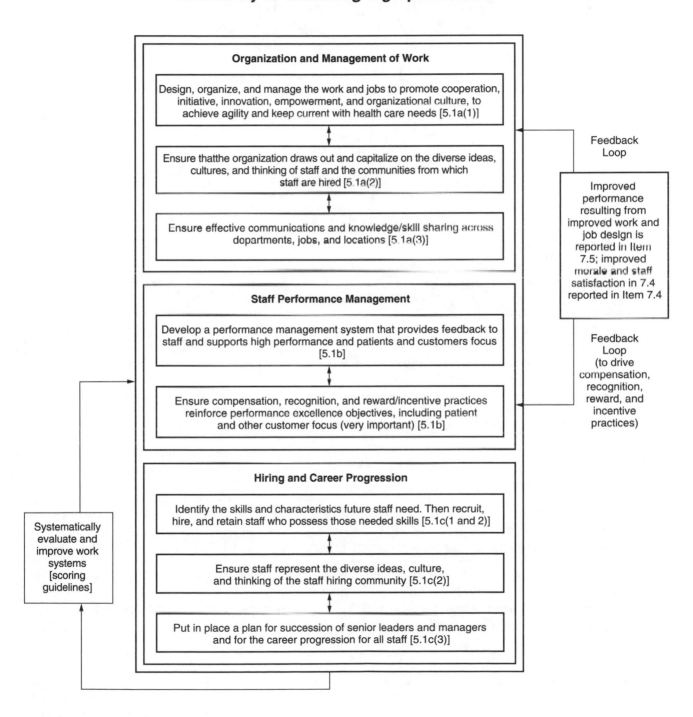

Organization and Management of Work

Design, organize, and manage the work and jobs to promote cooperation, initiative, innovation, empowerment, and organizational culture, to achieve agility and keep current with health care needs [5.1a(1)]

Ensure thatthe organization draws out and capitalize on the diverse ideas, cultures, and thinking of staff and the communities from which staff are hired [5.1a(2)]

Ensure effective communications and knowledge/skill sharing across departments, jobs, and locations [5.1a(3)]

Staff Performance Management

Develop a performance management system that provides feedback to staff and supports high performance and patients and customers focus [5.1b]

Ensure compensation, recognition, and reward/incentive practices reinforce performance excellence objectives, including patient and other customer focus (very important) [5.1b]

Hiring and Career Progression

Identify the skills and characteristics future staff need. Then recruit, hire, and retain staff who possess those needed skills [5.1c(1 and 2)]

Ensure staff represent the diverse ideas, culture, and thinking of the staff hiring community [5.1c(2)]

Put in place a plan for succession of senior leaders and managers and for the career progression for all staff [5.1c(3)]

Feedback Loop

Improved performance resulting from improved work and job design is reported in Item 7.5; improved morale and staff satisfaction in 7.4 reported in Item 7.4

Feedback Loop (to drive compensation, recognition, reward, and incentive practices)

Systematically evaluate and improve work systems [scoring guidelines]

5.1 Work Systems Item Linkages

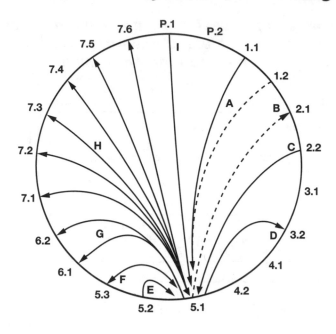

	NATURE OF RELATIONSHIP
A	Senior leaders (and subsequently leaders at all levels) [1.1a(2)] create an environment for staff empowerment, innovation, learning, and organizational agility; set related policies; and role model appropriate behaviors essential to improving work and job design to optimize performance and productivity [5.1a(1)].
B	Staff diversity, innovation, and related skills [5.1] affect staff strengths and weaknesses—important elements of the planning process [2.1a(2)].
C	Staff development plans and goals [2.2a(3)] are used to organize and manage work and jobs [5.1a(1)], align reward and recognition [5.1b], and decide which potential staff need to be recruited to close skill gaps [5.1c(1)].
D	Flexibility, initiative, [5.1a(1)] and communication and knowledge sharing [5.1a(3)] are essential to enhance the effectiveness and ability of patient and other customer-contact staff to resolve patient and other customer concerns promptly [3.2a(3)].
E	Effective training that contributes to achieving action plans [5.2a(1)] with appropriate feedback from staff and supervisors about their training needs [5.2a(3)] is critical to enable staff/managers at all levels to improve skills and improve their ability to manage, organize, and design better work processes [5.1a(1)] and retain key staff [5.1c(2)] .
F	A safe, secure work climate [5.3a] enhances staff motivation, participation, self-direction, and initiative [5.1a], and vice-versa.

Continued

	NATURE OF RELATIONSHIP	*Continued*
G	High-performance, flexible work systems [5.1a(1)] and effective recognition [5.1b] are essential to adding value and improving related health care processes [6.1].Effective performance feedback, compensation, and recognition [5.1b] are essential to improving health care and support processes [6.1 and 6.2].	
H	Compensation, incentives, recognition, and rewards [5.1b] are based in part of performance results [Category 7]. Improvements in work and job design, innovation, empowerment, [5.1a(1)] sharing, and communication [5.1a(3)] can result in improved performance and health care results [Category 7]. Processes to improve initiative and empowerment [5.1a(1)] can enhance all performance results [Category 7].	
I	Staff characteristics such as educational levels, workforce and job diversity, the existence of bargaining units, the use of contract staff, and other special requirements [P.1a(3)] help set the context for determining the requirements for knowledge and skill sharing across work units, jobs, and locations [5.1a(3)], and skills needed of potential staff [5.1c(1)].	

	IF YOU DON'T DO WHAT THE CRITERIA REQUIRE...
Item Reference	**Possible Adverse Consequences**
5.1a(1)	The alignment of strategic objectives and the work to accomplish them is vital to the success and optimum performance of the organization. Once strategic objectives, timelines [Item 2.1b(1)], and related actions [Item 2.2a(1)] have been identified and deployed to all levels of the organization, leaders and managers can more effectively organize staff (or they can organize themselves) to carry out the necessary work. In addition, appropriate responsibilities, authorities, and other tasks should be defined to ensure the actions are aligned (consistent) at all levels and effectively carried out. If the organization and management of work and jobs are not aligned to support strategic objectives and related actions, the organization may waste resources by failing to optimize the work that is done.
5.1a(2)	The failure to capitalize on diverse ideas, cultures, and thinking may limit the organization's ability to be innovative [Item 5.1a(1). This in turn, may limit the organization's ability to meet the challenges of today's highly competitive environment.
5.1a(3)	The failure to promote cooperation among work units often contributes to redundancy and working at cross-purposes. The failure to promote knowledge and skill sharing often forces the organization to duplicate efforts in the search for more effective and efficient processes. The failure to share knowledge also contributes to isolationism within an organization and prevents "pockets of excellence" from spreading. Frequently, staff organized in a hierarchical, command-and-control environment find individual initiative, empowerment, and innovation stifled, reducing morale and further eroding productivity and responsiveness.
5.1b	In order to optimize performance, work throughout the organization must be fully aligned to support strategic objectives and timelines [Item 2.1b(1)] and related action plans [Item 2.2a(1)]. The action plans should be deployed fully throughout the organization at all levels with appropriate quantitative measures developed to monitor progress [Item 2.2a(4)]. The work of individual staff, when taken together, should enable the organization to achieve its strategic objectives. There are two questions that are fundamental to the work endeavors that staff feedback should address: (1) are the right things being done (the vital few); and (2) are they being done right (correctly). 　　　The failure to provide feedback to staff about their performance may make it more difficult for them to determine if they are doing the right thing in support of the health care strategy, or if they are doing things in the right way (process discipline). It forces them to decide for themselves if they are doing a good job or not. In addition, the failure to provide feedback causes the organization to miss an opportunity to reinforce a patient and other customer and health care focus. After all, "What gets measured gets done." The alignment of what is "expected" and what is "rewarded" sends very strong messages throughout the organization about what is really important. Failing to align appropriate compensation, recognition, rewards, and incentives with the strategic objectives may also contribute to a lack of focus among the workforce, allowing staff to substitute their own ideas instead of being driven/guided by the reinforcement of management. Many staff equate

Continued

	IF YOU DON'T DO WHAT THE CRITERIA REQUIRE... *Continued*
Item Reference	**Possible Adverse Consequences**
5.1b	compensation with the activities that the organization wants to achieve. For example, if achieving profitability is critical for organization success, the organization typically rewards people for achieving financial goals. Everyone clearly understands the importance of "profit" because their own compensation and rewards are tied to it. Similarly, the failure to provide rewards, recognition, or compensation that supports a patient and other customer focus may cause staff to believe that patients and other customers are unimportant. Rewards (or the absence of them) drive behavior and motivate people to respond in certain ways.
5.1c(1)	Skill mapping is a process that many high-performing organizations practice to compare the skills it needs to achieve strategic objectives with the skills its workforce currently possesses. When a skill gap is identified, it enables organizations to more effectively make decisions as to whether they need to recruit, hire, and/or train appropriate staff. The failure to identify characteristics and skills needed by potential staff increases the likelihood of not having appropriate staff in the right places when needed.
5.1c(2)	In a competitive labor market, slowness in recruiting and inefficiencies in hiring may introduce delays that allow competitors to hire the best before your organization can act. Inefficient recruitment and bureaucratic bungling in the hiring process also provides a glimpse of the true management system and can scare off the best prospective staff. In addition, the hiring process represents a terrific opportunity to attract and hire staff with diverse ideas and cultures, without which it will be difficult to capitalize on diverse ideas, cultures, and thinking which may limit the organization's ability to be innovative and empowered [Item 5.1a(1)]. This, in turn, may limit the organization's ability to meet the challenges of today's highly competitive environment.
5.1c(3)	In the face of worldwide shortages of highly skilled medical staff, an organization's failure to conduct effective succession planning (both for senior leaders and for key positions throughout the organization) could threaten organizational stability in the long term and create immediate performance problems in the short term. When critical personnel shortages exist within an organization, it is frequently unable to carry out key objectives. If succession planning does not look ahead at least as far as it might take to acquire or train replacement personnel, the organization may lack the talent it needs to fulfill its promises to patients, other customers or other key stakeholders.

5.1 WORK SYSTEMS—SAMPLE EFFECTIVE PRACTICES

A. Organization and Management of Work

- Fully using the talents of all staff is a basic organizational value.

- Managers use cross-functional work teams to break down barriers, improve effectiveness, and meet goals.

- Teams have access to data and are authorized to make decisions about their work (not just make recommendations).

- Staff opinion is sought (and obtained) regarding work design and work processes.

- Prompt and regular feedback is provided to teams and individuals regarding their performance. Feedback covers both results and processes.

- Although lower-performing organizations use teams for special improvement projects (while the "regular work" is performed using traditional approaches), higher-performing organizations use teams and self-directed staff as the way regular work is done.

- Self-directed or self-managed work teams are used throughout the organization. They have authority over matters such as budget, hiring, and team membership and roles.

- A systematic process is used to evaluate and improve the effectiveness and extent of staff involvement.

- Many indicators of staff involvement effectiveness exist, such as the improvements in time or cost reduction produced by teams.

B. Staff Performance Management System

- The performance management system provides feedback to staff that supports their ability to contribute to a high-performing organization.

- Compensation, recognition, and rewards/incentives are provided for generating improvement ideas. In addition, a system exists to encourage and provide rapid reinforcement for submitting improvement ideas.

- Compensation, recognition, and rewards/incentives are provided for results, such as for reduction in cycle time and exceeding target schedules with error-free products or services at less-than-projected cost.

- Staff, as well as managers, participate in creating the compensation, recognition, and rewards/incentives practices and help monitor its implementation and systematic improvement.

- The organization evaluates its approaches to staff performance and compensation, recognition, and rewards to determine the extent to which staff are satisfied with them, the extent of staff participation, and the impact of the system on improved performance (reported in Item 7.4).

- Evaluations are used to make improvements. The best organizations have several improvement cycles. (Multiple improvement cycles can occur within one year.)

- Performance measures exist for staff involvement, self-direction, and initiative. Goals for these measures are expressed in measurable terms. These measurable goals form at least a good part of the basis for performance recognition.

- Recognition, reward/incentives, and compensation are influenced by patient and other customer satisfaction ratings as well as other performance measures.

C. Hiring and Career Progression

- Staff skill mapping is in place to define current skills of staff and compare to skills that are needed now and in the future. The resulting gap or surplus drives decisions to retrain, relocate, or recruit.

- The need for diverse ideas and cultures among staff is specifically considered during the skill mapping and recruitment process to ensure staff are able to provide the perspective needed to drive innovation and creativity.

- A formal system is in place to develop future leaders. This includes providing training and practice in high-performance leadership techniques. Leaders receive specific training and practice using Baldrige Criteria and performance improvement systems.

- Demonstrated proficiency in the use of the Baldrige Performance Excellence Criteria is a prerequisite to leadership advancement.

- Future leaders serve as examiners in the Baldrige process, state quality award process, or internal award process.

- Although not required to meet EEOC requirements, the organization has elected to do so. This shows a commitment to go "beyond compliance" to support corporate values.

- Service Recovery processes have been integrated into hiring, training, and empowerment of staff at all levels.

- A "no secrets, no excuses" culture has been integrated into the organization. While initially leading to higher reported medication errors, this culture has led to discovery of root cause and elimination of many medication errors.

- An annual Nursing Sharing Conference brings nurses from all locations together to share improvement and best practices.

- Managers motivate employees primarily through two non-monetary methods—coaching and recognition. This supports the organization's belief that a worker's primary motivation comes from an intrinsic desire to perform well in his or her work.

- Temporary and contract employees are used to allow flexibility in staffing because of changing patient volumes.

5.2 STAFF LEARNING AND MOTIVATION (25 pts.)   Approach/Deployment

Describe how your organization's staff education, training, and career development support the achievement of your overall objectives and contribute to high performance. Describe how your organization's education, training, and career development build staff knowledge, skills, and capabilities.

Within your response, include answers to the following questions:

a. Staff Education, Training, and Development

(1) How do staff education and training contribute to the achievement of your action plans? How do your staff education, training, and development address your key needs associated with organizational performance measurement, performance improvement, and technological change? How does your education and training approach balance short- and longer-term organizational objectives with staff needs, including licensure and recredentialing requirements, development, learning, and career progression?

(2) How do staff education, training, and development address your key organizational needs associated with new staff orientation, diversity, ethical health care and business practices, and management and leadership development? How do staff education, training, and development address your key organizational needs associated with staff, workplace, and environmental safety?

(3) How do you seek and use input from staff and their supervisors and managers on education and training needs? How do you incorporate your organizational learning and knowledge assets into your education and training?

(4) How do you deliver education and training? How do you seek and use input from staff and their supervisors and managers on options for the delivery of education and training? How do you use both formal and informal delivery approaches, including mentoring and other approaches, as appropriate?

(5) How do you reinforce the use of new knowledge and skills on the job?

(6) How do you evaluate the effectiveness of education and training, taking into account individual and organizational performance?

b. Motivation and Career Development

How do you motivate staff to develop and utilize their full potential? How does your organization use formal and informal mechanisms to help staff attain job- and career-related development and learning objectives? How do managers and supervisors help staff attain job- and career-related development and learning objectives?

Notes:

Education and training delivery [5.2a(4)] might occur inside or outside your organization and involve on-the-job, classroom, computer-based, distance learning, and other types of delivery (formal or informal).

This Item [5.2] looks at the organization's system for workforce education, training, and on-the-job reinforcement of knowledge and skills, as well as systems for motivation and staff career development with the aim of meeting ongoing needs of staff and a high-performance workplace.

To help the organization achieve its high-performance objectives, education and training must be effectively designed, delivered, reinforced on the job, evaluated, and improved. To optimize organization effectiveness, the education and training system should place special emphasis on meeting individual career progression and organizational health care needs.

Education and training needs might vary greatly depending on the nature of the organization's work, staff responsibility, and stage of organizational and personal development. These needs might include knowledge-sharing skills, communications, teamwork, problem solving, interpreting and using data, meeting patient and other customer requirements, process analysis and simplification, waste and cycle-time reduction, and priority setting based on strategic alignment or cost/benefit analysis. Education needs also might include basic skills, such as reading, writing, language, and arithmetic.

Organizations should consider job and organizational performance in education and training design and evaluation. Education and training should tie to action plans, and balance short- and longer-term individual and organizational objectives. Staff and their supervisors should help determine training needs and contribute to the design and evaluation of education and training, because these individuals frequently are best able to identify critical needs and evaluate success.

Education and training delivery might occur inside or outside the organization and could involve on-the-job, classroom, computer-based, distance learning (including Web-based instruction), or other types of delivery. Training also might occur through developmental assignments (including mentoring and apprenticeship) within or outside the organization.

When evaluating education and training, leaders should identify specific measures of effectiveness as a critical component of evaluation. Such measures might address impact on individual, unit, and organizational performance, impact on health care, patient and other customer-related performance, and cost/benefit analysis of the training. Training evaluation should at least cover the extent of knowledge and skills transfer (whether the staff learned anything) and the extent to which they use these new skills and knowledge on the job.

Although this Item does not require specific training for patient and other customer-contact staff, the Item does require that education and training "keep current with health care and individual needs" and "address performance excellence." If an objective of the organization is to enhance patient and other customer satisfaction and loyalty, it may be critical to identify job requirements for patient and other customer-contact staff and then provide appropriate training to staff. Such training is increasingly important and common among high-performing organizations. It frequently includes: acquiring critical knowledge and skills with respect to health care services, and patients and other customers; skills on how to listen to patients and other customers; recovery from problems or failures; and learning how to manage patient and other customer expectations effectively.

Organizations should ensure that training and education contribute to high performance. This may require organizations to provide training in the use of performance excellence tools.

- This training may be similar to the "quality" training organizations provided in the past. Training may focus on the use of performance measures, skill standards, quality control methods, benchmarking, problem-solving processes, and performance improvement techniques.

- This training should also address high-priority needs such as technological change, ethical health care practices, management and leadership development, orientation of new staff, safety, diversity, and performance measurement and improvement. Succession planning and leadership development [examined in Item 5.1c(3)] typically require organizations to provide specialized training and development to key individuals identified as possible successors.

Unless knowledge and skills acquired in training are reinforced on the job, they are quickly and easily forgotten—even after a few days. Accordingly, leaders, managers, and supervisors throughout the organization must promptly ensure that staff actually use the skills acquired through recent training. In fact, one of the measures of leadership effectiveness may consider the extent to which they reinforce these skills among their staff.

Finally, to help staff realize their full potential, many organizations prepare individual development plans with staff to address his or her career and learning objectives. In order to achieve optimum staff productivity, factors promoting and inhibiting motivation should be understood and addressed. A better understanding of these factors could be developed through exit interviews with departing staff and from feedback through staff satisfaction surveys.

5.2 Staff Learning and Motivation

How the organization's education, training, and career development support the achievement of overall objectives, contribute to high performance, and build staff knowledge, skills, and capabilities

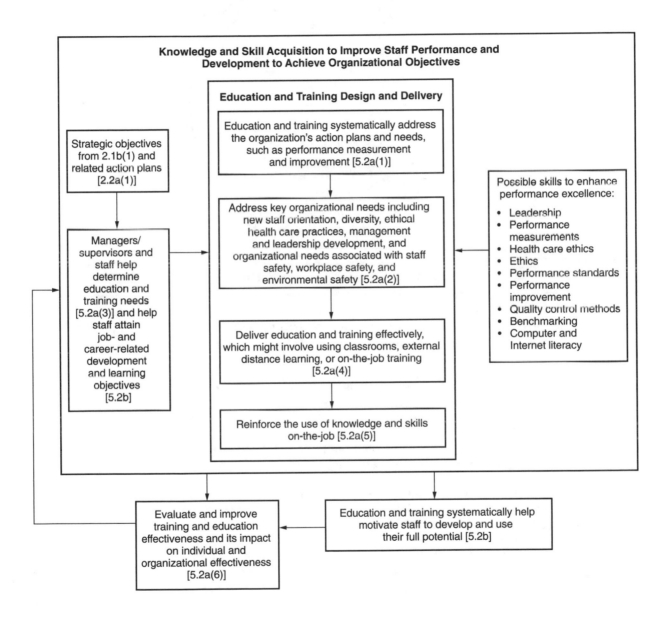

Knowledge and Skill Acquisition to Improve Staff Performance and Development to Achieve Organizational Objectives

Education and Training Design and Delivery

Education and training systematically address the organization's action plans and needs, such as performance measurement and improvement [5.2a(1)]

Address key organizational needs including new staff orientation, diversity, ethical health care practices, management and leadership development, and organizational needs associated with staff safety, workplace safety, and environmental safety [5.2a(2)]

Deliver education and training effectively, which might involve using classrooms, external distance learning, or on-the-job training [5.2a(4)]

Reinforce the use of knowledge and skills on-the-job [5.2a(5)]

Strategic objectives from 2.1b(1) and related action plans [2.2a(1)]

Managers/ supervisors and staff help determine education and training needs [5.2a(3)] and help staff attain job- and career-related development and learning objectives [5.2b]

Possible skills to enhance performance excellence:

- Leadership
- Performance measurements
- Health care ethics
- Ethics
- Performance standards
- Performance improvement
- Quality control methods
- Benchmarking
- Computer and Internet literacy

Evaluate and improve training and education effectiveness and its impact on individual and organizational effectiveness [5.2a(6)]

Education and training systematically help motivate staff to develop and use their full potential [5.2b]

5.2 Staff Learning and Motivation
Item Linkages

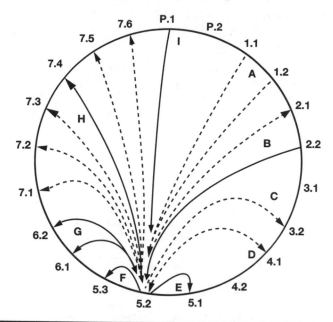

	NATURE OF RELATIONSHIP
A	Leaders [1.1a(2)] are responsible for supporting appropriate skill development of all staff through training and development systems and reinforcing learning on the job [5.2a(5)]. In addition, specific training may be required to ensure staff understand ethical and regulatory requirements [1.2a and b].
B	Staffing plans [2.2a(3)] (which were developed to support strategic objectives [2.1b(1)]) are used to help align training [5.2a(1)] to ensure staff and managers possess appropriate knowledge, skills, and ability.
C	Training [5.2] can enhance capabilities of patient and other customer-contact staff and strengthen patient and other customer relationships [3.2a(2 and 3)].
D	Key measures and benchmarking data [4.1] are used to improve training [5.2]. Information regarding training effectiveness [5.2] is analyzed [4.1b] to support planning and operational decision making.
E	Effective training [5.2a] enables managers at all levels to improve their ability to design, organize, and manage better work processes that promote empowerment, innovation [5.1a(1)] creativity, and sharing [5.1a(3)]; make performance feedback and recognition and reward more relevant [5.1b]; enhance succession planning [5.1c(3)]; and recruit and retain the best staff [5.1c(2)].
F	Effective environmental safety training [5.2a(2)] is critical to maintaining and improving a safe, healthful work environment [5.3a] and staff motivation and well-being [5.3b].

Continued

	NATURE OF RELATIONSHIP	*Continued*
G	Training [5.2a(2)] is essential to managing change and improving work effectiveness and innovation [6.1 and 6.2]. In addition, training requirements [5.2] are defined in part by process requirements [6.1 and 6.2].	
H	Results of improved training and development [5.2] are reported in 7.4. In addition, results pertaining to patient and other customer satisfaction [7.2], health care results [7.1], financial and market performance [7.3], organizational effectiveness [7.5], and social responsibility [7.6] reflect, in part, and are monitored to assess training effectiveness [5.2a(6)].	
I	Staff characteristics such as educational levels, workforce and job diversity, and other special requirements [P.1a(3)] help set the context for determining appropriate training needs by staff segment [5.2a(1)].	

IF YOU DON'T DO WHAT THE CRITERIA REQUIRE...	
Item Reference	**Possible Adverse Consequences**
5.2a(1)	Strategic objectives [Item 2.1b] define what the organization must achieve to be successful in the future. Action plans [Item 2.2a(1)] define the things the organization must do to achieve the strategic objectives. If staff lack the necessary skills to carry out required actions, the strategic plan may fail. Education and training that do not contribute to the achievement of action plans may be a waste of resources. Managers have a responsibility to help staff attain their job- and career-related learning and development objectives [Item 5.2b]. If managers fail to take advantage of appropriate education and training to help staff with work-related development, learning, and career progression, they run the risk of weakening morale and motivation as well as contributing to staff obsolescence. This may adversely impact staff job security and employability and undermine the organization's ability to maintain a viable workforce to compete effectively.
5.2a(2)	Today's best-performing organizations have found that the following four areas are instrumental in optimizing performance and winning in a highly competitive environment: (1) new staff orientation (acculturation); (2) diversity (capitalizing on diverse ideas and cultures); (3) ethical health care practices, and (4) management development. The failure to effectively address these factors as a part of staff education, training, and development may adversely affect the organization's ability to achieve its strategic objectives. The failure to provide effective staff orientation may make it difficult to get new staff to contribute to higher accident rates, higher compensation claims, and lost productivity. The failure to understand and take advantage of diverse ideas and cultures may limit the organization's creativity and innovation, and contribute to falling behind competitors. The failure to follow ethical health care practices gives rise to corruption, dishonesty, and ultimate health care failure. The failure to develop better managers and leaders may make it more difficult to develop strategic objectives, fully engage staff, and optimize individual or organizational performance.

	IF YOU DON'T DO WHAT THE CRITERIA REQUIRE... *Continued*
Item Reference	**Possible Adverse Consequences**
5.2a(3)	Staff and managers who are closest to the work usually understand best what skills are required (and missing) to do the work effectively. Failing to obtain and use input from these staff and their supervisors may result in the development of inappropriate or ineffective education and training opportunities. Providing ineffective or inappropriate training can waste resources in two ways: (1) the cost of paying staff salaries during training, the cost of facilities, and the cost of instruction; and (2) the cost to the organization of lost productivity while staff are participating in training.
5.2a(4)	The failure to deliver education and training using appropriate methods, consistent with the learning styles and needs of the students, usually suboptimizes the effectiveness of training. If students do not acquire relevant knowledge, skills, or abilities from education and training, the organization has wasted resources. If students learn new skills and acquire new abilities, but those new skills and abilities are not used on the job, the organization has also wasted resources. If the students use the new skills and abilities on the job and it makes no difference to organizational performance or career progression, the organization has again wasted resources.
5.2a(5)	If it is worth training staff to acquire new skills and abilities, it is worth reinforcing the use of those new skills when staff return to the job. The failure to reinforce the use of recently acquired knowledge and skills on the job may cause those new skills and abilities to become obsolete and quickly forgotten. Accordingly, the cost of training and the cost of lost productivity while the staff is receiving the training represent wasted resources. Most importantly, when the newly acquired skills are not utilized the value of those skills and potential productivity gains are lost. Losses of this nature can materially impact an organization's rate of growth and its ability to achieve strategy objectives.
5.2a(6)	The failure to evaluate and improve the effectiveness of training makes it difficult to optimize individual or organizational performance. Ineffective or inefficient training and education wastes resources directly (cost of training) and indirectly (cost of lost opportunity and productivity while staff is receiving training).
5.2b	An organization that fails to develop and use the full potential of its staff wastes significant resources. This waste can be classified into two categories: the failure to develop existing potential and take advantage of it; and the failure to use skills and abilities that already exist. This waste is equivalent to running an operation at less than optimum capacity; for example, paying staff for 40 hours of work but asking for only 20, or going out and hiring additional people when the potential for skills development already exists but goes unrecognized. To make matters worse, staff usually recognize when their skills are underused and their productivity suffers further erosion, or they seek job opportunities outside the organization where they can develop and advance more fully, or both.

5.2 STAFF LEARNING AND MOTIVATION—SAMPLE EFFECTIVE PRACTICES

A. Staff Education, Training, and Development

- Managers and staff conduct systematic needs analyses to ensure that skills required to perform work are routinely assessed, monitored, and maintained.

- Clear linkages exist between strategic objectives and education and training. Skills are developed based on work demands and staff needs.

- Training plans are developed based on staff input.

- Staff career and personal development options, including development for leadership, diversity, new staff orientation, and safety, are enhanced through formal education and training. Some development uses on-the-job training, including rotational assignments or job exchange programs.

- The organization uses various methods to deliver training to ensure that it is suitable for staff knowledge and skill levels.

- To minimize travel costs, all training is examined to determine if electronic or distance delivery options are viable.

- Training is linked to work requirements, which managers reinforce on the job. Just-in-time training is preferred (rather than just-in-case training) to help ensure that the skills will be used immediately after training.

- Staff feedback on the appropriateness of the training is collected and used to improve course delivery and content.

- The organization systematically evaluates training effectiveness on the job. Performance data are collected on individuals and groups at all levels to assess the impact of training.

- Staff satisfaction with courses is tracked and used to improve training content, training delivery, instructional effectiveness, and the effectiveness of supervisory support for the use of training on the job.

- Training design and delivery is systematically refined and improved based on regular evaluations.

B. Motivation and Career Development

- Formal career plans are in place for each staff. Progress against these plans is evaluated and adjustments are made to ensure they remain relevant.

- Staff receive incentives for developing additional career-enhancing skills such as bonuses or other rewards.

- Training strategy is derived from the organization's overall strategy, and benefit is measured against corporate goals.

- All employees receive an orientation to Continuous Quality Improvement (CQI) as part of new employee orientation. Principles of CQI are discussed, as well as why every employee is expected to be continuously improving their work.

5.3 STAFF WELL-BEING AND SATISFACTION (25 PTS.)   Approach/Deployment

Describe how your organization maintains a work environment and staff support climate that contribute to the well-being, satisfaction, and motivation of all staff.

Within your response, include answers to the following questions:

a. Work Environment

(1) How do you improve workplace health, safety, security, and ergonomics? How does staff take part in improving them? What are your performance measures or targets for each of these key workplace factors? What are the significant differences in workplace factors and performance measures or targets if different staff groups and work units have different work environments?

(2) How do you ensure workplace preparedness for emergencies or disasters? How do you seek to ensure health care service and business continuity for the benefit of your patients, other customers, and staff?

b. Staff Support and Satisfaction

(1) How do you determine the key factors that affect staff well-being, satisfaction, and motivation? How are these factors segmented for a diverse workforce and for different categories and types of staff?

(2) How do you support your staff via services, benefits, and policies? How are these tailored to the needs of a diverse workforce and different categories and types of staff?

(3) What formal and informal assessment methods and measures do you use to determine staff well-being, satisfaction, and motivation? How do these methods and measures differ across a diverse workforce and different categories and types of staff? How do you use other indicators, such as staff retention, absenteeism, grievances, safety, and productivity, to assess and improve staff well-being, satisfaction, and motivation?

(4) How do you relate assessment findings to key organizational performance results to identify priorities for improving the work environment and staff support climate?

Continued

Notes: *Continued*

N1. Specific factors that might affect your staff's well-being, satisfaction, and motivation [5.3b(1)] include effective staff problem or grievance resolution; safety factors; staff's views of management; staff training, development, and career opportunities; staff preparation for changes in technology or the work organization; the work environment and other work conditions; management's empowerment of staff; information sharing by management; workload; cooperation and teamwork; recognition; services and benefits; communications; job security; compensation; and equal opportunity.

N2. Approaches for staff support [5.3b(2)] might include providing counseling, career development and employability services, recreational or cultural activities, nonwork-related education, day care, job rotation or sharing, special leave for family responsibilities or community service, home safety training, flexible work hours and location, outplacement, and retirement benefits (including extended health care).

N3. Measures and indicators of well-being, satisfaction, and motivation [5.3b(3)] might include data on safety and absenteeism, the overall turnover rate, the turnover rate for patient/ customers contact staff, staff members' charitable contributions, grievances, strikes, other job actions, insurance costs, workers' compensation claims, and results of surveys. Survey indicators of satisfaction might include staff knowledge of job roles, staff knowledge of organizational direction, and staff perception of empowerment and information sharing. Your results relative to such measures and indicators should be reported in Item 7.4.

N4. Identifying priorities [5.3b(4)] might draw upon your staff and work system results presented in Item 7.4 and might involve addressing staff problems based on their impact on your organizational performance.

This Item [5.3] looks at the organization's work environment, the staff support climate, and how staff satisfaction is determined, for the purpose of enhancing the well-being, satisfaction, and motivation of all staff, while recognizing their diverse needs.

The first part of this Item [5.3a] looks at systems the organization has in place to provide a safe, secure, and healthful work environment for all staff, taking into account their differing work environments and associated requirements. Staff should help identify and improve factors important to workplace safety and security. The organization should identify appropriate measures and targets for key workplace factors so that status and progress can be tracked.

The organization should be able to show how it includes such factors in its planning and improvement activities. Important factors in this area include establishing appropriate measures and targets for staff safety, security, and health. Organizations should also recognize that staff groups might experi-

ence very different environments and need different services to ensure workplace safety.

Organizations should also have a workplace preparedness plan in place in case of emergencies or disasters. Part of the plan should focus on ensuring health care continuity for the benefit of both staff and patients and other customers. Such plans should provide for rapid recovery and minimize disruption to the work of staff and the services, and programs delivered to patients and other customers.

The second part of this Item [5.3b] looks at how the organization determines key factors that affect staff well-being, satisfaction, and motivation. The organization must provide appropriate services, benefits, and policies to enhance staff well-being, satisfaction, and motivation. The best organizations develop a holistic view of staff as key stakeholders. Most organizations, regardless of size, have many opportunities to contribute to staff well-being, satisfaction, and motivation. These organizations place special emphasis on the variety of approaches used to satisfy a diverse workforce with differing needs and expectations in order to reduce attrition and increase motivation.

Examples of services, facilities, activities, and other opportunities are: personal and career counseling; career development and employability services; recreational or cultural activities; formal and informal recognition; non-work-related education; day care; special leave for family responsibilities and/or for community service; home safety training; flexible work hours and benefits packages; outplacement services; and retiree benefits, including extended health care and access to staff services. Also, these services might include career enhancement activities such as skills assessments, helping staff develop learning objectives and plans, and conducting employability assessments.

As the workforce becomes more diverse (including staff that may work in other countries for multinational companies), it becomes more important to consider and support the needs of those staff with different services.

High-performing organizations also used both formal and informal assessment methods and measures to determine staff well-being, satisfaction, and motivation. These methods and measures are tailored to assess the differing needs of a diverse workforce. In addition, indicators other than staff opinion surveys (for example, staff turnover, grievances, complaints, and absenteeism) are used to support the assessment. Taken together, these methods and measures ensure that assessment findings are relevant and relate to key health care results in order to identify key priorities for improvement.

Many factors might affect staff motivation, well-being, and satisfaction. Although satisfaction with pay and promotion potential is important, these fac-

tors might not be adequate to understand the factors that contribute to the overall climate for motivation and high performance.

For this reason, high-performing organizations usually consider a variety of factors that might affect well-being, satisfaction, and motivation, such as effective staff problem and grievance resolution; safety; staff development and career opportunities; staff preparation for changes in technology or work organization; work environment and management support; workload; communication, cooperation and teamwork; job security; appreciation of the differing needs of diverse staff groups; recognition; benefits; compensation; and organizational support for serving patient and other customers.

In addition to direct measurement of staff satisfaction and well-being through formal or informal surveys, some other indicators of satisfaction and well-being include: absenteeism, turnover, grievances, strikes, accidents, lost-time injuries, and worker's compensation claims. Information and data on the well-being, satisfaction, and motivation of staff are actually used in identifying improvement priorities. Priority setting might draw upon staff results reported in Item 7.4 and might involve addressing staff problems based on the impact on organizational performance. Factors inhibiting motivation need to be prioritized and addressed. The failure to address these factors is likely to result in even greater problems, which may not only impact human resource results (Item 7.4), but adversely affect patient and other customer satisfaction (Item 7.2), health care results (Item 7.1), financial performance (Item 7.3), organizational effectiveness (7.5), and public responsibility (Item 7.6).

5.3 Staff Well-Being and Satisfaction

How the organization maintains a work environment and staff support climate that supports the well-being, satisfaction, and motivation of staff

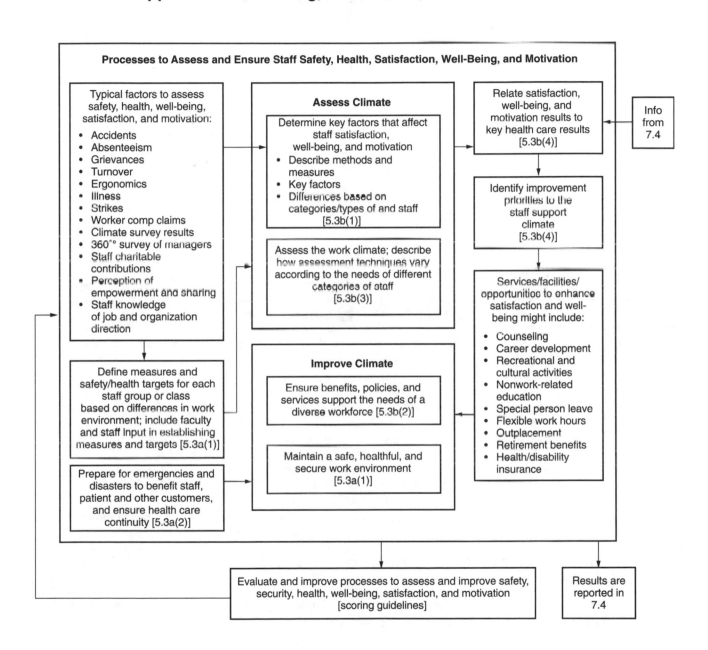

5.3 Staff Well-Being and Satisfaction Item Linkages

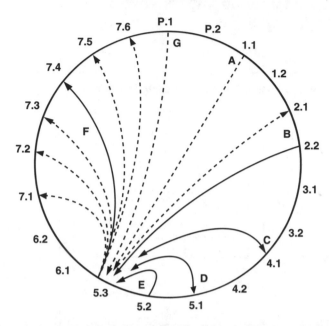

NATURE OF RELATIONSHIP	
A	Leaders [1.1a(2)] are responsible for creating an environment that fosters staff empowerment, innovation and organizational agility, consistent with effective systems to enhance staff health, safety, security, satisfaction, well-being, and motivation [5.3a].
B	Staff development plans [2.2a(3)] typically address or set the context for safety, security, motivation, satisfaction, and well-being systems [5.3]. Staff motivation and satisfaction, safety, security, and disaster recovery processes [5.3] may be important to consider in the process of developing strategy [2.1a(2)].
C	Key benchmarking data [4.1a(2)] are sued to design processes to enhance staff motivation and well-being [5.3b]. Information regarding staff well-being and motivation [5.3b(3)] is used to gain a better understanding of problems and performance capabilities to support strategic planning [4.1b(1)].
D	High motivation [5.3] enhances staff empowerment, initiative (self-direction), and innovation [5.1a(1)], and vice versa.
E	Effective training [5.2] is critical to maintaining and improving safety, security, and health of the work environment and providing an appropriate emergency or disaster response [5.3a], and improved staff motivation, satisfaction, and well-being [5.3b].
F	Systems that enhance staff motivation, satisfaction, and well-being [5.3] can boost financial and market productivity [7.5], and social responsibility [7.6]. Specific results of staff well-being and satisfaction systems are reported in 7.4.

Continued

NATURE OF RELATIONSHIP	*Continued*
G	Staff characteristics, such as educational levels, workforce and job diversity, the existence of bargaining units, the use of contract staff, and other special requirements [P.1a(3)] may help set the context for tailoring benefits, services, and satisfaction assessment methods for staff according to various types and categories [5.3a and b(1, 2, and 3)].

IF YOU DON'T DO WHAT THE CRITERIA REQUIRE...

Item Reference	Possible Adverse Consequences
5.3a	The failure to improve workplace health, safety, security, and ergonomics may increase staff accidents and illness, reduce staff effectiveness, and negatively impact morale and motivation. Poor working conditions can distract staff, reduce productivity, and increase errors, rework, cycle time, and waste, to name a few. Failing to involve staff in the identification of potential health, safety, security, and ergonomics issues may cause the organization to overlook and fail to correct those problems. If significant variation exists in the work environment for different staff groups or work units, staff are likely to face different workplace health, safety, security, and ergonomic issues. For example, carpal tunnel syndrome (repetitive stress injuries) may be a problem for those who do substantial keypunching, but not for certain staff on the floor. Those staff may be more concerned with injury from lifting heavy objects. Accordingly, the failure to define performance measures and establish targets for each key environmental factor and each distinct staff group increases the likelihood the problems will go unnoticed and those staff will be distracted from their work, suboptimizing performance.

In addition, the failure to plan and prepare for emergencies and disasters makes the organization vulnerable to serious disruptions of service, which may hurt both staff and patients and other customers, and damage the stability of health care service. |
| 5.3b(1) | Factors that affect staff well-being, satisfaction, and motivation can vary significantly from organization to organization, or within an organization from site to site, or among different groups of staff in the same organization. The failure to determine the key factors affecting staff well-being, satisfaction, and motivation for each staff or segment may make it difficult to identify key problems and take appropriate corrective action. The inability to identify and correct these problems can reduce staff morale and motivation which, in turn, hurts productivity and, ultimately, patient and other customer satisfaction. |

Continued

	IF YOU DON'T DO WHAT THE CRITERIA REQUIRE... *Continued*
Item Reference	**Possible Adverse Consequences**
5.3b(2)	Just as different staff groups may have different needs for safety, different groups of staff may need different support services and benefits to keep them from being distracted in their work. For example, in one health care organization, staff located in an extremely rural area lost an entire day of work traveling to a dentist or physician to deal with a toothache or a minor medical problem. Locating a trailer with dental and health professionals near the plant entrance minimized the time staff had to be absent from work due to a medical problem. A sister plant in the same company, located near a major metropolitan area, had plenty of dentists nearby and determined that its staff would be better served by an in-house exercise and wellness program. When an organization fails to identify and tailor benefits and services to the needs of its diverse workforce, it may increase distractions and reduce optimum staff participation and performance. Suboptimum staff performance hurts productivity.
5.3b(3)	Because the factors that affect staff well-being, satisfaction, and motivation can vary significantly among the diverse groups of staff, if an organization fails to differentiate assessment methods and measures it may not be able to determine accurately the existence of problems and take appropriate corrective action. The failure to identify and correct a problem that adversely affects staff well-being, satisfaction, and motivation can contribute to operational inefficiency, waste resources, and reduce product and service quality and patient and other customer satisfaction. Failing to consider data that relate to staff well-being and satisfaction, such as absenteeism, grievances, and undesired staff attrition, may also prevent a problem from being identified and corrected. Finally, the "one size fits all" method of assessing staff well-being and satisfaction (such as the *annual* climate survey) may fail to take into account parts of the organization that may be undergoing change and face more turmoil than other parts of the organization. For organizations that are relatively stable, an annual survey may be appropriate. However, for organizations (or parts of organizations) that face a more volatile, unstable health care environment, more frequent assessments may be required. The failure to ask the right questions, at the right time, and in the right manner, may prevent the organization from learning about and correcting serious problems that can adversely affect performance and productivity.
5.3b(4)	When deciding what actions to take to improve the work environment (based on the results of appropriate surveys and related data), organizations may waste resources if they do not set priorities for improvement that are likely to optimize health care results. In the example above [5.3b(2)], the supervisor could have installed a workout room and shower facilities rather than a dental health services trailer. However, analysis revealed that exercise facilities would have minimum impact on productivity, whereas the dental-health-care trailer would save hundreds of days each year in lost time due to staff absenteeism. Organizations risk wasting resources if they fail to understand the likely impact on results of the improvement priorities they set in response to staff satisfaction assessment findings.

5.3 STAFF WELL-BEING AND SATISFACTION—SAMPLE EFFECTIVE PRACTICES

A. Work Environment

- Issues and concerns relating to staff health, safety, security, and workplace environment are used to design the work environment for all groups of staff. Plans exist and processes are in place to optimize working conditions and eliminate adverse conditions.

- Root causes for health, safety, and security problems are systematically identified and eliminated. Corrective actions are communicated widely to help prevent the problem in other parts of the organization.

- Targets are set and reviewed for all key health, safety, security, and ergonomic factors affecting the staff work environment. Staff are directly involved in setting these targets.

- A documented and tested emergency recovery plan is in place and all staff are trained and understand the processes they will follow.

- Disaster recovery processes are in place and serious tests (drills) are conducted to simulate emergency response to minimize problems and risks to staff and patients and other customers in the event of a real crisis. These procedures were developed based on benchmarking other organizations that face crises.

B. Staff Support and Satisfaction

- Special activities and services are available for staff. These are quite varied, depending on the needs of different staff categories. Examples include the following:

  - Flexible benefits plan including: health care; on-site day care; dental; portable retirement; education (both work and non-work-related); maternity, paternity, and family illness leave.

  - Group purchasing power programs, where the number of participating merchants is increasing steadily.

  - Special facilities for staff meetings to discuss their concerns.

- Senior leaders build a work climate that addresses the needs of a diverse workforce. Recruitment and training are tools to enhance the work climate.

- Key staff satisfaction opinion indicators are gathered periodically based on the stability of the organization (organizations in the midst of rapid change conduct assessments more frequently). Supervisors, managers, and leaders take consistent and prompt action to improve conditions identified through these staff satisfaction surveys.

- On-demand electronic surveys are available for quick response and tabulations any time managers need staff satisfaction feedback. Whenever the survey is completed, managers always follow-up promptly to make improvements identified by the survey that relate to key health care results.

- Satisfaction data are derived from staff focus groups, staff satisfaction survey results, turnover, absenteeism, and other data that reflect staff satisfaction.

- Managers use the results of these surveys to focus improvements in work systems and enhance staff satisfaction. Actions to improve satisfaction are clearly tied to assessments so staff understand the value of the assessment, and the improvement initiatives do not appear random or capricious.

- Staff satisfaction indicators are correlated with drivers of health care success to help identify where resources should be placed to provide maximum health care benefit.

- Methods to improve how staff satisfaction is determined are systematically evaluated and improved. Techniques to actually improve staff satisfaction and well-being are, themselves, evaluated and refined consistently.

- The organization recognizes and measures the alignment of staff satisfaction, patient satisfaction, and organizational results.

  - A fundamental belief is that employee well-being and satisfaction is directly correlated to patient and physician satisfaction.

- Key factors that drive employee satisfaction, motivation, and well-being are determined through an annual staff survey.

- To address the challenge of losing experienced staff, a phased retirement option has been put in place that encourages retention of older employees who may be considering retirement.

- Each facility supports at least three community-based outreach activities.

6 Process Management—85 Points

*The **Process Management** Category examines the key aspects of the organization's process management, including key health care, business, and other support processes for creating value for patients, other customers, and the organization. This Category encompasses all key processes and all departments and work units.*

Process Management is the focal point within the Criteria for all key work processes—health care processes and those processes that support the delivery of health care. Key processes might include the conduct of health care research and/or the teaching of medical/nursing students or allied health care professionals as appropriate to an organization's mission. Built into the Category are the central requirements for efficient and effective process management: effective design; a prevention orientation; linkage to patients/customers, suppliers, and partners and a focus on creating value for all key stakeholders; operational performance; cycle time; and evaluation, continuous improvement, and organizational learning.

Agility, cost efficiencies, and cycle-time reduction are increasingly important in all aspects of process management and organizational design. In the simplest terms, "agility" refers to your ability to adapt quickly, flexibly, and effectively to changing requirements. Depending on the nature of the organization's strategy and markets, agility might mean rapid changeover to a new technology or treatment protocol, rapid response to changing payor requirements, or the ability to produce a wide range of patient-focused services. Agility also increasingly involves shared facilities, decisions to outsource, agreements with key suppliers, and novel partnering arrangements. Flexibility might demand special strategies, such as sharing facilities, cross training, and providing specialized training.

Cost and cycle-time reduction often involves agile process management strategies. It is crucial to utilize key measures for tracking all aspects of your overall process management.

Health Care Processes

(Considered to be core processes and key health care processes required to deliver the organization's main services and deliver value to patients and customers and other key stakeholders, and improve market, operational and financial position)

- Design, develop, and introduce health care services to meet customer requirements, operational performance requirements, and market requirements

- Use customer feedback, supplier feedback, and in-process measures to control and improve the performance of these processes

- Ensure a rapid, efficient, trouble-free introduction

- Manage and continuously improve health care design, development, and delivery processes

Support Processes

(Provide support to key business and health care processes)

- Design, develop, and provide services to meet internal customer requirements

- Use internal customer feedback and in-process measures to control and improve the performance of these processes

- Manage and continuously improve support processes

6.1 HEALTH CARE PROCESSES   (50 PTS.)   Approach/Deployment

Describe how your organization identifies and manages its key processes for delivering patient health care services.

Within your response, include answers to the following questions:

a. Health Care Processes

(1) How does your organization determine its key health care services and service delivery processes? What are your organization's key health care processes? How do these processes create value for the organization, your patients and other customers, and your other key stakeholders? How do they contribute to improved health care service outcomes?

(2) How do you determine key health care process requirements, incorporating input from patients and other customers, suppliers, and partners, as appropriate? What are the key requirements for these processes?

(3) How do you design these processes to meet all the key requirements, including patient safety, regulatory, accreditation, and payor requirements? How do you incorporate new technology and organizational knowledge into the design of these processes? How do you incorporate improved health care outcomes, cycle time, productivity, cost control, and other efficiency and effectiveness factors into the design of these processes? How do you implement these processes to ensure they meet design requirements?

(4) How are patients' expectations addressed and considered? How is health care service delivery processes and likely outcomes explained to set realistic patient expectations? How are patient decision making and patient preferences factored into the delivery of health care services?

(5) How does your day-to-day operation of your health care processes ensure meeting key process requirements, including patient safety, regulatory, accreditation, and payor requirements? What are your key performance assessments and measures or indicators used for the control and improvement of your health care processes? How are in-process measures used in managing these processes? How are patient and other customer, supplier, and partner input used in managing your health care processes, as appropriate?

(6) How do you minimize overall costs associated with inspections, tests, and process or performance audits, as appropriate? How do you prevent errors and rework?

(7) How do you improve your health care processes to achieve better performance, to reduce variability, to improve health care services and health care outcomes, and to keep the processes current with health care service needs and directions? How are improvements shared with other organizational units and processes?

Continued

Notes: *Continued*

N1. "Health care processes" refers to patient and community service processes for the purpose of prevention, maintenance, health promotion, screening, diagnosis, treatment/therapy, rehabilitation, recovery, palliative care, or supportive care. This includes services delivered to patients through other providers (e.g., laboratory or radiology studies). Responses to Item 6.1 should be based upon the most critical requirements for successful delivery of your services.

N2. Key processes for the conduct of health care research and/or a teaching mission should be reported in either Item 6.1 or 6.2, as appropriate to your organization's mission.

N3. Process requirements should include all appropriate components of health care service delivery. In a group practice, this might be the making of appointments, presentation, evaluation of risk factors, health education, and appointment closures. Depending upon the health care service, this might include a significant focus on technology and patient-specific considerations.

N4. To achieve better process performance and reduce variability, you might implement approaches such as the PDSA process, six sigma methodology, use of ISO 9000:2000 standards, or other process improvement tools.

This Item [6.1] looks at the management and improvement of key health care processes—both key design processes for services and their related delivery processes that create value for the organization, its patients and customers, and stakeholders. Descriptions must be provided of the key processes, their specific requirements, and an explanation of how performance relative to these requirements is determined and maintained. Increasingly, these requirements might include the need for agility—speed and flexibility—to adapt to change.

Design processes might address the following:

- Modifications and variants of existing health care services that might result from the shift of a service from an inpatient to an outpatient setting, the introduction of new technology for an existing service, or the institution of critical pathways

- New health care services resulting from research

- New/modified facilities to meet performance requirements

- Significant redesigns of processes to improve patient focus, productivity, or both (consistent with the key requirements for health care services)

Factors that might need to be considered in design include safety and risk management; timeliness, access, coordination, and continuity of care; patient involvement in care decisions; measurement capability; process capability; variability in customer expectations requiring health care service options; availability or scarcity of staff with critical skills; availability of referral sources; technology; facility capacity or utilization; supplier capability; regulatory requirements; and documentation. Effective design also must consider cycle time and productivity of health care service delivery processes. This might involve detailing critical pathways and redesigning ("reengineering") those delivery processes to achieve efficiency, as well as to meet changing requirements.

New technology, including e-technology, should be incorporated into the design of services. The use of e-technology might include new ways of electronically sharing information with suppliers/partners, communicating with patients and customers and giving them continuous (24/7) access, and automated information transfer.

Frequently, effective design processes require organizations to capture information from patient and customer complaint data using the processes described in Item 3.2a. Immediate access to complaint data allows the organization to make design changes quickly to prevent problems from occurring or recurring.

The best-performing organizations consider requirements of suppliers and/or health care partners at the design stage. This minimizes the chances that important design issues are not achievable because of supplier and/or partner limitations. Similarly, effective design systems take into account all stakeholders in the value chain.

To enhance design process efficiency, all related design activities should be coordinated within the organization. Coordination of design and delivery processes involves all work units and/or individuals who take part in delivery and whose performance materially affects overall process outcome. This might include researchers, health care providers, facilities engineering, and administration or processes, such as research marketing, design, product/process engineering, and key suppliers. Design processes should cover all key health care performance requirements and appropriate coordination and testing to ensure effective product/service launch without need for rework.

This Item also looks at how the organization ensures its delivery processes meet key performance requirements consistently. The best-performing organizations accurately and completely define key production/delivery processes, their key performance requirements, and key performance measures. These requirements and measures provide the basis for maintaining and improving products, services, and delivery processes. These organizations also define how performance relative to these requirements is determined and maintained. Increasingly, these requirements usually include the need for agility—speed and flexibility—to adapt to change.

Top organizations minimize the need for inspections, tests, and audits to avoid rework costs because they have implemented processes to prevent problems from occurring in the first place. Sometimes these processes involve error proofing, which make it impossible to do the wrong thing the wrong way. (For example, electrical cords on today's appliances have one plug blade wider than the other to prevent it from being inserted incorrectly into a wall outlet.)

Effective organizations also use key in-process measurements at critical points in processes to mini-

mize problems and costs. These activities should occur at the earliest points possible in processes to minimize problems and costs that may result from deviations in performance. Achieving expected performance frequently requires setting performance levels or standards to guide decision making. When deviations occur, corrective action is required to restore the performance of the process to its design specifications. Depending on the nature of the process, the corrective action could involve technical and/or human considerations. Proper corrective action involves changes at the source (root cause) of the deviation. Effective corrective action minimizes the likelihood of this type of variation occurring again or anywhere else in the organization.

The best-performing organizations have a system in place to evaluate and improve service delivery processes to achieve better process efficiency and better services. Better performance means not only better service quality from the patient and customer perspective but also better financial and operational performance—such as productivity. A variety of process improvement approaches are commonly used. These approaches include:

- Sharing successful strategies across the organization

- Process analysis and research (for example, process mapping, optimization experiments, and error proofing)

- Technical and health care research and development

- Benchmarking

- Using alternative technology

- Using information from patients and customers of the processes—within and outside of the organization

New process improvement approaches might also involve the use of cost data to evaluate alternatives and set improvement priorities. Taken together, these approaches offer a wide range of possibilities, including complete redesign of key processes to achieve new levels of operational excellence.

The effective design and delivery of health care services must take into account regulatory and payor requirements, in-process measurements or assessments, and patient/customer and supplier interactions. These measurements and interactions typically require the identification of critical points in processes for measurement, observation, or interaction. These activities should occur at the earliest points possible in design and delivery processes to minimize problems and costs that may result from deviations from expected performance.

Achieving expected performance frequently requires setting performance levels or standards to guide decision making. When deviations occur, corrective action is required to restore the performance of the process to its design specifications. Depending on the nature of the process, the corrective action could involve technical and human considerations. Proper corrective action involves changes at the source (root cause) of the deviation. Such corrective action should minimize the likelihood of this type of variation occurring again or elsewhere in your organization. When patients'/customers' interactions are involved, differences among patients/customers must be considered in evaluating how well the process is performing. This might entail allowing for specific or general contingencies, depending on the patient/customer information gathered.

Critical to health care service delivery are the consideration of patient expectations, the setting of realistic patient expectations relative to likely health care outcomes, and the opportunity for patients to participate on an informed basis in decision making relative to their own health care.

6.1 Health Care Processes

How the organization identifies and manages its key health care service design and delivery processes for creating patient and customer value and achieving health care success and growth

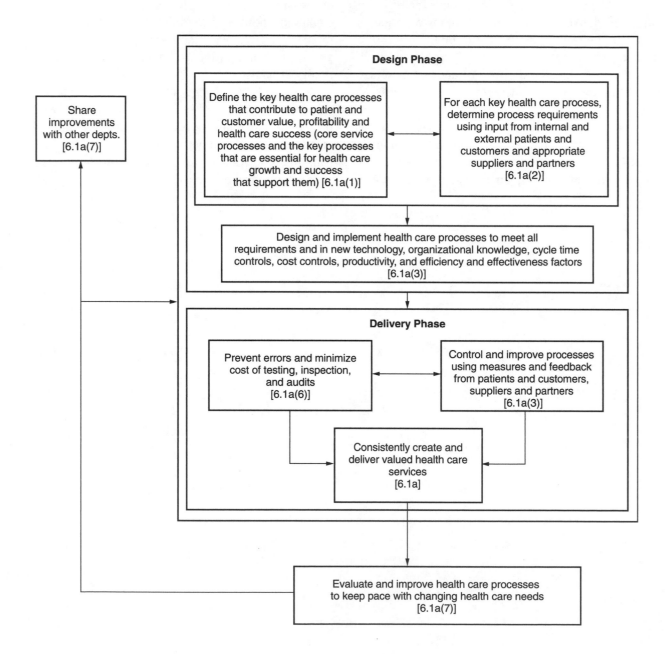

6.1 Health Care Processes Item Linkages

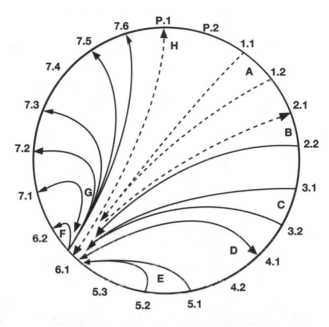

	NATURE OF RELATIONSHIP
A	Senior leaders and the governance system [1.1] have a responsibility for ensuring that health care processes critical for growth and success are designed [6.1a(1 and 2)] consistent with organizational objectives, including those relating to social responsibility and good corporate citizenship [1.2a].
B	Organizational heath care process strengths and weaknesses [6.1] are considered as part of the planning process [2.1a(2)]. Action plans, deployed to the workforce [2.2a], are used to align actions to design [6.1a(1, 2, and 3] and perform critical health care services [6.1a(3 and 4)].
C	Patient and customer requirements and preferences [3.1a(2)], customer questions [3.2a(2)], complaints/complaint resolution [3.2a(3)], and satisfaction/dissatisfaction [3.2b(1, 2, and 3)] are used to identify requirements for critical value creation and health care processes [6.1a(2)].
D	Key health care processes such as research, knowledge management, and information technology [6.1] are used to help identify and prioritize benchmarking targets [4.1a(2)]. Benchmarking data [4.1a(2)] are used to improve key value creation and health care processes [6.1].
E	High-performance, flexible work systems [5.1a(1)], effective recognition [5.1b], and training [5.2] are essential to improving health care processes [6.1].
F	Health care processes [6.1] help define requirements and set priorities for support processes [6.2].
G	Information about health care results [7.1] is used to target improvement efforts in key health care processes [6.1]. Improved health care processes [6.1] can be reflected in better health care results [7.1] and better patient and customer satisfaction [7.2], better financial results [7.3], operational efficiency [7.5a(1, 2)] and social responsibility/regulatory compliance [7.6].

Continued

	NATURE OF RELATIONSHIP	*Continued*
H	Information in P.1a(1) derives from the health care processes [6.1] and helps set the context for examiner review of these processes.	

IF YOU DON'T DO WHAT THE CRITERIA REQUIRE...

Item Reference	Possible Adverse Consequences
6.1a(1 and 3)	The requirements of design processes can vary significantly within an organization based on the nature of the services being delivered to patients and customers. Design processes may also vary based on whether the services are new or only involve minor variations to current product and service offerings. In any event, a design process that fails to consider the key requirements for services, and other factors, such as environmental impact, process capability, measurement capability, patient and customer service expectations, supplier capability, and customer documentation requirements, may make it difficult or impossible for the organization to achieve desired results (health care outcomes that satisfy patients and customers) in an efficient and profitable manner. In an effort to ensure the design process is consistent and effective, organizations frequently develop elaborate checkpoints or "gates" that must be passed as part of bringing a new service into the marketplace. The gates serve a two fold purpose: (1) assuring the focus on patient and customer requirements is maintained throughout the design process and responds to changing patient, customer and market demands and (2) assuring design maturity is on track. The first deals with fully responding to patient and customer requirements by providing value in the eyes of the patient/customer. The second addresses the ability of the organization to do this in an efficient, effective, and profitable manner. Design processes that are not capable of incorporating changing patient, customer or market requirements into services in a timely fashion may find it difficult to remain agile and competitive. For example, an organization that receives patient and customer change requirements at a faster pace than they can implement the changes can be virtually paralyzed. For example, consider a new procedure that replaces arteries or joints capable of lasting ten years instead of five years. The demand for this procedure, when FDA approved, will be large and the organization that is ready will benefit, yielding patient and physician positive regard. Unwieldy design systems often lead to frustrated staff, excessive delay, and ultimately, dissatisfied patients and customers and lost health care opportunities. When faced with rapidly changing technology, patient/customer requirements, or market demands, an inflexible, cumbersome design processes can render a once good design obsolete before it ever gets to market.
6.1a(2)	An organization that fails to accurately identify the performance requirements of its key health care processes may find it difficult to design and optimize those processes to meet patient and customer expectations. Design flaws produce undesired results and nonconforming services. This, in turn, requires even more rework or more people-intensive services, which can add significant delay and prevent the organization from achieving its objectives. When these processes fail to meet requirements, resources are wasted and the objectives of the organization may be jeopardized.

Continued

	IF YOU DON'T DO WHAT THE CRITERIA REQUIRE... Continued
Item Reference	**Possible Adverse Consequences**
6.1a(3)	Organizations that fail to take into account all key operational performance requirements when designing key health care processes frequently find that the system they designed is not optimum. Design flaws produce undesired results, as well as nonconforming products and services. These, in turn, require even more rework. The failure to consistently meet the requirements of patients and customers may increase the likelihood of downstream problems with the design and delivery of core services. 　　In today's highly competitive and fast-changing economy, speed and agility are important factors that distinguish the best-performing organizations from the rest. The best-performing organizations provide their patients and customers with value faster (speed) and across a wider range of health care areas (agility) than their competition. The speed and agility offered by new technologies enhance that value. As a consequence, the leaders are able to distinguish their organizations in chosen markets, keeping their current patients and customers and acquiring new ones. Increasingly, the failure to use the appropriate technologies limits the organization's ability to keep pace with aggressive competitors. These organizations may have the latest computers but those computers may not be used effectively to accelerate delivery of the services that are important to patients and customers. One large health care organization, learning that its patients and customers placed a premium on accurate test results being delivered on time, acquired and implemented new technology to dramatically speed up its reporting cycle. Unfortunately, the process itself was not capable of rendering an accurate and timely report. Patients and customers received their inaccurate reports faster than ever. Using technology to accelerate a bad process only produces unsatisfactory results faster. The failure to incorporate the *appropriate* technologies can have significant adverse affects on an organization's ability to bring value to its patients and customers, and to operate in an efficient and effective manner. 　　Eliminating unnecessary steps in any work process tends to reduce variation (increasing quality), reduce cycle time, and reduce cost. In addition, learning from the successes and mistakes of others helps prevent staff from repeating the same problems (which add rework, waste, and delay). When designing new services and related delivery systems, the failure to consider factors such as cost control, new technology, variability, and ways to enhance productivity and efficiency typically adds unnecessary cost, delay, and rework, making it more difficult to meet increasing demands of patients, customers and the marketplace.
6.1a(4 and 5)	The best-performing organizations are able to consistently deliver services that meet key performance requirements. They do this by identifying key processes, monitoring them regularly, and improving then continuously. The failure to ensure consistent day-to-day operation of delivery processes increases the likelihood of defects, which contribute to rework, waste, delay, and excessive cost.

	IF YOU DON'T DO WHAT THE CRITERIA REQUIRE... *Continued*
Item Reference	**Possible Adverse Consequences**
6.1a(4 and 5)	Organizations can always tell if a process is producing desired results by waiting for those results and checking to see if the end result meets customer and operational requirements. Unfortunately, waiting for the end of the process to learn that it has not produced desired results is time consuming and expensive. Most costs have already been incurred by the end of the process. The earlier an organization can determine if a process is not likely to produce desired results, the earlier it can take corrective action to minimize rework, scrap, delay, and unnecessary cost. In addition, the failure to collect and analyze in-process data makes it more difficult for staff to know when to adjust a process to make it work better. Inappropriate or unnecessary adjustments can actually increase variation and decrease productivity quality. Patients and customers can usually determine quickly if the services they receive meet (or exceed) their requirements. They are in a good position to provide near real-time feedback that will enable staff to make adjustments to meet requirements. The failure to gather and use this information makes it more difficult for organizations to make timely changes to reduce rework costs and increase patient and customer satisfaction.
6.1a(5 and 6)	High-performing organizations do not rely on excessive inspection and testing to determine if health care process requirements are likely to be met. Conceptually, the only time to inspect is when the outcome is not known. Instead, these organizations design process controls that let them know how well the process is performing during each of its critical steps. They develop processes that prevent problems using tools and techniques such as error proofing. The best that testing or inspection can hope to accomplish is to uncover and correct a problem before the patient/customer service is disrupted. Although this is better than causing problems for patients and customers, it is still more costly to fix the problem than to prevent it from happening in the first place.
6.1a(6 and 7)	Organizations that fail to systematically evaluate and improve delivery systems and processes often seem to lag behind the competition. Consider two comparable organizations, each using similar processes to develop and deliver similar services. Let's also assume that the organizations are equally competitive today. However, one organization has embedded into its work processes an ongoing evaluation and improvement of its design, and delivery systems; the other has not. As time passes, the first organization begins to see the impact of improved work processes. It is able to deliver services faster, better, and cheaper than its competitor. It has been able to pass a portion of its cost savings on to its patients and customers (lowering prices), keeping the rest as increased profit. As a result of better, more timely, and less expensive services, it is acquiring greater market share—at the expense of its competitor—and making its stakeholders and stockholders exceedingly happy as its market share increases. In addition, the first organization has been able to accelerate performance by sharing improvements with other organizational units so they can get better as well. The organization that does not systematically improve continues to fall further and further behind in a highly competitive environment. As the popular adage claims: if you're standing still (not continuously improving), you're falling behind.

IF YOU DON'T DO WHAT THE CRITERIA REQUIRE...	*Continued*

Item Reference	Possible Adverse Consequences
6.1a(6 and 7)	The failure to share effective practices with other organizational support units may cause them to waste time and other resources in redundant work—work that adds cost but not value.

6.1 HEALTH CARE PROCESSES—SAMPLE EFFECTIVE PRACTICES

A. Health Care Processes

- A systematic, iterative process (such as quality function deployment) is used to maintain a focus on the voice of the patient and customer and convert requirements into service design and delivery.

- Design requirements are systematically translated into process specifications, with measurement plans to monitor process consistency.

- The work of various functions is coordinated to bring the service through the design-to-delivery phases. Functional barriers between units have been eliminated organizationwide.

- All design activities are closely coordinated through effective communication and teamwork.

- Internal process capacity and supplier capability, using measures such as Cpk, are reviewed and considered before delivery process designs or plans are finalized.

- Market, design service, and delivery reviews occur at defined intervals or as needed.

- Steps are taken (such as design testing or prototyping) to ensure that the delivery process will work as designed, and will meet patient/ customer requirements.

- Design processes are evaluated and improvements have been made so that future designs are developed faster (shorter cycle time), at lower cost, and with higher quality, relative to key service characteristics that predict patient/customer satisfaction.

- Performance requirements and patient/customer requirements are set using facts and data and are monitored using statistical or other process control techniques.

- Health care delivery processes are measured and tracked. Measures (quantitative and qualitative) should reflect or assess the extent to which patient/customer requirements are met, as well as service consistency.

- For processes that produce defects (out-of-control processes), root causes are quickly and systematically identified and corrective action is taken to prevent their recurrence.

- Corrections are monitored and verified. Improvements are shared throughout the organization.

- Processes are systematically reviewed to improve productivity, reduce cycle time and waste, and increase quality.

- Performance improvement tools—such as flowcharting, work redesign, and reengineering—are used throughout the organization to improve work processes.

- Benchmarking, competitive comparison data, or information from patients and customers of the process (in or out of the organization) are used to gain insight to improve processes.

- Information about patient and customer requirements, complaints, concerns, and reactions to services are captured "near real-time" and used directly by workers to improve the value and delivery processes.

- All key health care processes are subject to continuous review and improvements in performance and patient/customer satisfaction.

- Key health care processes are systematically reviewed to improve productivity, reduce cycle time and waste, and increase quality. Improvements in these processes are shared throughout the organization.

- In order to reduce medication errors, bar-coding technology is used to ensure correct medication and blood transfusion products at the patient's bedside.

- An organization sharing conference is used to bring together representatives from all facilities to highlight best practices. Best practices are also shared at an annual leadership conference.

- A collaborative process is used across disciplines to improve understanding and ensure rapid improvements in clinical outcomes.

- A suggestion program drives employees to submit at least four ideas per year.

- A process to develop new health care services is based on the Plan-Do-Check-Act approach. Development teams spend significant time analyzing need before committing to new health care services.

6.2 SUPPORT PROCESSES (35 pts.)   Approach/Deployment

Describe how your organization manages its key business and other support processes.

Within your response, include answers to the following questions:

a. Business and Other Support Processes

(1) How does your organization determine its key business and other support processes? What are your key processes for supporting your health care processes?

(2) How do you determine key support process requirements, incorporating input from internal and external customers, and suppliers and partners, as appropriate? What are the key requirements for these processes?

(3) How do you design these processes to meet all the key requirements? How do you incorporate new technology and organizational knowledge into the design of these processes? How do you incorporate improved cycle time, productivity, cost control, and other efficiency and effectiveness factors into the design of the processes? How do you implement these processes to ensure they meet design requirements?

(4) What are your key performance measures or indicators used for the control and improvement of your support processes? How does your day-to-day operation of key support processes ensure meeting key performance requirements? How are in-process measures used in managing these processes? How are patient and other customer, supplier, and partner input used in managing these processes, as appropriate?

(5) How do you minimize overall costs associated with inspections, tests, and process or performance audits, as appropriate? How do you prevent errors and rework?

(6) How do you improve your support processes to achieve better performance, to reduce variability, and to keep the processes current with health care service needs and directions? How are improvements shared with other organizational units and processes?

Notes:

N2. Your key business processes are those non-health care service processes that are considered most important to business growth and success by your organization's senior leaders. These might include processes for innovation, technology acquisition, information and knowledge management, supply chain management, supplier partnering, outsourcing, mergers and acquisitions, project management, and sales and marketing. The key business processes to be included in Item 6.2 are distinctive to your organization and how you operate.

N2. Your other key support processes are those that are considered most important for support of your organization's health care service design and delivery processes, staff, and daily operations. These might include key patient support processes (e.g., housekeeping and medical records) and key administrative support processes (e.g., finance and accounting), facilities management, legal, human resource, and project management.

N3. The results of improvements in your key business and other support processes and their performance results should be reported in Item 7.5.

This Item [6.2] looks at the organization's key business and other support processes in order to improve overall operational performance. The organization must ensure its key support processes are designed to meet all internal operational and customer requirements.

The requirements of this Item are similar to the requirements in Items 6.1.

- Key business processes are those non-health care service processes that are considered most important to growth and success by your senior leaders. These processes frequently relate to an organization's strategic objectives and critical success factors. Key business processes might include processes for innovation, technology acquisition, information and knowledge management, supply-chain management, supplier partnering, outsourcing, mergers and acquisitions, project management, and sales and marketing. Given the diverse nature of these processes, the requirements and performance characteristics might vary significantly for different processes.

- Key support processes are those that support your daily operations and health care service delivery, but are not usually designed in detail with the health care services. The support process requirements usually do not depend significantly on health care service characteristics. Support process design requirements usually depend significantly on internal requirements and must be coordinated and integrated to ensure efficient and effective linkage and performance. Support processes might include housekeeping, medical records, finance and accounting, facilities management, legal services, human resource services, public relations, community relations, and other administrative services.

As with value-creation processes, described in Item 6.1, the organization must ensure that the day-to-day operation of its key business and support processes consistently meet the key performance requirements. To do this, in-process measures are defined to permit rapid identification and correction of potential problems. As with other work processes, key business and support processes should incorporate mechanisms to obtain and use customer feedback to help identify problems and take prompt corrective action. The organization should also minimize costs associated with inspection, tests, and audits through use of prevention-based processes, as in Item 6.1.

Finally, organizations should systematically evaluate and improve their key business and support processes to achieve better performance and to keep them current with changing health care needs and directions. Top organizations evaluate and improve the performance of key support processes. Four approaches to evaluating and improving support processes are frequently used:

1. Process analysis and research

2. Benchmarking

3. Use of alternative technology

4. Use of information from patients and customers of the processes

As with core health care processes, a systematic, fact-based approach to improving support processes presents a wide range of possibilities, including complete redesign of key processes or steps within the processes.

6.2 Support Processes

How the organization identifies and manages its key business and other support processes

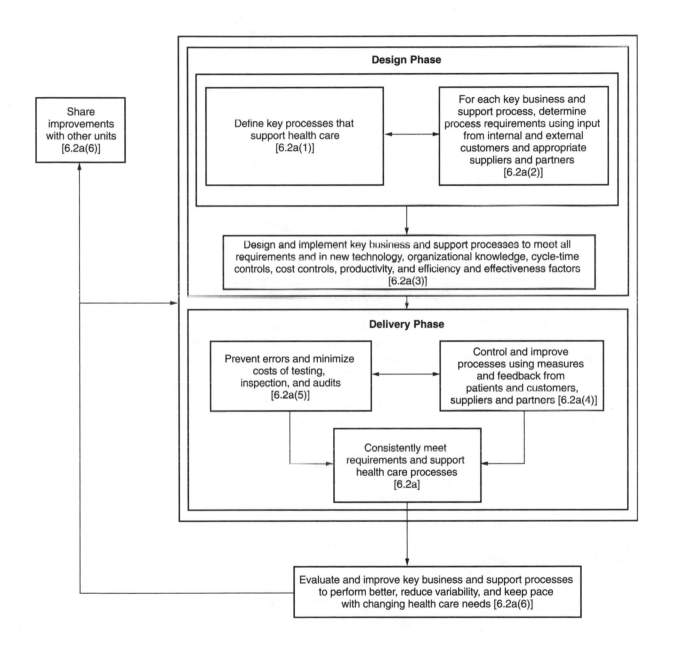

6.2 Support Processes Item Linkages

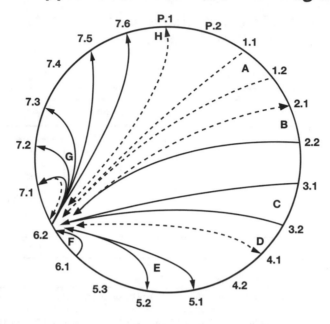

	NATURE OF RELATIONSHIP
A	Senior leaders and the governance system [1.1] have a responsibility for ensuring that key business and support processes are designed [6.2a(2)] consistent with organizational objectives, including those relating to social responsibility and good corporate citizenship [1.2a].
B	Key business and support process strengths and weaknesses [6.2] are considered as part of the planning process [2.1a(2)]. Action plans, deployed to the workforce [2.2a], are used to align actions to help ensure that support services [6.2] meet the requirements needed to carry out the action plans.
C	Patient and other customer complaints [3.2a(3)] and satisfaction/dissatisfaction [3.2b(1 and 2)] may be used to identify requirements for key business and support processes [6.2a(2)], or provide feedback to help manage those processes [6.2a(4)].
D	Key business and support processes [6.2a] may be used to help identify and prioritize benchmarking targets [4.1a(2)]. Benchmarking data [4.1a(2)] are used to improve key business and support work processes [6.2].
E	High-performance work systems [5.1a(1)] and effective recognition [5.1b] and training [5.2a] are essential to improving key business and support work processes [6.2]. In addition, effective design and delivery of key business and support services [6.2] can help promote cooperation and strengthen agility [5.1a(1)] and training [5.2a].
F	Health care processes [6.1] help define requirements and set priorities for key business and support processes, as do patients and customers of key business and support processes [6.2].
G	Information about patient and customer satisfaction [7.2] can be used to target improvement efforts in support processes [6.2]. Improved support processes [6.2] can be reflected in better patient and customer satisfaction [7.21], health care results [7.1], financial results [7.3], operational efficiency [7.5], and social responsibility/regulatory compliance [7.6].

Continued

NATURE OF RELATIONSHIP	*Continued*
H	Information in P.1a(1) derives in part from the support processes [6.2] and helps set the context for Examiner review of these processes.

IF YOU DON'T DO WHAT THE CRITERIA REQUIRE...

Item Reference	Possible Adverse Consequences
6.2a(1)	The requirements of key business and support processes can vary significantly within an organization based on the nature of the core health care services that these business processes must support. If a work process has not been identified as a key health care process, it is a key business or support process, reviewed under the requirements of Item 6.2.
6.2a(2)	An organization that fails to accurately identify the performance and operational requirements of its key business and support processes may find it difficult to design those processes to meet internal or external customer expectations. When key business and support processes fail to meet requirements, resources are wasted and the achievement of objectives may be jeopardized.
6.2a(3)	Organizations that fail to take into account all key operational performance requirements when designing key business and support processes frequently find that the system they design does not meet internal customer requirements. Design flaws produce undesired results and nonconforming support services. This, in turn, usually requires even more rework and disrupts core health care delivery processes.
6.2a(4)	The failure to consistently meet the requirements of key business and support process requirements of patients and other customers may increase the likelihood of downstream problems with the design and delivery of core health care services. Without key measures or indicators of process performance, it is difficult for staff to determine if a process is working as it should. Without in-process measures, staff must generally wait until they get the results at the end of the line to determine if the support processes worked as intended. The failure to collect and analyze in-process data makes it more difficult for staff to know when to adjust a process to make it work better. Inappropriate or unnecessary adjustments can actually increase variation and decrease quality. Patients and other customers can usually determine quickly if the products and services they receive meet requirements. The failure to gather and make timely use of feedback from patients and other customers makes it more difficult for organizations to reduce rework costs and increase customer satisfaction.
6.2a(5)	High-performing organizations do not rely on excessive inspection and testing to determine if key business and support process requirements are likely to be met. Instead, these organizations develop processes that prevent problems using tools and techniques. The best that testing or inspection can hope to accomplish is to uncover and correct a problem before the internal customer is disrupted. However, it is still more costly to fix the problem than to prevent it from happening in the first place.

Continued

IF YOU DON'T DO WHAT THE CRITERIA REQUIRE...	*Continued*
Item Reference	**Possible Adverse Consequences**
6.2a(6)	Key business and support processes that do not improve may cause the business or support function to become so ineffective that it becomes a target for outsourcing. These business or support process units may not be able to effectively provide critical support to core health care delivery units within the parent organization and may contribute to the erosion of overall capability in the parent organization. The failure to share effective practices with other organizational support units may cause them to waste time and other resources in redundant work—work that adds cost but not value.

6.2 SUPPORT PROCESSES— SAMPLE EFFECTIVE PRACTICES

A. Support Processes

- A formal process exists to understand internal customer requirements for all key business and support processes, translate those requirements into efficient service delivery, and measure their effectiveness.

- Specific improvements in key business and support services are made with the same rigor and concern for the internal and external customer as improvements in health care processes.

- All key business and support services are subject to continuous review and improvements in performance and customer satisfaction.

- Systems are in place to ensure process performance is maintained and customer requirements are met. In-process measures are defined and monitored to ensure early alert of problems.

- Root causes of problems are systematically identified and corrected for processes that produce defects.

- Corrections are monitored and verified. Processes used and results obtained should be systematic and integrated throughout the organization.

- Key business and support processes are systematically reviewed to improve productivity, reduce cycle time and waste, and increase quality. Improvement ideas are routinely implemented and shared throughout the organization.

- Work process simplification and performance improvement tools are applied to key business and support processes with measurable sustained results.

- Measurable goals and related actions are used to drive higher levels of key business and support process performance.

- Benchmarking, competitive comparison data, or other information from patients and customers of the key business and support processes (in or out of the organization) are used to gain insight to improve processes.

- Quarterly reviews are held with key suppliers to conduct a formal business review and planning session. This ensures supplier alignment with the organization's vision and mission.

7 Organizational Performance Results—450 Points

*The **Organizational Performance Results** Category examines the organization's performance and improvement in key areas—health care delivery and outcomes, patient and other customer satisfaction, financial and marketplace performance, staff and work system results, operational performance, and governance and social responsibility. Also examined are performance levels relative to those of competitors and other organizations providing similar health care services.*

The Organizational Performance Results Category provides a results focus for meeting the organization's mission as a health care provider. This focus encompasses health care results, patients'/customers' evaluation of health care services, overall financial and health care market performance, staff and work system results, the results of all key processes and process improvement activities, and results for effective governance and social responsibility.

Through this focus, the Criteria's purposes—superior health care quality and value as viewed by patients/customers and the marketplace; superior organizational performance as reflected in clinical, operational, legal, ethical, and financial indicators; and organizational and personal learning—are maintained. Category 7 thus provides "real-time" information (measures of progress) for evaluation and improvement of health care outcomes and all key processes, in alignment with overall organizational strategy. (Note that Item 4.1 calls for analysis of health care results data and information to determine overall organizational performance.)

Historically, many health care organizations have been far too preoccupied with financial performance. Many performance reviews focused almost exclusively on achieving (or failing to achieve) expected levels of financial performance. As such, the results were considered "unbalanced."

- Financial results are considered "lagging" indicators of health care success. Financial results are the net of all the good processes, bad processes, satisfied patients and customers, dissatisfied patients and customers, motivated staff, disgruntled staff, effective suppliers, and sloppy suppliers, to name a few. By the time financial indicators become available, bad products and dissatisfied patients and customers have already occurred.

- The second most lagging indicator is patient and customer satisfaction. By definition, patients and customers must experience the service before they are in a position to comment on their satisfaction with that service. As with financial results, patient and customer satisfaction is affected by many variables including process performance, staff motivation and morale, and supplier performance.

- On the other hand, leading indicators help organizations predict subsequent patient and customer satisfaction and financial performance. Leading indicators include operational effectiveness and staff well-being and satisfaction. Supplier and partner performance, because it affects an organization's own operating performance, is also a leading indicator of patient and customer satisfaction and financial performance.

Taken together, these measures represent a balance between leading and lagging indicators and enable decision makers to identify problems early and take corrective action.

Category 7 requires organizations to report current levels and improvement trends for the following:

- Health care results, including health care outcomes, service delivery results, and patient safety and functional status

- Patient- and other customer-focused results, including satisfaction and dissatisfaction and perceived value and other customer loyalty and retention, positive referral and relationship building, broken out by appropriate patient and customer groups and market segments

- Financial and marketplace performance

- Staff and work system results

- Operational performance

- Governance and social responsibility

For all of these areas, organizations must include appropriate comparative data to enable examiners to define what "good" means. Otherwise, even though performance may be improving, it is difficult to determine whether the level of performance is good or not.

7.1 HEALTH CARE RESULTS (75 pts.)   **Results**

Summarize your organization's key health care performance results. Segment your results by patient and customer groups and market segments, as appropriate. Include appropriate comparative data. Indicate those measures that are mandated by regulatory, accreditor, or payor requirements.

Provide data and information to answer the following questions:

a. Health Care Results

What are your current levels and trends in key measures or indicators of health care outcomes, health care service delivery results, patient safety, and patients' functional status that are important to your patients and other customers? How do these results compare to the performance of your competitors and other organizations providing similar health care services?

Notes:

N1. Health care results reported in this Item should include the key health care service features identified as patient and other patient and customer requirements or expectations in P.1b(2), based on information gathered in Items 3.1 and 3.2. The measures or indicators should address factors that affect patient and other patient and customer preference, such as those included in P.1, Note 3, and Item 3.1, Note 3.

N2. Key health care results should be tailored to your organization and might include both mandated and nonmandated results.

Item 7.1 looks at the organization's health care outcomes to demonstrate how well the organization has been delivering health care services. The Item addresses those measures that best reflect the organization's success in delivering on its mission as a health care provider.

The Item calls for the use of key data and information to establish the organization's performance in delivering health care. This is a critically important Item in the Criteria, as it focuses on demonstrating improved health care results over time and demonstrating superior results relative to other organizations that provide similar health care services. (Risk-adjusted data for the patient population provide a useful basis for demonstrating superior performance and improving performance over time.)

This Item places an emphasis on measures of health care service performance that serve as indicators of patients' and other customers' views and health care decisions relative to continuing interactions with your organization and/or positive referral. These measures of service performance are derived from patient- and other customer-related information gathered in Items 3.1 and 3.2.

Organizations must provide data to demonstrate current levels, trends, and appropriate comparisons for key measures and/or indicators of health care outcomes, service delivery, patient safety, and patient functional status. The correlation between health care service performance and patient/customer indicators is a critical management tool with multiple uses:

(1) Defining and focusing on key quality and patient/customer requirements;

(2) Identifying service differentiators in the health care marketplace; and

(3) Determining cause-effect relationships between health care services' attributes and evidence of customer satisfaction and loyalty, as well as positive referrals.

The correlation might reveal emerging or changing market segments, the changing importance of requirements, or even the potential obsolescence of health care and other patient/customer services.

7.1 Health Care Results

Key health care results segmented by groups, patient and customer groups, and market segments

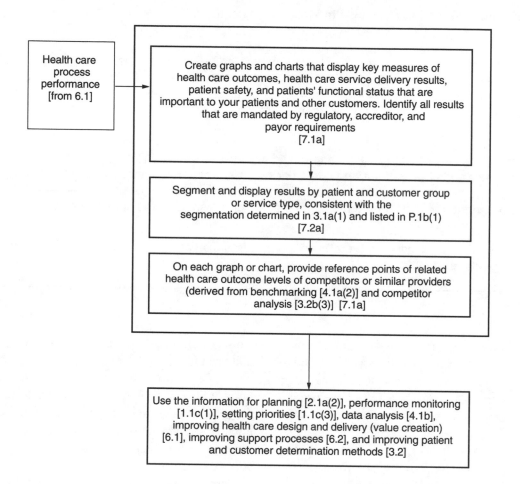

Health care
process
performance
[from 6.1]

Create graphs and charts that display key measures of
health care outcomes, health care service delivery results,
patient safety, and patients' functional status that are
important to your patients and other customers. Identify all results
that are mandated by regulatory, accreditor, and
payor requirements
[7.1a]

Segment and display results by patient and customer group
or service type, consistent with the
segmentation determined in 3.1a(1) and listed in P.1b(1)
[7.2a]

On each graph or chart, provide reference points of related
health care outcome levels of competitors or similar providers
(derived from benchmarking [4.1a(2)] and competitor
analysis [3.2b(3)] [7.1a]

Use the information for planning [2.1a(2)], performance monitoring
[1.1c(1)], setting priorities [1.1c(3)], data analysis [4.1b],
improving health care design and delivery (value creation)
[6.1], improving support processes [6.2], and improving patient
and customer determination methods [3.2]

7.1 Health Care Results Item Linkages

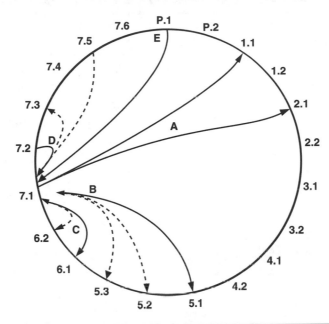

	NATURE OF RELATIONSHIP
A	Data on health care outcomes [7.1] are monitored by senior leaders [1.1c(1)] and are used for strategic planning [2.1a(2)].
B	Recognition and rewards [5.1a] should be based, in part, on service quality results [7.1]. Innovation, empowerment, and initiative developed by effective work systems [5.1a] can foster better health care service quality [7.1]. Health care quality data [7.1] are monitored, in part, to assess training effectiveness [5.2]. In addition, results pertaining to health care service quality [7.1] can be improved with effective training [5.2]. Systems to enhance staff motivation, satisfaction, and well-being (including disaster prevention and recovery systems) [5.3] can produce higher levels of health care service quality [7.1]. Improved health care service quality can affect the morale and motivation of patient- and customer-contact staff.
C	Data on service quality [7.1] may be used to help design and improve value creation [6.1] and support [6.2] processes. These processes [6.1 and 6.2] can have a direct effect on service quality [7.1].
D	Better health care service quality [7.1] results can enhance patient- and customer-focused results [7.2]. Better service quality [7.1] can improve financial and market performance [7.3].
E	The information in P.1b(1) helps examiners identify the kind of health care service quality results, broken out by patient and customer and market segment, that should be reported in Item 7.1.

IF YOU DON'T DO WHAT THE CRITERIA REQUIRE...	
Item Reference	**Possible Adverse Consequences**
7.1	Failing to provide comparison data makes it difficult for leaders (or Baldrige Examiners) to determine if the level of performance reported is good or not. Failing to provide results data for at least most areas of importance to the organization makes it difficult to determine if performance is getting better in key areas. Finally, the failure to provide this information as part of a Baldrige Award assessment is likely to reduce the score and may even prevent an organization from receiving a site visit (during which time additional results data are usually obtained).

7.1 HEALTH CARE RESULTS— SAMPLE EFFECTIVE RESULTS

A. Health Care Results

- Data are presented for the most relevant health care service quality indicators collected through the processes described in Item 3.2 (some of which may be referenced in the Organizational Profile).

- Operational data are presented that correlate with, and help predict, patient and customer satisfaction. These data show consistently improving trends and levels that compare favorably with competitors.

- All indicators show steady improvement. (Indicators include health care outcomes data collected in Item 6.1. For example, "Unplanned Readmission Rates" may be a key indicator of high-performance clinical outcomes.)

- All or most indicators compare favorably to competitors or similar providers.

- Graphs and information are accurate and easy to understand.

- Data are not missing.

7.2 PATIENT- AND OTHER CUSTOMER-FOCUSED RESULTS (75 PTS.) Results

Summarize your organization's key patient- and other customer-focused results, including patient satisfaction and patient-/customer-perceived value. Segment your results by customer groups and market segments, as appropriate. Include appropriate comparative data.

Provide data and information to answer the following questions:

a. Patient- and Other Customer-Focused Results

    (1) What are your current levels and trends in key measures or indicators of patient and other customer satisfaction and dissatisfaction? How do these compare with satisfaction relative to competitors and other organizations providing similar health care services?

    (2) What are your current levels and trends in key measures or indicators of patient- and other customer-perceived value, including patient and other customer loyalty and retention, positive referral, and other aspects of building relationships with patients and other customers, as appropriate?

Notes:

N1. Patient and other customer satisfaction and dissatisfaction results reported in this item should relate to determination methods and data described in Item 3.2.

N2. There may be several different dimensions of patient satisfaction, such as satisfaction with quality of care, satisfaction with provider interaction, satisfaction with the long-term health outcome, and satisfaction with ancillary services. All of these areas are appropriate satisfaction indicators.

N3. Measures and indicators of your patients' and other customers' satisfaction relative to satisfaction with competitors or other organizations providing similar health care services might include objective information and data from your customers and from independent organizations.

7.2 Patient- and Other Customer-Focused Results

Key patient- and customer-focused results, patient and customer satisfaction, and patient- and customer-perceived value.

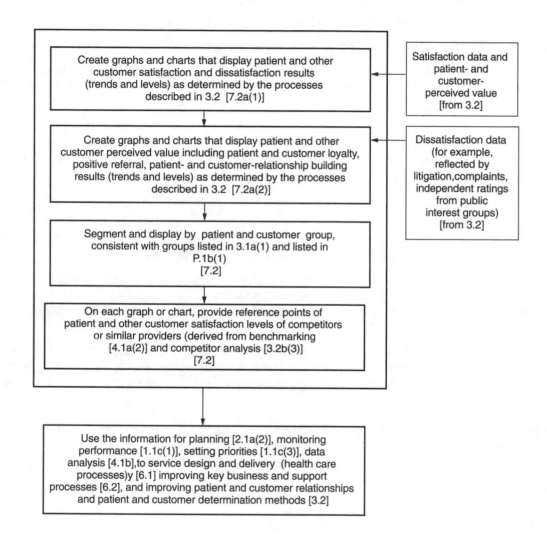

Create graphs and charts that display patient and other customer satisfaction and dissatisfaction results (trends and levels) as determined by the processes described in 3.2 [7.2a(1)]

Satisfaction data and patient- and customer-perceived value [from 3.2]

Create graphs and charts that display patient and other customer perceived value including patient and customer loyalty, positive referral, patient- and customer-relationship building results (trends and levels) as determined by the processes described in 3.2 [7.2a(2)]

Dissatisfaction data (for example, reflected by litigation,complaints, independent ratings from public interest groups) [from 3.2]

Segment and display by patient and customer group, consistent with groups listed in 3.1a(1) and listed in P.1b(1) [7.2]

On each graph or chart, provide reference points of patient and other customer satisfaction levels of competitors or similar providers (derived from benchmarking [4.1a(2)] and competitor analysis [3.2b(3)] [7.2]

Use the information for planning [2.1a(2)], monitoring performance [1.1c(1)], setting priorities [1.1c(3)], data analysis [4.1b],to service design and delivery (health care processes)y [6.1] improving key business and support processes [6.2], and improving patient and customer relationships and patient and customer determination methods [3.2]

7.2 Patient- and Other Customer-Focused Results Item Linkages

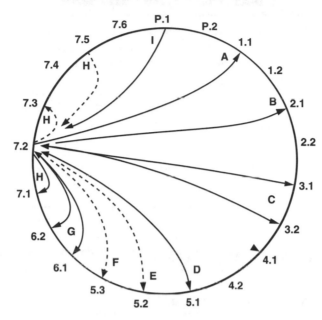

NATURE OF RELATIONSHIP	
A	Data on levels of satisfaction of patients and customers [7.2] are monitored by senior leaders [1.1c(1)].
B	Data on patient and customer satisfaction and loyalty [7.2a(2)] are used for strategic planning [2.1a(2)].
C	Processes used to gather intelligence about current patient and customer requirements [3.1a(2)], strength of patient and customer relations [3.2a(1)], and to determine patient and customer satisfaction [3.2b(1)] produce patient and customer satisfaction results data [7.2a]. In addition, patient and customer satisfaction results [7.2] are used to help set patient- and customer-contact requirements (service standards) [3.2a(2)] and better understand patient and customer requirements and preferences [3.1a(2)].
D	Recognition and rewards [5.1b] should be based, in part, on patient and other customer satisfaction results [7.2]. Innovation, empowerment, and initiative developed by effective work systems [5.1a] can foster better patient and customer satisfaction [7.2].
E	Patient and other customer satisfaction data [7.2] are monitored, in part, to assess training effectiveness [5.2a(6)]. In addition, results pertaining to patient and other customer satisfaction [7.2] can be improved with effective training [5.2].
F	Systems to enhance staff motivation, satisfaction, and well-being (including disaster prevention and recovery systems) [5.3] can produce higher levels of patient and other customer satisfaction [7.2]. Improved patient and customer satisfaction can affect the morale and motivation of patient- and customer-contact staff.

NATURE OF RELATIONSHIP	
G	Data on satisfaction and dissatisfaction of patients and other customers [7.2a(1)] are used to help design and improve value creation [6.1] and key business and support [6.2] processes. These processes [6.1 and 6.2] have a direct effect on patient and other customer satisfaction/dissatisfaction and loyalty [7.2].
H	Better health care outcomes [7.1] and operational [7.5a] results can enhance patient and other customer results [7.2]. Better patient and customer satisfaction [7.2] can improve financial and market performance [7.3].
I	The information in P.1b(1) helps examiners identify the kind of results, broken out by patient and customer and market segment, that should be reported in Item 7.2.

IF YOU DON'T DO WHAT THE CRITERIA REQUIRE...	
Item Reference	**Possible Adverse Consequences**
7.2	Failing to provide comparison data makes it difficult for leaders (or Baldrige Examiners) to determine if the level of performance achieved is good or not. Failing to provide results data for at least most areas of importance to the organization makes it difficult to determine if performance is getting better in key areas. Finally, the failure to provide this information as part of a Baldrige Award assessment is likely to reduce the score and may even prevent an organization from receiving a site visit (during which time additional results data are usually obtained).

7.2 PATIENT- AND OTHER CUSTOMER-FOCUSED RESULTS—SAMPLE EFFECTIVE RESULTS

A. Patient- and Other Customer-Focused Results

- Trends and indicators of patient and customer satisfaction and dissatisfaction (including complaint data), segmented by patient and customer groups, are provided in graph and chart form for all key measures. Multiyear data are provided.

- All indicators show steady improvement. (Indicators include data collected in Area 3.2b, such as patient and customer assessments of products and services, patient and customer awards, and patient and customer retention.)

- All indicators compare favorably to competitors or similar providers.

- Graphs and information are accurate and easy to understand.

- Data are not missing.

- Results data are supported by patient and customer feedback and their overall assessments of products and services, patient and customer awards, and indicators from design and production/delivery processes of products and services.

- Patient Loyalty Index has increased during the past three years, and ranks in the top 10 percent of health care systems in the country.

7.3 FINANCIAL AND MARKET RESULTS (75 PTS.)   Results

Summarize your organization's key financial and health care marketplace performance results by market segments, as appropriate. Include appropriate comparative data.

Provide data and information to answer the following questions:

a. Financial and Market Results

  (1) What are your current levels and trends in key measures or indicators of financial performance, including aggregate measures of financial return and economic value, as appropriate?

  (2) What are your current levels and trends in key measures or indicators of health care marketplace performance, including market share or position, business growth, and new markets entered, as appropriate?

Notes:

Responses to 7.3a(1) might include aggregate measures such as return on investment (ROI), asset utilization, operating margins, profitability (if relevant), profitability by market or customer segment, liquidity, debt to equity ratio, value added per staff member, bond ratings (if appropriate), and financial activity measures.

Item 7.3 looks at the organization's financial and market results to provide a complete picture of financial and marketplace success and challenges.

Organizations should provide data demonstrating levels, trends, and appropriate comparisons for key financial, market, and health care indicators. Measures reported in this Item are used by senior leaders to assess organization-level performance.

Appropriate financial measures and indicators might include:

- Revenue

- Profits

- Market position

- Service-to-cash cycle time

- Earnings per share

- Returns

Appropriate measures of marketplace performance might include:

- Market share

- Measures of growth

- New markets entered

- Entry into e-services for patients/customers

- New populations served

- The percentage of income derived from new health care services.

Organizations should provide appropriate comparisons for key measures and/or indicators to permit the assessment of the strength or "goodness" of the organization's performance

7.3 Financial and Market Results

Results of improvement efforts using key measures and/or indicators of financial and market performance

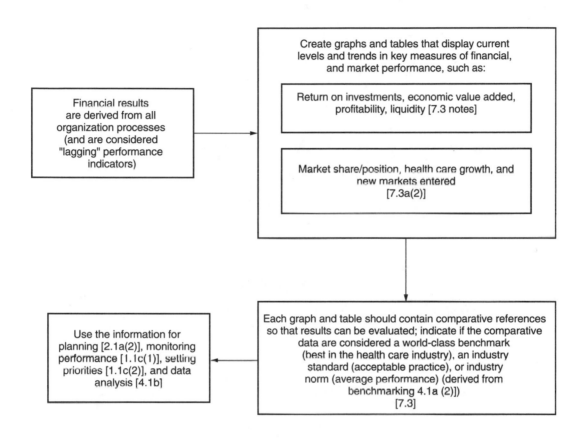

Financial results are derived from all organization processes (and are considered "lagging" performance indicators)

Create graphs and tables that display current levels and trends in key measures of financial, and market performance, such as:

Return on investments, economic value added, profitability, liquidity [7.3 notes]

Market share/position, health care growth, and new markets entered [7.3a(2)]

Each graph and table should contain comparative references so that results can be evaluated; indicate if the comparative data are considered a world-class benchmark (best in the health care industry), an industry standard (acceptable practice), or industry norm (average performance) (derived from benchmarking 4.1a (2)]) [7.3]

Use the information for planning [2.1a(2)], monitoring performance [1.1c(1)], setting priorities [1.1c(2)], and data analysis [4.1b]

7.3 Budgetary, Financial, and Market Results Item Linkages

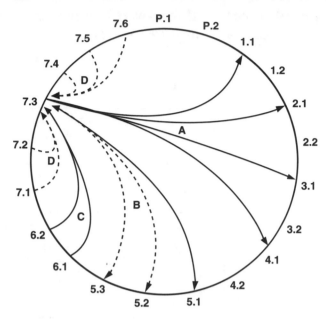

	NATURE OF RELATIONSHIP
A	Financial [7.3a] and market results are used for strategic planning [2.1a(2)]; understanding market requirements and patient and customer preferences [3.1a(2)]; leadership monitoring [1.1c(1)]; priority setting [1.1c(3)]; analysis [4.1b]; and could be used as a partial basis for compensation, recognition, and reward [5.1b].
B	Financial results [7.3a] are monitored, in part, to assess training effectiveness [5.2]. In addition, results pertaining to financial and market performance [7.3a] reflect, in part, training effectiveness [5.2]. Staff motivation and well-being [5.3] affect financial-performance results [7.3], and vice versa.
C	Financial [7.3a] and market results are enhanced by improvements in value-creation processes [6.1] and support processes [6.2]. Those processes may be modified or improved based on financial and market performance.
D	Better financial [7.3a] and market results (lagging indicators) can be driven by better health care results [7.1], patient and other customer satisfaction [7.2], staff motivation and morale [7.4], operational effectiveness [7.5] results, and compliance with laws and regulations and good ethical behavior [7.6].

IF YOU DON'T DO WHAT THE CRITERIA REQUIRE...	
Item Reference	**Possible Adverse Consequences**
7.3	Failing to provide comparison data makes it difficult for leaders (or Baldrige Examiners) to determine if the level of performance reported is good or not. Failing to provide results data for at least most areas of importance to the organization makes it difficult to determine if performance is getting better in key areas. Finally, the failure to provide this information as part of a Baldrige Award assessment is likely to reduce the score and may even prevent an organization from receiving a site visit (during which time additional results data are usually obtained).

7.3 FINANCIAL AND MARKET RESULTS—SAMPLE EFFECTIVE RESULTS

A. Financial and Market Results

- Key measures and indicators of organization market and financial performance address the following areas:

  - Effective use of materials, energy, capital, and assets

  - Asset utilization

  - Market share, health care growth, new markets entered, and market shifting

  - Return on equity

  - Operating margins

  - Pre-tax profit

  - Earnings per share

  - Generating enough revenue to cover expenses (not for profit and public sector)

  - Operating within budget (government sector)

- Measures and indicators show steady improvement.

- All key financial and market data are presented.

- Comparative data include industry best, best competitor, and other appropriate benchmarks.

- The health care system earned AA Credit Rating (the highest rating given to health care systems).

7.4 STAFF AND WORK SYSTEM RESULTS (75 PTS.)   **Results**

Summarize your organization's key staff and work system results, including work system performance and staff learning, development, well-being, and satisfaction. Segment your results to address the diversity of your workforce and the different types and categories of staff, as appropriate. Include appropriate comparative data.

Provide data and information to answer the following questions:

a. Staff and Work System Results

  (1) What are your current levels and trends in key measures or indicators of work system performance and effectiveness?

  (2) What are your current levels and trends in key measures of staff learning and development?

  (3) What are your current levels and trends in key measures or indicators of staff well-being, satisfaction, and dissatisfaction?

Notes:

N1. Results reported in this item should relate to activities described in Category 5. Your results should be responsive to key process needs described in Category 6 and to your organization's action plans and human resource plans described in Item 2.2.

N2. Appropriate measures and indicators of work system performance and effectiveness [7.4a(1)] might include job and job classification simplification, job rotation, work layout improvement, staff retention and internal promotion rates, and changing supervisory ratios.

N3. Appropriate measures and indicators of staff learning and development [7.4a(2)] might include innovation and suggestion rates, courses completed, learning, on-the-job performance improvements, credentialing, and cross-training rates.

N4. For appropriate measures of staff well-being and satisfaction [7.4a(3)], see Item 5.3, Notes.

Item 7.4 looks at the organization's staff and work system results to demonstrate how well the organization has created, maintained, and enhanced a positive, productive, learning, and caring work environment.

Organizations should provide data demonstrating current levels, trends, and appropriate comparisons for key measures and/or indicators of staff well-being, satisfaction, dissatisfaction, and development.

The best-performing organizations also provide data and information on the organization's work system performance and effectiveness, showing favorable comparisons with industry leaders. Results reported might include generic or organization-specific factors.

• Generic factors might include: safety, absenteeism, turnover, satisfaction, and complaints (grievances). For some measures, such as absenteeism and turnover, local or regional comparisons may be most appropriate.

• Organization-specific factors are related to the staff results of staff well-being and satisfaction. These factors might include: the extent of training or cross-training, and the extent and success of systems that promote self-directed and empowered staff.

Organizations should provide appropriate comparisons for key measures and/or indicators to permit the assessment of the strength or "goodness" of the organization's performance.

7.4 Staff and Work System Results

Results of staff and work systems improvement efforts using key measures and/or indicators of such performance

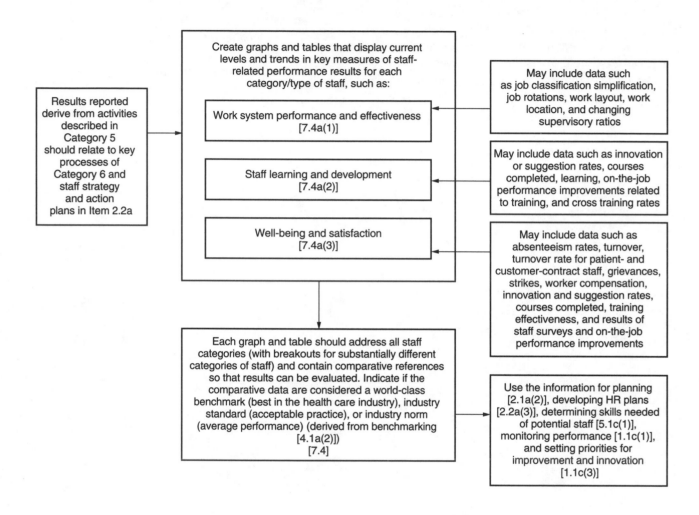

Results reported derive from activities described in Category 5 should relate to key processes of Category 6 and staff strategy and action plans in Item 2.2a

Create graphs and tables that display current levels and trends in key measures of staff-related performance results for each category/type of staff, such as:

Work system performance and effectiveness [7.4a(1)]

Staff learning and development [7.4a(2)]

Well-being and satisfaction [7.4a(3)]

May include data such as job classification simplification, job rotations, work layout, work location, and changing supervisory ratios

May include data such as innovation or suggestion rates, courses completed, learning, on-the-job performance improvements related to training, and cross training rates

May include data such as absenteeism rates, turnover, turnover rate for patient- and customer-contract staff, grievances, strikes, worker compensation, innovation and suggestion rates, courses completed, training effectiveness, and results of staff surveys and on-the-job performance improvements

Each graph and table should address all staff categories (with breakouts for substantially different categories of staff) and contain comparative references so that results can be evaluated. Indicate if the comparative data are considered a world-class benchmark (best in the health care industry), industry standard (acceptable practice), or industry norm (average performance) (derived from benchmarking [4.1a(2)])
[7.4]

Use the information for planning [2.1a(2)], developing HR plans [2.2a(3)], determining skills needed of potential staff [5.1c(1)], monitoring performance [1.1c(1)], and setting priorities for improvement and innovation [1.1c(3)]

7.4 Staff and Work System—Item Linkages

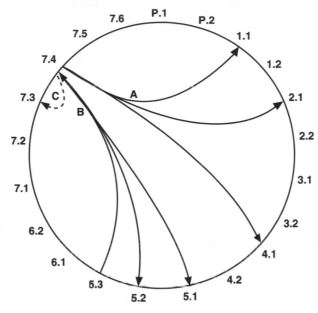

	NATURE OF RELATIONSHIP
A	Staff and work system results [7.4] are reported and used for planning [2.1a(2)], for monitoring organizational performance [1.1c(1)], and analysis [4.1b].
B	Staff and work system results derive from and are enhanced by improving work systems and enhancing flexibility, and by strengthening staff recognition systems [5.1b], training [5.2], and well-being and satisfaction [5.3]. In addition, staff results data [7.4] are monitored, in part, to assess training effectiveness [5.2].
C	Better financial and market results [7.3] (lagging indicators) can be affected by better staff motivation and morale [7.4].

IF YOU DON'T DO WHAT THE CRITERIA REQUIRE...	
Item Reference	**Possible Adverse Consequences**
7.4	Failing to provide comparison data makes it difficult for leaders (or Baldrige Examiners) to determine if the level of performance reported is good or not. Failing to provide results data for at least most areas of importance to the organization makes it difficult to determine if performance is getting better in key areas. Finally, the failure to provide this information as part of a Baldrige Award assessment is likely to reduce the score and may even prevent an organization from receiving a site visit (during which time additional results data are usually obtained).

7.4 STAFF AND WORK SYSTEM RESULTS—SAMPLE EFFECTIVE RESULTS

A. Staff Results

The results reported in Item 7.4 derive from activities described in Category 5 and the staff plans from Item 2.2a(3).

- Multiyear data are provided to show sustained performance.

- All results show steady improvement.

- Data are not missing. If staff results are declared important, related data are reported.

- Comparison data for benchmark or competitor organizations are reported, and the organization compares favorably.

- Trend data are reported for staff satisfaction with working conditions, safety, retirement package, and other staff benefits. Satisfaction with management is also reported.

- Trends for declining absenteeism, grievances, staff turnover, strikes, and worker compensation claims are reported.

- Data reported are segmented for all staff categories.

- Staff turnover decreased significantly.

- Total training hours per staff member are significantly higher than the health care benchmark.

- Medical staff satisfaction is equal to or better than the best in the U. S. for the past three years

7.5 ORGANIZATIONAL EFFECTIVENESS RESULTS (75 PTS.)   Results

Summarize your organization's key operational performance results that contribute to the achievement of organizational effectiveness. Segment your results by health care services and market segments, as appropriate. Include appropriate comparative data.

Provide data and information to answer the following questions:

a. Organizational Effectiveness Results

(1) What are your current levels and trends in key measures or indicators of the operational performance of your key health care processes? Include productivity, cycle time, supplier and partner performance, and other appropriate measures of effectiveness and efficiency.

(2) What are your current levels and trends in key measures or indicators of the operational performance of your key support and business processes? Include productivity, cycle time, supplier and partner performance, and other appropriate measures of effectiveness and efficiency.

(3) What are your results for key measures or indicators of accomplishment of organizational strategy and action plans?

Notes:

N1. Results reported in Item 7.5 should address your key operational requirements and progress toward accomplishment of your key organizational performance goals as presented in the organizational profile and in Items 1.1, 2.2, 6.1, and 6.2. Include results not reported in Items 7.1–7.4.

N2. Results reported in Item 7.5 should provide key information for analysis [Item 4.1] and review of your organizational performance [Item 1.1] and should provide the operational basis for health care results [Item 7.1], patient- and other customer-focused results [Item 7.2], and financial and market results [Item 7.3].

Item 7.5 looks at the organization's key operational performance results to demonstrate organizational effectiveness in both value creation and support processes, and the achievement of key goals and strategic objectives. Organizations should provide data in this item if it does not belong in other Category 7 Items (7.1, 7.2, 7.3, 7.4, or 7.6).

This Item encourages the organization to develop and include unique and innovative measures to track health care development and operational improvement. However, all key areas of health care and operational performance should be covered by measures that are relevant and important to the organization.

Measures and/or indicators of operational effectiveness and efficiency might include:

- Reduced emission levels, waste stream reductions, by-product use, and recycling

- Internal responsiveness indicators, such as reduced cycle times, reduced the incidence of repeat diagnostic tests; reduced operational costs

- Increased innovation rates and increased use of e-technology, six sigma initiative results, and delivery performance

- Supply chain indicators such as reductions in inventory and inspections, increases in quality and productivity, improvements in electronic data exchange, and reductions in supply chain management costs

- Third-party assessment results, such as JHACO assessments

- Indicators of strategic goal achievement

Organizations should provide appropriate comparisons for key measures and/or indicators to permit the assessment of the strength or "goodness" of the organization's performance.

7.5 Organizational Effectiveness Results

Results of improvement efforts that contribute to achievement of organizational effectiveness

Organizational Effectiveness Results

Create graphs and tables that display current levels of sustained trends of key operational performance results that contribute to strategic objectives

Key process performance improvement results are derived from *health care* processes in Items 6.1, including productivity, cycle time, and other efficiency and effectiveness measures important to the organization [7.5a(1)]

Key process performance improvement results are derived from *key business and support* processes in Items 6.2, including productivity, cycle time, supplier and partner performance, and other efficiency and effectiveness measures important to the organization [7.5a(2)]

Results supporting accomplishment of strategy and action plans [7.5a(3)]

Each graph and table should contain comparative references so that results can be evaluated; indicate if the comparative data are considered a world-class benchmark (best in the health care industry), industry norm (average performance) (derived from benchmarking [4.1a(2)]) [7.5]

Results provide data for analysis [4.1b] and performance review [1.1c(1)]

7.5 Organizational Effectiveness Results Item Linkages

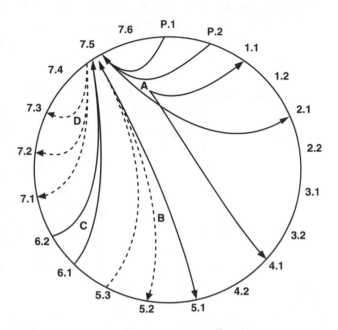

	NATURE OF RELATIONSHIP
A	Organizational effectiveness results [7.5] are reported and used for planning [2.1a(2)], management improvement, performance monitoring and priority setting [1.1c], and analysis [4.1b]. Progress in addressing strategic challenges, as described in P.2b, and strategic objectives listed in 2.1b(1), should be reported in Item 7.5a(3). [Note that the strategic challenges identified in P.2b should be consistent with the strategic objectives in 2.1b(1).] Performance related to the key suppliers and partners listed in P.1b(2) should be reported in 7.5a(2)].
B	Organizational effectiveness results [7.5] are used to provide staff feedback and to drive rewards and recognition [5.1b] and training and staff development [5.2]. Processes to improve staff initiative and flexibility [5.1a(1)], and staff safety, security, morale, motivation, and well-being [5.3], and better align recognition and reward to desired performance outcomes [5.1b] may enhance performance results [7.5].
C	Designing value creation health care processes to meet patient and other customer requirements [6.1a(3)] and to improve design and service delivery and consistency [6.1a(4)] and key business and support service processes [6.2] should affect organizational effectiveness performance outcomes [7.5].
D	Organizational effectiveness results [7.5] contribute to financial and market results [7.3], health care results [7.1], and patient- and customer-focused results [7.2].

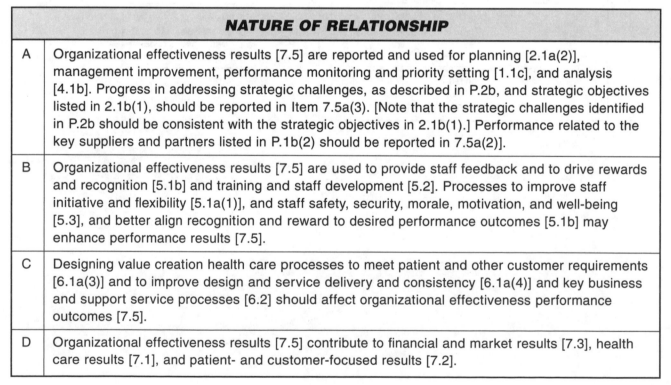

IF YOU DON'T DO WHAT THE CRITERIA REQUIRE...	
Item Reference	**Possible Adverse Consequences**
7.5	Failing to provide comparison data makes it difficult for leaders (or Baldrige Examiners) to determine if the level of performance reported is good or not. Failing to provide results data for at least most areas of importance to the organization makes it difficult to determine if performance is getting better in key areas. Finally, the failure to provide this information as part of a Baldrige Award assessment is likely to reduce the score and may even prevent an organization from receiving a site visit (during which time additional results data are usually obtained).

7.5 ORGANIZATIONAL EFFECTIVENESS RESULTS— SAMPLE EFFECTIVE RESULTS

A. Organizational Effectiveness Results

- Indices and trend data are provided in graph and chart form for all operational performance measures identified in 1.1, 6.1, and 6.2, relevant organizational goals (2.2) and strategic objectives (2.1b), and the key health care factors identified in the Organizational Profile and not reported elsewhere in Category 7. Multiyear data are reported.

- Most to all indicators show steady improvement.

- Design service delivery quality measures and indicators address requirements such as accuracy, timeliness, and reliability. Examples include defect levels, repeat services, meeting service delivery or response times, and availability levels. However, if these measures predict patient and customer satisfaction, they should be moved to Item 7.2.

- Operational performance measures address:

  – Productivity, efficiency, and effectiveness, such as productivity indices and service design improvement measures

  – Cycle-time reductions

- Comparative data include industry best, best competitor, industry average, and appropriate benchmarks. Data are also derived from independent surveys, studies, laboratory testing, or other sources.

- Data are not missing. (For example, do not show a steady trend from 1998 to 2002, but leave out 2001.)

- Data are not aggregated since aggregation tends to hide poor performance by blending it with good performance. Charts and graphs break out and report trends separately.

- Results, such as average Acute Length of Stay, are below the comparison data for top hospital systems. Paid Hours per Adjusted Patient Day results have been better than top benchmark figures for the last three years.

7.6 GOVERNANCE AND SOCIAL RESPONSIBILITY RESULTS (75 pts.)

Results

Summarize your organization's key governance and social responsibility results, including evidence of fiscal accountability, ethical behavior, legal compliance, and organizational citizenship. Segment your results by organizational units, as appropriate. Include appropriate comparative data.

Provide data and information to answer the following questions:

a. Governance and Social Responsibility Results

(1) What are your key current findings and trends in key measures or indicators of fiscal accountability, both internal and external, as appropriate?

(2) What are your results for key measures or indicators of ethical behavior and of stakeholder trust in the governance of your organization?

(3) What are your results for key measures or indicators of organizational accreditation, assessment, and regulatory and legal compliance?

(4) What are your results for key measures or indicators of organizational citizenship in support of your key communities, including contributions to the health of your community?

Notes:

N1. Responses to 7.6a(1) might include financial statement issues and risks, important internal and external auditor recommendations, and management's response to these matters.

N2. For examples of measures of ethical behavior and stakeholder trust [7.6a(2)], see Note 2 to Item 1.2.

N3. Regulatory and legal compliance results [7.6a(3)] should address requirements described in 1.2a. If your organization has received sanctions or adverse actions under law (including malpractice), regulation, accreditation, or contract during the past three years, briefly describe the incident(s) and current status. If settlements have been negotiated in lieu of potential sanctions or adverse actions, give explanations.

N4. Organizational citizenship and community health results [7.6a(4)] should address support for the key communities discussed in 1.2c.

Item 7.6 looks at key results in the area of societal responsibility that reflect the behavior of an ethical organization that is a good citizen in its communities. In this Item, provide data and information on key measures or indicators of organizational accountability, stakeholder trust, and ethical behavior, as well as regulatory and legal compliance and citizenship.

Although there is an increased focus nationally on issues of governance, ethics, and board and leadership accountability, the best-performing organizations practice and demonstrate high standards of overall conduct. The failure to do so may threaten an organization's public trust, which may threaten its long-term success, if not its survival. Boards and senior leaders should track performance measures that relate to governance and social responsibility on a regular basis and emphasize this performance in stakeholder communications.

Results reported should include key accreditation and regulatory review findings, patient safety data, staff licensure and re-credentialing, certification, and accreditation determinations, external audits, proficiency testing results, and utilization review results, as appropriate.

Results reported should include environmental and regulatory compliance and highlight noteworthy achievements in these areas, as appropriate. Results also should include indicators of support for key communities and other public purposes.

Summarize and report any sanctions or adverse findings (including independent audit findings) under law, regulation, or contract the organization has received during the past three years, including the nature of the incidents and their current status.

Organizations should provide appropriate comparisons for key measures and/or indicators to permit the assessment of the strength or "goodness" of the organization's performance.

7.6 Governance and Social Responsibility Results

Results of improvement efforts that contribute to achievement of key governance and social responsibility results, including fiscal accountability ethical behavior, legal compliance, and organizational citizenship

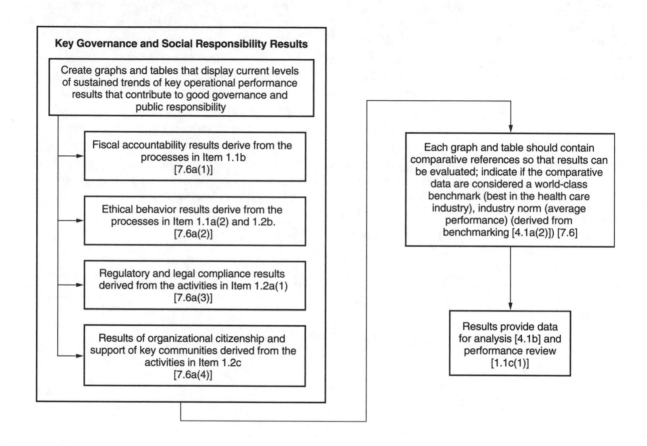

7.6 Governance and Social Responsibility Results Item Linkages

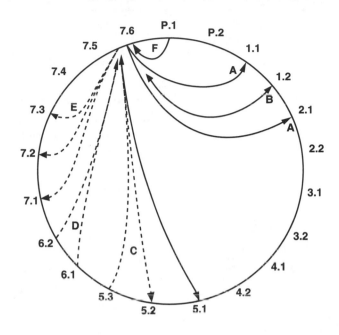

NATURE OF RELATIONSHIP	
A	Governance and social responsibility results that relate to fiscal accountability, ethical behavior, and regulatory compliance [7.6a(1, 2, 3)] are used for planning [2.1a(2)], management improvement, performance monitoring and priority setting [1.1c].
B	Results for regulatory and legal compliance and citizenship, related to the activities in Item 1.2, should be reported in 7.5a(3). In addition, these results are monitored to determine if process changes are needed.
C	Staff motivation, satisfaction, and well-being [5.3] affect governance and social responsibility results of ethical behavior and regulatory compliance [7.6a(2& 3)]. In addition, results pertaining to these key areas [7.6] should be reflected, in part, in staff feedback [5.1b] and are monitored to assess training effectiveness [5.2].
D	Design and service delivery and consistency [6.1], and key business and support service processes [6.2] affect regulatory compliance and possible ethical results [7.6a(2 and 3)].
E	Governance and social responsibility results [7.6a(1 and 4)] may affect financial and market results [7.3], health care results [7.1], and patient- and customer-focused results [7.2].
F	The regulatory requirements described in P.1a(5) define the related performance results that should be reported in 7.6a(3).

IF YOU DON'T DO WHAT THE CRITERIA REQUIRE...	
Item Reference	**Possible Adverse Consequences**
7.6	Failing to provide comparison data makes it difficult for leaders (or Baldrige Examiners) to determine if the level of performance reported is good or not. Failing to provide results data for at least most areas of importance to the organization makes it difficult to determine if performance is getting better in key areas. Finally, the failure to provide this information as part of a Baldrige Award assessment is likely to reduce the score and may even prevent an organization from receiving a site visit (during which time additional results data are usually obtained).

7.6 GOVERNANCE AND SOCIAL RESPONSIBILITY RESULTS— SAMPLE EFFECTIVE RESULTS

A. Governance and Social Responsibility Results

- Indices and trend data are provided in graph and chart form for all regulatory and legal compliance requirements identified in Item 1.2(1) and P.1a(5).

- Results address public responsibilities, such as environmental improvements and the increased use of technologies, materials, and work processes that are environmentally friendly.

- Ethical behavior is demonstrated by a large percentage of independent board members. In addition, independent audits demonstrate full compliance with ethics rules established by the organization.

- Areas of community support demonstrate increasing efforts to strengthen local community services, education, and health care; the environment; and related trade and health care associations.

- Data indicate most measures of regulatory compliance exceed requirements. Performance is leading the industry. No sanctions or violations have been reported.

- Data show sustained improvements in waste reduction and energy efficiency.

- Resources allocated to support key communities, consistent with health care strategy, demonstrate positive desired results, increasing in effectiveness over time.

- Most to all indicators show steady improvement.

- Comparative data include industry best, best competitor, industry average, and appropriate benchmarks. Data are also derived from independent surveys, studies, laboratory testing, or other sources.

- Data are not missing. (For example, do not show a steady trend from 1998 to 2002, but leave out 2001.)

- Data are not aggregated since aggregation tends to hide poor performance by blending it with good performance. Charts and graphs break out and report trends separately.

- Contributions to community health care have increased over the past four years.

- Senior leaders commit extensive time (40 hours or more each year) serving on community or industry boards.

Tips on Preparing a Baldrige Award Application

Applications are put together by every conceivable combination of teams, committees, and individual efforts, including consultants. There is no "right" or "best" way to do it. There are, however, lessons that have been learned and are worth considering because they contribute to people and organizations growing and improving.

Author's Note: Gathering process information from across the organization is essential to prepare an accurate and complete Baldrige application. Over the past several years, I have helped many organizations conduct assessments and apply for awards. During this time, Mark Blazey prepared a Microsoft® Word template to help writing teams gather information and prepare to write. The application template—provided on a CD that is included with this book—facilitates the collection of critical information and makes it easier to write a Baldrige application. The thoughts that follow are intended to generate conversation and learning. They are not intended to present a comprehensive treatment of the subject.

Getting the Fingerprints of the Organization on the Application

How do we put together a "good" application? To be "good" from a technical perspective, it must be both accurate and respond fully to the multiple requirements of the criteria.

To be effective, the application must be more than technically accurate. The organization must reflect a sense of commitment and ownership for the application. Ownership requires a role for people throughout the organization as well as top leadership. The actual "putting of words on paper" can be accomplished in a variety of ways. However, ignoring this larger question of ownership exposes the organization to developing a sterile, disjointed, or unrecognizable document that diminishes its value as a vehicle of growth.

The Spirit and Values in an Application

Like it or not, the team or individual that is responsible for developing an application will be closely watched by everyone in the organization. The people coordinating the development of the application need to be perceived as "walking the talk." They need to be seen as believers and role models for what is being written. In the midst of the pressure of putting together an application, a few values have to be continuously brought to the forefront:

- Continuous improvement must be fully embedded into all management processes and work processes.

- The application describes the system used to run the business. This includes not just a description of the pieces, but also the linkages among the activities that make the organization function effectively.

- Put your best foot forward, but do not exaggerate.

Core Values and Recurring Themes

In a document as complex and fact-filled as a Baldrige Award application, make sure key messages are clearly communicated. There are 11 Core Values and the application must address all of them. The organization needs to decide at the onset what key messages reflect the drivers of health care success. These key messages should be reflected in each category and tie together the entire application. This is one of the reasons it becomes so important to design and write the Organizational Profile early and well. Too many applicants ignore the importance of the Organizational Profile as an organizing tool. An effective Organizational Profile clearly identifies those things that are important to the business, important to its patients and customers and stakeholders, and important to the future of the health care organization. These selected themes guide the development of the application. We are often asked, "How many themes should an organization focus on?" The answer really depends on how many the organization actually uses. Try focusing on three

Tests for Reasonableness

During the development of an application, there are "tests" that need to be conducted periodically with two groups of people: the senior executive team and patient/customer-contact or frontline staff.

With senior executive teams the issue is the rate of growth of those items undergoing intensive improvement efforts and under the direct sponsorship of senior executives. Every Baldrige application effort should use the occasion to drive significant business process improvements throughout the organization. The development of an application offers an opportunity to review and improve these initiatives. Each improvement of an existing process is a candidate for inclusion in an application to demonstrate progress.

At the patient/customer-contact or front line staff level, conduct a "reality check." Determine whether the application as written reflects the way the health care organization is run. When people are given the opportunity to review an application during the developmental stages, several things happen:

- Frontline people can comment on how closely the write-up reflects reality. It provides the writer(s) an opportunity to calibrate those words with reality.

- The review forces the patient/customer-contact staff to take a top level view, which can be a learning experience in itself.

- It forces the writer to walk in the shoes of the individual contributor, another learning experience.

Test the Application

As an application comes together, a question asked by everyone—particularly the leadership team—is, "How well are we doing, what's the score?" Although the real value of an application is continuous improvement, the competitive nature of people also comes to the forefront. After all, that spirit helps drive people to higher levels of excellence. Nurture that spirit.

The best means of getting an objective review is to have people familiar with the Baldrige process, but unbiased with respect to the organization and its processes, examine the application. It is surprising how differently outsiders view the workings of the business. The important aspect of this review is obviously the skill of the reviewers or examiners. The value to the organization is threefold:

- An early assessment, which sets expectations and eliminates surprises

- An opportunity for an early start on improvement initiatives

- A test of understandability by outsiders, which every application ultimately has to pass

Take Time to Celebrate/ Continuously Improve

Developing an application is tough work. At the end of the day, the application represents:

- A document highlighting the accomplishments and future aspirations of the organization

- A plan for getting there

- An operations manual for new people entering the business

At key milestones in the development of an application, it is important to take time to celebrate the accomplishments just completed. The celebration should be immediate, inclusive, and visible. Such a celebration raises questions within the organization, and it raises expectations—all of which are critical when trying to change and improve the overall performance of the organization. It also presents a perfect opportunity to promote improvement initiatives.

In the words of David Kearns, former CEO of Xerox and one of the greatest leaders of performance excellence in the world, "Quality is a journey without an end." Every company today is faced with the struggle to bring about change—and the pace quickens each year. Baldrige is a mechanism that can help focus the energy for change in a most productive manner. Used properly it can help organizations breakout of restrictive paradigms and continue on the journey to top levels of performance excellence.

2003 CRITERIA RESPONSE GUIDELINES

The guidelines given in this section are offered to assist Criteria for Performance Excellence users in responding most effectively to the requirements of the 19 Criteria Items. Writing an application for the Baldrige Award involves responding to these requirements in 50 or fewer pages.

The guidelines are presented in three parts:

1. General Guidelines regarding the criteria booklet, including how the Items are formatted

2. Guidelines for Responding to Approach/Deployment Items

3. Guidelines for Responding to Results Items

General Guidelines

Read the entire Criteria booklet

The main sections of the booklet provide an overall orientation to the criteria, including how responses are to be evaluated for self-assessment or by Award Examiners. You should become thoroughly familiar with the following sections:

- Criteria for Performance Excellence

- Scoring Information

- Glossary of Key Terms

- Category and Item Descriptions

Review the Item format and understand how to respond to the Item requirements

The Item format shows the different parts of Items, the significance of each part, and where each part is placed. It is especially important to understand the Areas to Address and the Item Notes. Each Item is classified as either Approach/Deployment or Results depending on the type of information required.

Item requirements are presented in question format, sometimes with modifying statements. Responses to an Item should contain answers to all questions and modifying statements; however, each question need not be answered separately. Responses to multiple questions within a single Area to Address may be grouped as appropriate to the organization. The CD accompanying this book contains a restatement of the Criteria in declarative sentences, not questions. Many have found this makes it easier to understand the different requirements that are embedded in the Criteria.

Start by preparing the Organizational Profile

The Organizational Profile is the most appropriate starting point for initiating a self-assessment or for writing an application. The Organizational Profile is intended to help everyone—including Criteria users, application writers, and reviewers—to understand what is most relevant and important to the organization's business and to its performance.

In addition, read the information describing the linkages, sample effective practices, and process flow diagrams presented in this book. In particular, be certain to understand how the various requirements of the Criteria are integrated into a comprehensive management system. Then gather data using the electronic application template provided with this book.

Guidelines for Responding To Approach/Deployment Items

The Criteria focus on key performance results. However, results by themselves offer little diagnostic value. For example, if some results are poor or are improving at rates slower than the competition's, it is important to understand why this is so and what might be done to accelerate improvement.

The purpose of Approach/Deployment Items is to permit diagnosis of the organization's most important processes—the ones that enable fast-paced performance improvement and contribute to key business results. Diagnosis and feedback depend heavily upon the content and completeness of Approach/Deployment Item responses. For this reason, it is important to respond to these Items by providing key process information.

Understand the Meaning of "How"

Items requesting information on approach and deployment include questions that begin with the word "how." Responses should outline key process information, such as methods, measures, deployment, evaluation, improvement, and learning factors. Responses lacking such information, or merely providing an example, are referred to in the Scoring Guidelines as anecdotal information and are worth little to nothing

Understand the Meaning of "What"

Two types of questions in Approach/Deployment Items begin with the word "what." The first type of question requests basic information on key processes and how they work. Although it is helpful to include who performs the work, merely stating who does not permit diagnosis or feedback. The second type of question requests information on what your key findings, plans, objectives, goals, or measures are. These questions set the context for showing alignment in your performance management system. For example, when you identify key strategic objectives, your action plans, staff development plans, some of your results measured, and results reported in Category 7 should be expected to relate to the stated strategic objectives.

Describe your system for meeting the requirements of each item. Ensure that methods, processes, and practices are fully described. Use flowcharts to help examiners visualize your key processes.

Show That Activities Are Systematic

Ensure that the response describes a systematic approach, not merely an anecdotal example. Systematic approaches are repeatable, predictable, and involve the systematic use of data and information for evaluation,

subsequent improvement, and learning. In other words, the approaches are consistent over time, build in learning and evaluation, and show maturity. Scores above 50 percent rely on clear evidence that approaches are systematic, evaluated, and refined.

Show Deployment

Ensure that the response gives clear and sufficient information on deployment. For example, one must be able to distinguish from a response whether an approach described is used in one, some, most, or all parts of the organization. If the process you describe is widely used in the organization be sure to state where it is deployed.

Deployment can be shown compactly by using summary tables that outline what is done in different parts of the organization. This is particularly effective if the basic approach is described in a narrative.

Show Focus, Consistency, and Integration

The response demonstrates that the organization is focused on key processes and on improvements that offer the greatest potential to improve business performance and accomplish organization action plans. There are four important factors to consider regarding integration:

1. The Organizational Profile should make clear what is important.

2. The Strategic Planning Category, including the strategic objectives and action plans, should highlight areas of greatest focus and describe how strategy alignment is accomplished.

3. Descriptions of organizational-level analysis and review (Items 4.1 and 1.1) should show how the organization analyzes and reviews performance information to set priorities.

4. The Process Management Category should highlight product, service, support, and supplier processes that are key to overall performance.

Integrating systems required in the Approach/Deployment Items and tracking corresponding measures in the Results Items should improve business performance.

Respond Fully to Item Requirements

Ensure that the response fully addresses all important parts of each Item and each Area to Address. Missing or incomplete information will be interpreted by examiners as a system deficiency—a gap in approach and/or deployment. All areas should be addressed and checked in final review. Individual components of an Area to Address may be addressed individually or together.

Cross-Reference When Appropriate

Each Item response should be, as much as possible, self-contained. However, some responses to different Items might be mutually reinforcing. It is then appropriate to refer to the other responses, rather than to repeat information. In such cases, key process information should be given in the Item requesting this information. For example, staff education and training should be described in detail in Item 5.2. References elsewhere to education and training would then reference, but not repeat, this detail.

Use a Compact Format

Applicants should make the best use of the 50 application pages permitted. Use flowcharts, tables, and "bulletized" presentation of information.

Refer to the Scoring Guidelines

The evaluation of item responses is accomplished by consideration of the Criteria Item requirements and the maturity of the organization's approaches, breadth of deployment, and strength of the improvement process relative to the scoring guidelines. Therefore, applicants need to consider both the criteria and the Scoring Guidelines in preparing responses. *In particular, remember that in order to score over 50 percent, organizations must have in place a fact-based evaluation process and corresponding improvements at least for the key Item requirements. The Scoring Guidelines make this requirement applicable to all Items in Categories 1 through 6. Even if the Criteria questions for the Item do not ask for a description of techniques, it will help the examiners give you full credit for your*

processes if an explanation is provided to show how the processes are systematically evaluated and refined. List the process improvements that have been made during the last three to four years.

GUIDELINES FOR RESPONDING TO RESULTS ITEMS

The Baldrige Criteria place great emphasis (and 45 percent of the score) on results. All Results Items remain in Category 7 for 2002. Items 7.1, 7.2, 7.3, 7.4, 7.5 and 7.6 call for results related to all key requirements, patients, customers, stakeholders, and goals.

Focus on Reporting Critical Results

Results reported should cover the most important requirements for business success highlighted in the Organizational Profile and the Strategic Planning and Process Management Categories, and included in responses to other Items, such as Staff Focus (Category 5) and Process Management (Category 6).

Four key requirements for effective presentation of results data include the following:

1. Trends show directions of results and rates of change.

2. Performance levels show performance on some meaningful measurement scale.

3. Comparisons show how trends or levels compare with those of other, appropriately selected organizations.

4. Breadth and importance of results show that all important results are included.

No Minimum Time

No minimum period of time is required for trend data. However, results data might span five years or more for some results. Trends might be much shorter for some of the organization's more recent improvement activities. Because of the importance of showing deployment and focus, new data should be included even if trends and comparisons are not yet well established. However, it may be better to report four quarterly measures covering a one-year period than two measures for beginning and end of year. The four measures help to demonstrate a sustained trend (if one exists).

Compact Presentation

Many results can be reported compactly by using graphs and tables. Graphs and tables should be labeled for easy interpretation. Results over time or compared with others should be "normalized"—presented in a way (such as use of ratios) that takes into account various size factors. For example, reporting safety trends in terms of lost workdays per 100 staff would be more meaningful than total lost workdays, if the number of staff has varied over the time period or if you are comparing your results to organizations varying in size from yours.

Link Results with Text

Descriptions of results and the results themselves should be in close proximity in the application. Trends that show a significant positive or negative change should be explained. Use figure numbers that correspond to Items. For example, the third figure for Item 7.1 should be 7.1-3. (See Figure 33.)

Figure 33 illustrates data an applicant might present as part of a response to Item 7.1, Health Care Results. In the Organizational Profile, in Item 2.1b(1) and in Item 3.1, the applicant has indicated that

reducing the average length of stay is a key performance requirement.

Using the graph in Figure 33, the following characteristics of clear and effective data reporting are illustrated:

- A figure number is provided for reference to the graph in the text.

- Both axes and units of measure are clearly labeled.

- Trend lines report data for a key patient/customer requirement—average length of stay.

- Results are presented for several years.

- Appropriate comparisons are clearly shown.

- An arrow indicates desired direction of performance.

To help interpret the Scoring Guidelines, the following comments on the graphed results would be appropriate:

- The current overall organizational performance level is *excellent*. This conclusion is supported by the comparison with the best competitor and with a health care industry average.

- The organization shows excellent improvement trends.

Complete Data

Be sure that results data are displayed for all relevant patient and other customer, financial, market, staff, operational, supplier/partner and governance performance characteristics. If you identify relevant performance measures and goals in other parts of the analysis (for example, Categories 1 through 6), be sure to include the results of these performance characteristics in Category 7. As each relevant performance measure is identified in the assessment process, create a blank chart and label the axes. Define all units of measure, especially if they are industry-specific or unique to the applicant. As data are collected, populate the charts. If expected data are not provided in the application, examiners may assume that the trends or levels are not good.

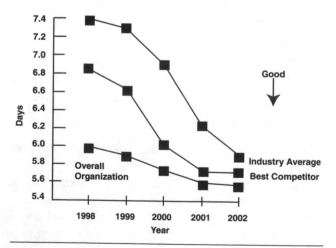

Figure 33 Sample results.

Missing data drive the score down in the same way that poor trends do.

After you complete all of the data in Category 7, review the Organizational Profile and the processes described in Categories 1 through 6. Make a list of all of the results that an examiner would expect to find in Category 7. Then cross-check this list with the data provided in Category 7. If any "Expected" data are missing, be sure to add the appropriate charts or graphs.

Break Out Data

This point, mentioned earlier, bears repeating: Avoid aggregating the data. Where appropriate, break data into meaningful components. If you serve several different customer groups, display performance and satisfaction data for each group. As Figure 34 demonstrates, only one of the three trends is positive, although the average is positive. Examiners will seek component data when aggregate data are reported. Presenting aggregate data instead of meaningful component data is likely to reduce the score.

Data and Measures

Comparison data are required for all items in Category 7. These data are designed to demonstrate how well the organization is performing. To judge performance excellence, one must possess comparison data. In Figure 35, performance is represented by the line connecting the squares. Clearly the organization is

improving, but how "good" is it? Without comparison data, answering that question is difficult.

Now consider the chart with comparison data added (Figure 36).

Note the position of three hypothetical comparisons, represented by the letters A, B, and C. Consider the following two scenarios:

1. If A represents the industry average and both B and C represent competitors, then examiners would conclude that your organization's performance was substandard, even though it is improving.

2. If A represents a best-in-class (benchmark) organization and B represents the industry average,

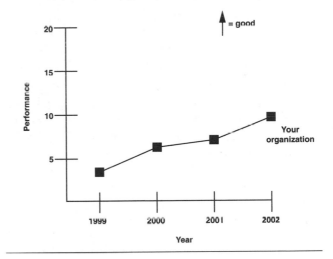

Figure 35 Getting better.

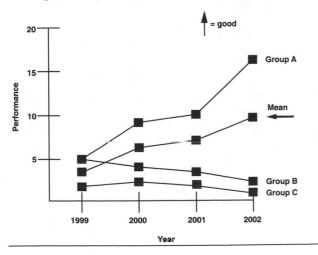

Figure 34 Break out group data.

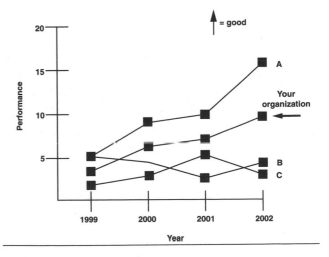

Figure 36 Comparison data.

then examiners would conclude that your organizational performance is very good.

In both scenarios, the organizational performance remained the same, but the examiner's perception of it changed based on comparison data.

Measures

Agreeing on relevant measures is a difficult task for organizations in the early phases of quality and performance improvement. The task is easier if the following guidelines are considered:

- *Clearly define patient and other customer requirements.* Clear requirements are easier to measure. Clearly defined requirements require probing and suggesting. For example, the patient and customer of a new heart monitor wants the equipment to be reliable. After probing to find what "reliable" means, we discover that the customer expects: (a) it to work all of the time; (b) prompt appearance by a repair technician at the site if it does stop working; (c) immediate access to parts; and (d) the ability to fix it right the first time.

- *For each of the four requirements defined, identify a measure.* For example, mean-time between failures is one indicator of reliability, but it does not account for all of the variation in patient and customer satisfaction. Since the customer is concerned with operational time, we must assess how long it took the repair technician to arrive at the site, diagnose the problem, and fix it. Measures include time in hours, days, weeks between failures, time in minutes between the service call and the monitor regaining capability (time to fix), time in minutes waiting for parts, and the associated costs in terms of lost patient business, cost, and staff time and effort.

- *Collect and report data.* Several charts might be required to display these factors, or one chart with several lines.

Scoring System

Scoring Dimensions are classified according to the kinds of information and/or data being reviewed. The two types of Items and their designations are:

1. Approach/Deployment (for the 13 Items in Categories 1–6)

2. Results (for the six Items in Category 7)

Applicants need to furnish information relating to these dimensions. Specific factors for these dimensions are described as follows:

Approach

Approach refers to how you address the Item requirements and what methods are used. The factors used to evaluate approaches include:

- Appropriateness of the methods to the requirements

- Effectiveness of use of the methods. Degree to which the approach:

  - Is repeatable, integrated, and consistently applied

  - Embodies evaluation/improvement/learning cycles

  - Is based on reliable information and data

- Alignment with organizational needs

- Evidence of beneficial innovation and change

Deployment

Deployment refers to the extent to which your approach is applied to all requirements of the Item. The factors used to evaluate deployment include:

- Use of the approach in addressing Item requirements relevant and important to your organization

- Use of the approach by all appropriate work units

Approach and Deployment are linked as Scoring Guidelines to emphasize that the strength or maturity of a process is related, in part, to the extent of use or deployment of the process—consistent with the specific requirements of the Item. Although Approach and Deployment dimensions are linked, feedback to award applicants may reflect strengths and/or opportunities for improvement in either or both dimensions.

Results

Results refers to outcomes in achieving the purposes given in the Item. The factors used to evaluate results include:

- Current performance

- Performance relative to appropriate comparisons and/or benchmarks

- Rate and breadth of performance improvements

- Linkage of results measures to important customer, market, process, and action plan performance requirements identified in the Organizational Profile and in Approach/ Deployment Items

Results Items call for data showing performance levels, relevant comparative data, and improvement trends for key measures/indicators of organizational performance. Results Items also call for data on breadth of performance improvements, that is, on how widespread your improvement results are. This is directly related to the Deployment dimension; if improvement processes are widely deployed, there should be corresponding results. A score for a Results Item is thus a composite based upon overall performance, taking into account the rate and breadth of improvements and their importance.

"Importance" as a Scoring Factor

Evaluation and feedback also consider the importance of the reported Approach, Deployment, and Results to the organization's key factors, which should be identified in the Organizational Profile and discussed in the narrative for Items, such as 2.1 (Strategy Development), 2.2 (Strategy Deployment), 3.1 (Patient, Other Customer and Market Knowledge), 3.2 (Patient and Other Customer Relationships and Satisfaction), 4.1 (Measurement and Analysis of Organizational Performance), 5.1 (Work Systems), 5.3 (Staff Well-Being and Satisfaction), 6.1 (Health Care Processes), 6.2 (Support Processes), and Category 7 (Organizational Performance Results). Your key patient and customer requirements and key strategic objectives and action plans are particularly important.

Assignment of Scores to Your Responses

Baldrige Award Examiners observe the following guidelines in assigning scores to applicants' responses:

- The multiple requirements of the Areas to Address should be included in the Item response. Also, responses should reflect what is important to the organization.

- In assigning a score to an Item, an Examiner first decides which scoring range (for example, 50 percent to 60 percent) best fits the overall Item response. Overall "best fit" does not require total agreement with each of the statements for that scoring range. The actual 10 percent score within the range that is assigned by

the Examiner depends upon an Examiner's judgment of the closeness of the Item response in relation to the statements in the next higher and next lower scoring ranges.

- An Approach/Deployment Item score of 50 percent represents an approach that meets the overall objectives of the Item and that is deployed to the principal activities and work units covered in the Item. In addition, the approach includes a fact-based process to evaluate the effectiveness of key Item requirements. A score of 60 percent represents an approach that meets the requirements at the 50 percent level described above plus evidence that at least one cycle of refinement was made in the process based on the fact-based evaluation. Higher scores reflect maturity (multiple cycles of improvement), integration, and broader deployment.

- A Results Item score of 50 percent represents a clear indication of improvement trends and/or good levels of performance in the principal results areas covered in the Item. Higher scores reflect better improvement rates and/or levels of performance, and better comparative performance as well as broader coverage and integration with business requirements.

Supplementary Scoring Guidelines

Author's note: Many examiners and organizations have found the official Scoring Guideline to be vague, although they have been improved considerably since the earlier years of the Award. The official Scoring Guidelines, presented in 20 percent increments, may increase the difficulty of reaching consensus on a score and increase scoring variation. To resolve this problem, I developed the following supplemental scoring guidelines. Many organizations and state award programs have used these guidelines for several years and found that they make the consensus process easier and produce comparable scores.

Approach/Deployment

1. For each Approach/Deployment Item, first determine the appropriate level on the approach scale. This sets the upper possible score the applicant may receive on the Item.

2. Then read the corresponding level on the deployment scale. For example, if the approach level is 40 percent, read the 40 percent standard on the deployment scale where one would expect "several work units are in the early stages of deployment," and "progress in achieving the primary purposes of the Item is not inhibited." If that is the case, the final score is 40 percent.

3. However, if the deployment score is lower than the approach score, then it establishes the lower range of possible final scores for the Item. The actual final score will be between the low and high scores. For example, if "many major gaps exist and progress is significantly inhibited," the lowest possible score would be 10 percent. This final score must be between 40 and 10 percent (for example, 10, 20, 30, or 40 percent).

4. Never increase an approach score based on better deployment.

5. Scoring Guidelines for Approach/Deployment Items are presented on the pages immediately following this scoring section.

Results

1. For Results Items, base your assessment only on the standards described on the results scale. Do not consider Approach or Deployment standards at all.

2. Determine the extent to which performance results are positive, complete, and at high levels relative to competitors or similar providers or an industry standard.

3. To determine the extent to which all important results are reported, examiners should develop a list of the key measures the applicant indicates are important. Start with the measures listed in the overview section. Then add to the key measures list based on key data reported in Item 2.1 and the goals in 2.2, as well as measures that may be mentioned in Categories 5 and 6. Key measures can be reported anywhere in an application.

CALIBRATION GUIDELINES

Defining scoring terms may help reduce unnecessary variability. I have frequently asked Examiners to define, in terms of percent, the meaning of "most." Some define "most" as 51 percent. Others have a higher standard, even up to 90 percent. Defining "good" and "very good" is even more difficult. To reduce this variability, the following guidelines are suggested:

Few:	Up to 15%
Some:	Greater than 15% to 30%
Many:	Greater than 30% to 50%
Most:	Greater than 50% to 80%
Nearly All:	Greater than 80% to less than 100%
All:	100%

Good:	For example, better than average for relevant competitors or similar providers; above industry average.
Very Good:	For example, in the top quartile of competitors or similar providers.
Excellent:	For example, at or near the top of competitors or similar providers; top 5 percent; best benchmark; better than best competitor.

Baldrige Scoring Guidelines	
Approach/Deployment	
0%	• No systematic approach evident; information is anecdotal.
10% to 20%	• The beginning of a systematic approach to the *basic* requirements of the Item is evident. • Major gaps exist in deployment that would inhibit progress in achieving the *basic* requirements of the Item. • Early stages of a transition from reacting to problems to a general improvement orientation are evident.
30% to 40%	• An effective, systematic approach, responsive to the *basic* requirements of the Item, is evident. • The approach is deployed, although some areas or work units are in early stages of deployment. • The beginning of a systematic approach to evaluation and improvement of key processes is evident.
50% to 60%	• An effective, systematic approach, responsive to the *overall* requirements of the Item and your key organizational requirements, is evident. • The approach is well deployed, although deployment may vary in some areas or work units. • A fact-based, systematic evaluation and improvement process is in place for improving the efficiency and effectiveness of key processes. • The approach is aligned with your basic organizational needs identified in the other Criteria Categories.
70% to 80%	• An effective, systematic approach, responsive to the *multiple* requirements of the Item and your current and changing educational service needs, is evident. • The approach is well deployed, with no significant gaps. • A fact-based, systematic evaluation and improvement process and organizational learning/sharing are key management tools; there is clear evidence of refinement, innovation, and improved integration as a result of organizational-level analysis and sharing. • The approach is well integrated with organizational needs identified in the other Criteria Categories.
90% to 100%	• An effective, systematic approach, fully responsive to *all* the requirements of the Item and all your current and changing educational service needs, is evident. • The approach is fully deployed without significant weaknesses or gaps in any areas or work units • A very strong, fact-based, systematic evaluation and improvement process and extensive organizational learning/sharing are key management tools; strong refinement, innovation, and integration, backed by excellent organizational-level analysis and sharing, are evident. • The approach is fully integrated with your organizational needs identified in the other Criteria Categories.

	Supplemental Approach/Deployment Scoring Guidelines	
Score	**Approach**	**Deployment**
0%	No systematic approach evident; anecdotal information	Anecdotal, undocumented.
10%	Early beginning of a systematic approach consistent with the *basic* purposes of the Item is somewhat evident. Mostly reactive approach to problems. Some basic requirements of the Item not addressed. In the earliest stages of transitioning from reacting to problems to a general improvement orientation.	Many major gaps exist in deployment. Progress in achieving basic purposes of Item is significantly inhibited.
20%	A partially systematic but beginning approach consistent with the *basic* purposes of the Item is evident. Generally reactive to problems. A few basic requirements of the Item not addressed. In the early stages of transitioning from reacting to problems to a general improvement orientation.	Some major gaps exist in deployment. Progress in achieving basic purposes of Item is noticeably inhibited.
30%	An effective, systematic approach is in place responsive to the *basic* purposes of the Item. No systematic approach to evaluation and improvement of basic Item processes is evident. Random improvements may have been made.	The approach is generally deployed although several units are in the earliest stages of deployment. Progress in achieving basic purposes of Item is minimally inhibited.
40%	An effective, systematic approach responsive to the *basic* purposes of the Item is in place. Several minor requirements of the Item are not addressed. Beginning of a systematic approach to evaluation and improvement of basic Item processes is evident. Random improvements may have been made.	The approach is deployed although several units are in the early stages of deployment. Progress in achieving basic purposes of Item is not inhibited.
50%	An effective, systematic approach is in place that is responsive to the *overall* purposes of the Item and educational service needs. Fact-based evaluation system is in place to evaluate the effectiveness and efficiency of basic Item processes (but no refinements based on this evaluation are in place). Random improvements may have been made. The approach is aligned with some basic organization needs identified in the Organizational Profile and other Criteria Categories.	No major gaps in deployment exist that inhibit progress in achieving overall purposes of Item, although deployment may vary in some areas or work units. Some work units still in the early stages of deployment.
60%	An effective, systematic approach is in place that is responsive to the *overall* purposes of the Item and educational service needs. Fact-based evaluation system is in place to evaluate the effectiveness and efficiency of basic Item processes, including some systematic refinement based on the evaluation. The approach is aligned with the most basic organization needs identified in the Organizational Profile and other Criteria Categories.	No major gaps in deployment exist that inhibit progress in achieving overall purposes of Item, although deployment may vary in some areas or work units. A few work units still are in the early stages of deployment.
70%	An effective, systematic approach is in place that is responsive to *many to most of the* multiple purposes of the Item and current and changing educational service needs. Organizational learning and sharing are frequently used management tools at many levels. Some cycles of systematic fact-based evaluation with evidence of refinements, improved integration, and organization-level analysis and learning. The approach is aligned and well-integrated with many overall organization needs identified in the Organizational Profile and other Criteria Categories.	Approach is well deployed with some work units in the middle to advanced stages. No significant gaps exist that inhibit progress in achieving many of the multiple purposes of Item.
80%	An effective, systematic approach is in place that is responsive to *most to nearly all of the* multiple purposes of the Item and current and changing educational service needs. Organizational learning and sharing are frequently used management tools at most levels. Many cycles of systematic fact-based evaluation with evidence of refinements, improved integration, and organization-level analysis and learning. The approach is aligned and well-integrated with most overall and many multiple organization needs identified in the Organizational Profile and other Criteria Categories.	Approach is well deployed with many work units in the advanced stages. No gaps exist that inhibit progress in achieving most of the multiple purposes of Item.
90%	An effective, systematic approach is in place that is responsive to *nearly all of the multiple* purposes of the Item and current and changing educational service needs. Extensive organizational innovation learning and sharing are key management tools at most levels. Considerable, systematic evaluation and extensive refinements; and improved organizational sharing and learning are key management tools at most levels. Some innovative processes are evident with strong refinement and integration supported by substantial organization-level analysis and sharing.	Approach is fully deployed with most work units in the advanced stages. No significant gaps or weaknesses exist in any areas or work units that inhibit progress in achieving nearly all of the multiple purposes of Item.
100%	An effective, systematic approach is in place that is responsive to *all of the multiple* purposes of the Item and all current and changing educational service needs, is clearly in place. Extensive organizational innovation, learning and sharing are key management tools at all levels. Considerable systematic evaluation; clear evidence of strong refinements; and improved organizational sharing and learning are key management tools at all levels.	Approach is fully deployed with nearly all to all work units in the advanced stages. No significant gaps or weaknesses exist in any areas or work units that inhibit progress in achieving all of the multiple purposes of Item.

Baldrige Scoring Guidelines	
Score	**Results**
0%	• There are no organizational performance results or poor results in areas reported.
10% to 20%	• There are some improvements and/or early good performance levels in a few areas. • Results are not reported for many to most areas of importance to your key organizational requirements.
30% to 40%	• Improvements *and/or* good performance levels are reported in many areas of importance to your key organizational requirements. • Early stages of developing trends and obtaining comparative information are evident. • Results are reported for many to most areas of importance to your key organizational requirements.
50% to 60%	• Improvement trends *and/or* good performance levels are reported for most areas of importance to your key organizational requirements. • No pattern of adverse trends and no poor performance levels are evident in areas of importance to your key organizational requirements. • Some trends *and/or* current performance levels—evaluated against relevant comparisons *and/or* benchmarks—show areas of strength *and/or* good to very good relative performance levels. • Organizational performance results address most key customer, market, and process requirements.
70% to 80%	• Current performance is good to excellent in areas of importance to your key organizational requirements. • Most improvement trends *and/or* current performance levels are sustained. • Many to most trends *and/or* current performance levels—evaluated against relevant comparisons *and/or* benchmarks—show areas of leadership and very good relative performance levels. • Organizational performance results address most key customer, market, process, and action plan requirements.
90% to 100%	• Current performance is excellent in most areas of importance to your key organizational requirements. • Excellent improvement trends *and/or* sustained excellent performance levels are reported in most areas. • Evidence of education sector and benchmark leadership is demonstrated in many areas. • Organizational performance results fully address key customer, market, process, and action plan requirements.

Supplemental Results Scoring Guidelines	
Score	**Results**
0%	No results or poor results in areas reported.
10%	Results not reported or evident for most areas of importance to the organization's key requirements. Limited positive results and/or limited good performance levels are evident for a few areas.
20%	Results not reported or evident for many areas of importance to the organization's key requirements. Some positive results and/or early good performance levels are evident for these areas.
30%	Results are reported or evident for many to most areas of importance to the key organizational requirements. Improvements or good performance levels are evident for many areas of importance to the organization's key requirements. Early stages of developing trends but no comparative data has been reported.
40%	Results are reported or evident for many to most areas of importance to the key organizational requirements. Improvements and good performance levels are evident for many areas of importance to the organization's key requirements. Some trend data and a little comparative information are reported.
50%	Results are reported or evident for most areas of importance to the key organizational requirements. Some positive trends and/or good performance levels—evaluated against relevant comparisons or benchmarks—show a few areas of strength or good relative performance levels. No poor performance levels are evident in areas of importance to key organization requirements.
60%	Results are reported or evident for most areas of importance to the key organizational requirements; they address most key customer, market, and process requirements. Some positive trends and/or good performance levels—evaluated against relevant comparisons and/or benchmarks—show areas of strength and/or good relative performance levels. No pattern of adverse trends and no poor performance levels in areas of importance to key organizational requirements. (A "pattern of adverse trends" is more than isolated declining or poor performance in a few areas.)
70%	Results are reported or evident for most areas of importance to the key organizational requirements; they address most key customer, market, process, and action plan requirements. Current performance is good (above average) in many areas important to key organizational requirements. Most improvement trends and/or current performance levels are sustained. Many trends and/or current performance levels—evaluated against relevant comparisons and/or benchmarks—show very good relative performance levels.
80%	Results are reported or evident for most areas of importance to the key organizational requirements; they address most key customer, market, process, and action plan requirements. Current performance is excellent in many areas important to key organizational requirements. Most improvement trends and/or current performance levels are sustained. Most trends and/or current performance levels—evaluated against relevant comparisons and/or benchmarks—show areas of leadership and very good relative performance levels.
90%	Results are reported or evident for most areas of importance to the key organizational requirements; they fully address nearly all key customer, market, process, and action plan requirements. Most performance trends and or sustained levels of performance in areas important to key organizational requirements are excellent. Improvement trends or current performance levels—evaluated against relevant comparisons or benchmarks—show areas of health care sector or benchmark leadership in many areas.
100%	Results are reported or evident for most areas of importance to the key organizational requirements; they fully address all key customer, market, process, and action plan requirements. Most current performance trends and or sustained levels of performance in areas important to key organizational requirements are excellent. Improvement trends or current performance levels—evaluated against relevant comparisons and/or benchmarks—show areas of health care sector and/or benchmark leadership in many areas.

APPROACH/DEPLOYMENT TERMS

Systematic

Look for evidence of a system—a repeatable, predictable process that uses data and information to promote improvement and learning—that is used to fulfill the requirements of the Item. Briefly describe the system. Be sure to explain how the system works. You must communicate the nature of the system to people who are not familiar with it. This is essential to achieve the 30 percent scoring threshold.

Integrated

Determine the extent to which the system is integrated or interconnected with other elements of the overall management system. Show the linkages across categories for key themes, such as those displayed earlier for each Item. Consider the extent to which the work of *senior leaders* is integrated. For example:

1. Senior executives (Item 1.1) are responsible for shaping and communicating the organization's values and performance expectations throughout the leadership system and workforce.

2. They develop relationships with patients and other key customers (Item 3.2) and monitor patient and customer satisfaction (Item 7.2), related health care results (Item 7.1), and other organization performance (Items 7.3, 7.4, 7.5, and 7.6).

3. Leaders must convert goals and strategic objectives into measurable milestones and timelines to serve as a basis for monitoring performance [Item 1.1c(1)] and setting improvement priorities [Item 1.1c(3)]. (Timelines [2.1b(1)] should be set to coincide with the review cycle of senior leaders. If they review progress quarterly, then quarterly timelines or milestones should be set.)

4. This information, when properly analyzed (Item 4.1), helps senior leaders plan and monitor progress better and make more informed decisions to optimize patient and customer satisfaction and operational and financial performance.

5. With this in mind, senior executives participate in strategy development (Item 2.1) and ensure the alignment of the workplace to achieve strategic objectives (Item 2.2).

6. Senior executives may also become involved in supporting new structures to improve staff performance and motivation (Item 5.1), training effectiveness (Item 5.2), and staff well-being and satisfaction (Item 5.3).

Similar relationships (linkages) exist between other items.

Prevention-Based

Prevention-based systems are characterized by actions to minimize or prevent the recurrence of problems. In an ideal world, all systems would produce perfect and flawless service. Since that rarely happens, high-performing organizations are able to act quickly to recover from a problem (fight the fire) and then take action to identify the root cause of the problem and prevent it from surfacing again. The nature of the problem, its root cause, and appropriate corrective action is communicated to all relevant staff so that they can implement the corrective action in their area before the problem arises.

Continuous Improvement

Continuous improvement is a bedrock theme. It is the method that helps organizations establish and keep their competitive edge. Continuous improvement involves the fact-based evaluation and improvement of processes crucial to organizational success. Evaluation and improvement completes the high-performance management cycle. Fact-based continuous improvement evaluations can be complex, statistical processes, or as simple as a focus group discussing *and recording* what went right, what went wrong, and how it could be done better. The key to optimum performance lies in the pervasive evaluation and improvement of all processes. By practicing systematic, pervasive, continuous improvement, time becomes the organization's ally. Consistent fact-based evaluation and refinement practices with correspondingly good deployment can drive the score to 60 percent or 70 percent, and higher.

Complete

Each Item contains one or more Areas to Address. Many Areas to Address contain several parts. Failure to address all areas and parts can push the score lower. If an Area to Address or part of an Area does not apply to your organization, it is important to explain why. Otherwise, examiners may conclude that the system is incomplete.

Anecdotal

If the application narrative describes a process or procedure that is random, ad hoc, or non-systematic and does not address the Criteria in a predictable, disciplined manner, it is worth very little (0 points).

Deployment

The extent to which processes are widely used by organization units affects scoring. For example, a systematic approach that is well-integrated, evaluated consistently, and refined routinely may be worth 70 percent to 90 percent. However, if that process is not in place in all key parts of the organization, the 70 percent to 90 percent score will be reduced, perhaps significantly, depending on the nature and extent of the deployment gap.

Major gaps are expected to exist at the 10 to 20 percent level. At the 30 percent and higher levels, no major gaps exist, although some units may still be at the early stages of development. At the 70 percent to 80 percent level, no major gaps exist and the approach is well-integrated with organizational needs identified in other parts of the criteria.

Summary

For each Item examined, the process is rated as follows:

- Anecdotal: 0 percent to 10 percent

- Beginnings of a systematic approach to meet *basic* Item requirements (perhaps recently piloted or implemented process): 10 percent or 20 percent

- Effective, systematic approach in place to meet *basic* Item requirements: 30 percent

- Effective, systematic approach in place to meet *basic* Item requirements with the beginnings (planned or piloted) of a process to evaluate and improve: 40 percent

- Effective, systematic approach in place to meet *overall* Item requirements with fact-based evaluation process in place: 50 percent

- Effective, systematic approach in place to meet *overall* Item requirements with fact-based evaluation process in place and at least one cycle of refinements based on the evaluation: 60 percent

- Effective, systematic approach in place to meet *multiple* Item requirements with fact-based evaluation process in place and multiple cycles of refinement, innovation, and integration based on the evaluation: 70 percent or 80 percent

- Integrated: 70 percent to 100 percent

- Refined: 60 percent to 100 percent

- Widely used, with no significant gaps in deployment: 70+ percent

Systematic, integrated, prevention-based, and continuously improved systems that are widely used are generally easier to describe than undeveloped systems. Moreover, describing activities or anecdotes does not convince examiners that an integrated, prevention-based system is in place. In fact, simply describing activities and anecdotes suggests that an integrated system does not exist. However, by tracing critical success threads through the relevant Items in the Criteria, the organization demonstrates that its system is integrated and fully deployed.

To demonstrate system integration, pick several critical success factors and show how the organization manages them. For example, trace the leadership focus on performance.

- Identify performance-related data that are collected to indicate progress against goals [Item 4.1].

- Show how performance data are analyzed [Item 4.1], reviewed by senior leaders [Item 1.1c(1)], and used to set priorities work for work and resources [Item 1.1c(3)].

- Show how performance effectiveness is considered in the planning process [Item 2.1a] and how work at all levels is aligned to increase performance [Item 2.2a].

- Demonstrate the impact of staff management [Item 5.1] and training [Item 5.2] on performance and show how both tie to the strategy and staff plans [Item 2.2a(3)].

- Show how health care and support processes [Items 6.1 and 6.2] are enhanced to improve results.

- Report the results of improved performance [Items 7.1, 7.2, 7.3, 7.4, 7.5, and 7.6] and be sure all key results are reported with key comparative or benchmark data included.

- Determine how improved health care results quality [7.1] affects patient and customer satisfaction levels [Item 7.2].

- Show how patient and other customer requirements and preferences [Item 3.1] and concerns [3.2] are used to drive the selection of key measures [Item 4.1] and to impact design and delivery processes [Item 6.1 and 6.2].

Note that the application is limited to 50 pages, not including the five-page Organizational Profile. This may not be sufficient to describe in great detail the approach, deployment, results, and systematic integration of all of your critical success factors, goals, or key processes. Thus, you must pick the most important few, indicate them as such, and then thoroughly describe the threads and linkages throughout the application.

Clarifying the Requirements for Basic-, Overall-, and Multiple-Level Scoring

INTRODUCTION

The Baldrige Criteria, together with the Scoring Guidelines, are supposed to help Examiners identify the key strengths and vital few areas needing improvement to help leaders focus their resources on the steps needed to get to the next developmental level. Unfortunately, for several years, national and State Examiners have tended to "nit-pick" applicants by citing minute, inconsequential opportunities for improvement—even when basic or fundamental processes were not in place. Because of the tendency to "nit-pick," scores were inappropriately low and comments were not properly focused.

To avoid this problem, the Baldrige Award office redefined the Scoring Guidelines to focus attention on a hierarchy of requirements moving from "basic" to "overall" to "multiple." The purpose of this hierarchy was to keep Examiners focused on the most important factors each applicant needed to put in place to get to the next level and not turn the examination process into a compliance checklist.

In other words, the strengths comments were supposed to describe the processes and systems an applicant had in place that supported or justified the score assigned. The opportunities for improvement were supposed to identify the processes or systems that were not in place that kept the organization from moving to the next higher level. By listing insignificant issues (nits) in the feedback report, an applicant might spend resources fixing a problem that had relatively low impact and overlook a key area essential for growth and improvement.

We believe that the Baldrige Award office was correct in identifying the need to prevent Examiners from "nit-picking" while getting them to focus on the vital few issues. To achieve this objective, *it is essential that all Examiners reviewing applications for a state, regional, or "in-house" Baldrige-based recognition program interpret the Criteria and Scoring Guidelines consistently.* Unfortunately, the process and definitions presented in the 2003 Criteria and Scoring Guidelines do not achieve this objective.

Based on extensive experience in training thousands of Examiners *each year* on the use of the Baldrige criteria, the greatest source of unacceptable variation is caused by Examiners focusing on different aspects of the Criteria during the review process. The lack of clarity in defining precisely what systems and/or processes are required for each scoring level and for each Item forces Examiners to decide for themselves the elements of each Item they deem more critical than others. With many different opinions of what constitutes basic and overall requirements, Examiners' comments and scores have not been consistent, either from team to team or Examiner to Examiner. For example, in each of six recent Examiner training classes conducted in 2003, I asked the Examiners to follow the Baldrige definitions and list the factors they would look for as a *basic* requirement of "Organizational Leadership" [Item 1.1]. Each class generated a list similar to the following.

The applicant organization and its senior leaders must have in place processes to:

- Set direction
- Set expectations
- Empower staff
- Focus on patients and customers
- Deploy values

- Set values

- Communicate values and directions to staff

- Engage in two-way communication with staff and patients and other customers

- Protect stakeholder and stockholder interests

- Hold leaders and managers accountable

- Review organizational performance

- Assess progress relative to goals

- Identify priorities for improvement

- Improve their personal leadership effectiveness

The list of "basic" requirements that the individual Examiners produced (required for a score of 10 percent to 40 percent) more accurately defines most of the "multiple" level requirements (needed for a score of 70 percent to 80 percent). With this kind of variation on one relatively straightforward Item, imagine the differences a team of six to 10 Examiners will have interpreting the requirements of the 13 Items in Categories 1 through 6 that use the Approach/ Deployment Scoring Guidelines. It is difficult to conduct a consistently accurate assessment when each Examiner's interpretation of the "basic" and "overall" requirements is so varied.

During the past year, several state and in-house organizational award programs pilot tested a new approach to help produce more consistently accurate assessments in both the government and private sectors. This technique provides Examiners with a more precise definition of "basic" and "overall" requirements for each Item (the multiple level requirements are already precise).

By providing consistent definitions of basic requirements, overall requirements, and multiple requirements, Examiners have been able to more accurately and consistently assess, score, and provide meaningful feedback to participating organizations or quality award applicants.

Official Baldrige Definitions

This section presents the actual definitions (in bold italic type) from the Baldrige Award office that created the confusion.

Basic Requirements

The term "basic requirements" refers to the most central concept of an Item. Basic requirements are the fundamental theme of that Item. In the Criteria, the basic requirements of each Item are presented as the Item title.

Meeting the basic requirements of the Item could result in a score at the 10 percent to 40 percent level depending on the level of development of the basic systems and on the extent of deployment of those systems.

Accordingly, for Item 1.1, an organization can meet the "basic" requirements by providing "Organizational Leadership" (the title of Item 1.1). For Item 2.1, the organization must have a process for "Strategy Development" (also undefined). What do these terms mean? What must "strategy development process" include? There is simply not enough information presented by these terms to ensure a consistent review, which is critical to ensure appropriate feedback and an accurate score.

Overall Requirements

The term "overall requirements" refers to the topics Criteria users need to address when responding to the central theme of an Item. Overall requirements address the most significant features of the Item requirements. In the Criteria, the overall requirements of each Item are presented as an introductory sentence(s) printed in bold.

Meeting the overall requirements of the Item could result in a score at the 50 percent or 60 percent level depending on the maturity of the overall systems, the extent of deployment of those systems, and the extent of systematic evaluation and refinement of those systems.

More detail is provided to define the "overall" level than is provided for the "basic" level. However, the explanation is still too limited to enable Examiners to provide a consistent review, appropriate feedback, and an accurate score.

For example, under the requirements of Item 1.1, senior leaders must "guide the organization" and "review organizational performance." The organization must also "describe its governance system." Under Item 2.1, the organization must have a system in place to establish "strategic objectives" and enhance its "competitive position." Ask any 10 people what systems might be needed to meet these requirements and you will receive 10 different answers.

Multiple Requirements

The term "multiple requirements" refers to the individual questions Criteria users need to answer within each Area to Address. These questions constitute the details of an Item's requirements. They are presented in black text under each Item's Area(s) to Address.

Meeting the multiple requirements of the Item could result in a score at the 70 percent to 100 percent level, depending on the maturity of the multiple systems, the extent of deployment of those systems, and the extent of systematic evaluation, refinement, innovation, and improved integration of those systems.

Unlike the "basic" and "overall" definitions, the "multiple" level definitions are quite clear. Sufficient detail is provided to enable Examiners to identify the elements of management systems and processes that must be in place to score at the 70 percent or higher level.

Importance as a Scoring Factor

Examiners must determine the extent to which the management systems and processes are responsive to the organization's *key health care requirements and changing health care service needs* (especially at the 50 percent and higher scoring bands). Accordingly, Examiners consider the extent to which processes in the application appear to support or respond to key health care organization needs that were expressed in the Organizational Profile and in Items such as:

- 2.1 Strategic objectives

- 2.2 Action plans and measures that derive from the strategic objectives and are deployed to all levels of the organization

- 3.1 The definition of patient and patient and customer segments, their requirements, and preferences for services that are most likely to drive loyalty

- 5.1 Work systems and systems to align staff feedback, reward, recognition and compensation with high performance, health care, and patient and customer-focused objectives

- 6.1 Key health care and key business and support processes critical to organizational success and growth

Clarifications for Scoring

The definitions on the following pages are intended to help improve consistency of interpretation and are offered as guidelines only. Prior to using these clarifying statements, the cognizant award program should reach consensus that the Basic, Overall, and Multiple requirements listed on the following pages appropriately capture the levels and meaning of the Criteria.

Examiners please remember that the notes at the end of each Item provide additional clarification about information that is expected as part of the review.

- The word "should" creates an expectation that the process is in place. For example, Note 2 for Item 1.1 indicates that "Senior leaders' organizational performance reviews [1.1c(1)] should be informed by organizational performance analyses described in 4.1b and guided by strategic objectives and action plans described in Items 2.1 and 2.2." This means that Examiners will be looking for, and expect to find, these linkages.

- The word "might" is meant to suggest alternatives or examples, but not establish the expectation that the process is required. For example, the same Note 2 in 1.1 indicates that "Senior leaders' organizational performance reviews *might* be informed by internal or external Baldrige assessments." This means that Examiners cannot require such reviews to be used to assess organizational performance or capabilities and should not write an Opportunity for Improvement comment or lower the score if the organization's senior leaders do not use such reviews.

To make the following clarifying tables more complete, the Scoring Guidelines are presented in the first column as a reminder of the key points in the scoring for each level.

Remember, the following analysis is presented only as a guideline that state, local, and in-house recognition programs may want to consider in order to help Examiners provide more consistent and meaningful scoring and feedback to applicants.

Scoring Guidelines	1.1 Organizational Leadership Expected Observations
10%–20% The beginning of a systematic approach to the *basic* requirements of the Item is evident. Major gaps exist in deployment that would inhibit progress in achieving the basic requirements of the Item. Early stages of a transition from reacting to problems to a general improvement orientation are evident.	*1.1 Organizational Leadership.* Senior leaders are in the beginning stages of establishing and implementing systems and/or processes to lead the organization and review organizational performance. *The values and approaches that guide the organization and its senior leaders are not widely or clearly understood. The organizational review processes are not uniform and may overlook many key measures important to organizational success.*
30%–40% An effective, systematic approach, responsive to the *basic* requirements of the Item, is evident. The approach is deployed, although some areas or work units are in early stages of deployment. The beginning of a systematic approach to evaluation and improvement of key processes is evident.	*1.1 Organizational Leadership.* Senior leaders have effective, systematic processes in place to lead the organization and review organizational performance. *The values and approaches that guide the organization and its senior leaders are generally understood. The organizational review processes generally consider key measures of organizational success, but a few measures may be overlooked. Senior leaders are beginning to evaluate and improve these processes.*
50%–60% An effective, systematic approach, responsive to the *overall* requirements of the Item and your key health care requirements, is evident. The approach is well deployed, although deployment may vary in some areas or work units. A fact-based, systematic evaluation and improvement process is in place for improving the efficiency and effectiveness of key processes. The approach is aligned with your basic organizational needs identified in the other Criteria Categories.	*1.1 Organizational Leadership.* Senior leaders have effective, systematic processes in place to do the following: a. *Senior Leadership Direction.* Communicate and reinforce directions and performance expectations with a focus on delivering value to patients and other key customers. b. *Organizational Governance.* Ensure management accountability for the organization's actions and the protection of stockholder and stakeholder interests. c. *Organizational Performance Review.* Review organizational performance and progress relative to goals/strategic objectives. *Some relatively minor gaps may exist in the deployment of these processes in some parts of the organization. However, there is a systematic, fact-based process in place to evaluate and improve the key elements of (a), (b), and (c) above.*

Continued

1.1 Organizational Leadership	*Continued*
Scoring Guidelines	**Expected Observations**

70%–80% An effective, systematic approach, responsive to the *multiple* requirements of the Item and your current and changing health care needs, is evident. The approach is well deployed, with no significant gaps. A fact-based, systematic evaluation and improvement process and organizational learning/sharing are key management tools; there is clear evidence of refinement, innovation, and improved integration as a result of organizational-level analysis and sharing. The approach is well integrated with organizational needs identified in the other Criteria Categories.

90%–100% An effective, systematic approach, fully responsive to *all* the requirements of the Item and all your current and changing health care needs, is evident. The approach is fully deployed without significant weaknesses or gaps in any areas or work units. A very strong, fact-based, systematic evaluation and improvement process and extensive organizational learning/sharing are key management tools; strong refinement, innovation, and integration, backed by excellent organizational-level analysis and sharing, are evident. The approach is fully integrated with your organizational needs identified in the other Criteria Categories.

1.1 Organizational Leadership. Senior leaders have well-deployed, effective, systematic processes in place to do the following:

a. *Senior Leadership Direction*
   (1) Senior leaders—
   - Set and deploy organizational values, short- and longer-term directions, and performance expectations
   - Include a focus on creating and balancing value for patients and customers and other stakeholders in their performance expectations
   - Communicate organizational values, directions, and expectations through the leadership system, to all staff, and to key suppliers and partners
   - Ensure two-way communication on these topics
   (2) Senior leaders create an environment—
   - For empowerment, innovation, and organizational agility
   - For organizational and staff learning
   - That fosters and requires legal and ethical behavior

b. *Organizational Governance.* The organization addresses the following key factors in your governance system.
   - Management accountability for the organization's actions
   - Budgetary and fiscal accountability
   - Independence in internal and external audits
   - Protection of stockholder and stakeholder interests, as appropriate

c. *Organizational Performance Review*
   (1) Senior leaders review organizational performance and capabilities and use these reviews to—
   - Assess organizational success, competitive performance, and progress relative to short- and longer-term goals.
   - Assess your organizational ability to address changing organizational needs.
   (2) Key performance measures regularly reviewed by senior leaders are defined and key recent performance review findings are reported.
   (3) Senior leaders translate organizational performance review findings into priorities for continuous and breakthrough improvement of key organizational results and into opportunities for innovation. These priorities and opportunities are deployed throughout your organization and, when appropriate, to affected suppliers and partners to ensure organizational alignment.
   (4) The performance of senior leaders, including the chief executive and, as appropriate, members of the board of directors is systematically evaluated. Senior leaders use organizational performance review findings to improve both their own leadership effectiveness and that of the board and leadership system, as appropriate.

The approach is well deployed with no significant gaps. In addition, there is a systematic, fact-based process in place to evaluate and improve (a), (b), and (c) above with clear evidence of innovation, learning, and organizational sharing, which results in refinements and improved integration.

Notes:

N1. Organizational directions [1.1a(1)] relate to creating the vision for the organization and to setting the context for strategic objectives and action plans described in Items 2.1 and 2.2.

N2. Senior leaders' organizational performance reviews [1.1c) *should* be informed by organizational performance analyses described in 4.1b and guided by strategic objectives and action plans described in Items 2.1 and 2.2. Senior leaders' organizational performance reviews also *might* be informed by internal or external Baldrige assessments.

N3. Leadership performance evaluation [1.1c(4)] *might* be supported by peer reviews, formal performance management reviews (5.1b), and formal and/or informal staff and other stakeholder feedback and surveys.

N4. Your organizational performance results *should* be reported in Items 7.1 – 7.6.

1.2 Social Responsibility	
Scoring Guidelines	**Expected Observations**
10%–20% The beginning of a systematic approach to the *basic* requirements of the Item is evident. Major gaps exist in deployment that would inhibit progress in achieving the basic requirements of the Item. Early stages of a transition from reacting to problems to a general improvement orientation are evident.	*1.2 Social Responsibility.* The organization is in the beginning stages of establishing systems and processes to address the organization's responsibilities to the public, such as complying with laws and regulations. *Major gaps exist where the processes do not cover many key regulatory or legal requirements in many parts of the organization.*
30%–40% An effective, systematic approach, responsive to the *basic* requirements of the Item, is evident. The approach is deployed, although some areas or work units are in early stages of deployment. The beginning of a systematic approach to evaluation and improvement of key processes is evident.	*1.2 Social Responsibility.* The organization has effective, systematic processes in place to address the organization's responsibilities to the public, such as complying with laws and regulations. *The processes cover most key regulatory or legal requirements in most parts of the organization.* *The organization is beginning to evaluate and make some improvements in the key elements of these processes.*
50%–60% An effective, systematic approach, responsive to the *overall* requirements of the Item and your key health care requirements, is evident. The approach is well deployed, although deployment may vary in some areas or work units. A fact-based, systematic evaluation and improvement process is in place for improving the efficiency and effectiveness of key processes. The approach is aligned with your basic organizational needs identified in the other Criteria Categories.	*1.2 Social Responsibility.* The organization has effective, systematic processes in place to do the following: a. *Responsibilities to the Public.* Address regulatory and other legal requirements; anticipate public concerns and address risks to the public. b. *Ethical Behavior.* Ensure ethical behavior in most parts of the organization. c. *Support of Key Communities.* Strengthen and support key communities important to the organization. *Some relatively minor gaps may exist in the deployment of these processes in some parts of the organization. However, there is a systematic, fact-based process in place to evaluate and improve the key elements of (a), (b), and (c) above.*

Continued

1.2 Social Responsibility	*Continued*
Scoring Guidelines	**Expected Observations**

70%–80% An effective, systematic approach, responsive to the *multiple* requirements of the Item and your current and changing health care needs, is evident. The approach is well deployed, with no significant gaps. A fact-based, systematic evaluation and improvement process and organizational learning/sharing are key management tools; there is clear evidence of refinement, innovation, and improved integration as a result of organizational-level analysis and sharing. The approach is well integrated with organizational needs identified in the other Criteria Categories.

90%–100% An effective, systematic approach, fully responsive to *all* the requirements of the Item and all your current and changing health care needs, is evident. The approach is fully deployed without significant weaknesses or gaps in any areas or work units. A very strong, fact-based, systematic evaluation and improvement process and extensive organizational learning/sharing are key management tools; strong refinement, innovation, and integration, backed by excellent organizational-level analysis and sharing, are evident. The approach is fully integrated with your organizational needs identified in the other Criteria Categories.

1.2 Social Responsibility. The organization has well-deployed, effective, systematic processes in place to do the following:

a. *Responsibilities to the Public*
 (1) Address the impacts on society of your programs, offerings, services, and operations. Put in place appropriate compliance processes, measures, and goals for achieving and surpassing accreditation, regulatory, and legal requirements. Put in place key processes, measures, and goals for addressing risks associated with programs, offerings, services, and operations.
 (2) Anticipate public concerns with current and future programs, offerings, services, and operations. Prepare for these concerns in a proactive manner.

b. *Ethical Behavior*
 Ensure ethical behavior in all stakeholder transactions and interactions. Put processes in place with appropriate measures or indicators for monitoring ethical behavior throughout the organization, with key partners, and in the governance structure.

c. *Support of Key Communities*
 Identify, support, and strengthen key communities and determine areas of emphasis for organizational involvement and support. Senior leaders and staff contribute to improving these communities.

The approach is well deployed with no significant gaps. In addition, there is a systematic, fact-based process in place to evaluate and improve (a), (b), and (c) above with clear evidence of innovation, learning, and organizational sharing, which results in refinements and improved integration.

Notes:

N1. Societal responsibilities in areas critical to your industry also *should* be addressed in Strategy Development [Item 2.1] and in Process Management [Category 6]. Key results, such as results of regulatory and legal compliance or environmental improvements through use of "green" technology or other means, *should be* reported as Governance and Social Responsibility Results [Item 7.6].

N2. Measures or indicators of ethical behavior [1.2b] *might* include the percentage of independent board members, measures of relationships with stockholder and nonstockholder constituencies, and results of ethics reviews and audits.

N3. Areas of community support appropriate for inclusion in 1.2c *might* include your efforts to strengthen local community services, education, and health; the environment; and practices of trade, health care, or professional associations.

N4. The health and safety of staff are not addressed in Item 1.2; you *should* address these staff factors in Item 5.3.

2.1 Strategy Development	
Scoring Guidelines	**Expected Observations**
10%–20% The beginning of a systematic approach to the *basic* requirements of the Item is evident. Major gaps exist in deployment that would inhibit progress in achieving the basic requirements of the Item. Early stages of a transition from reacting to problems to a general improvement orientation are evident.	*2.1 Strategy Development.* The organization is in the beginning stages of developing its strategic objectives. *Major gaps exist where the strategic planning process does not consider many business requirements or challenges (which may have been presented in the organizational profile) that are key to future business success and essential to effective strategic planning.*
30%–40% An effective, systematic approach, responsive to the *basic* requirements of the Item, is evident. The approach is deployed, although some areas or work units are in early stages of deployment. The beginning of a systematic approach to evaluation and improvement of key processes is evident.	*2.1 Strategy Development.* The organization has effective, systematic processes in place to develop its strategic objectives. *The planning and related strategic objectives cover some business requirements or challenges (which may have been presented in the organizational profile) that are key to future business success and essential to effective strategic planning. The organization is beginning to evaluate and make some improvements in the key elements of these processes.*
50%–60% An effective, systematic approach, responsive to the *overall* requirements of the Item and your key health care requirements, is evident. The approach is well deployed, although deployment may vary in some areas or work units. A fact-based, systematic evaluation and improvement process is in place for improving the efficiency and effectiveness of key processes. The approach is aligned with your basic organizational needs identified in the other Criteria Categories.	*2.1 Strategy Development.* The organization has effective, systematic processes in place to do the following: a. *Strategy Development Process.* Examine key organizational strengths, weaknesses, opportunities, and threats. b. *Strategic Objectives.* Develop clear strategic objectives to enhance competitive position, overall performance, and future success. *Some relatively minor gaps may exist in the process of planning and setting strategic objectives.* *However, there is a systematic, fact-based process in place to evaluate and improve the key elements of (a) and (b) above.*

Continued

2.1 Strategy Development		*Continued*
Scoring Guidelines	**Expected Observations**	

70%–80% An effective, systematic approach, responsive to the *multiple* requirements of the Item and your current and changing health care needs, is evident. The approach is well deployed, with no significant gaps. A fact-based, systematic evaluation and improvement process and organizational learning/sharing are key management tools; there is clear evidence of refinement, innovation, and improved integration as a result of organizational-level analysis and sharing. The approach is well integrated with organizational needs identified in the other Criteria Categories.

90%–100% An effective, systematic approach, fully responsive to *all* the requirements of the Item and all your current and changing health care needs, is evident. The approach is fully deployed without significant weaknesses or gaps in any areas or work units. A very strong, fact-based, systematic evaluation and improvement process and extensive organizational learning/sharing are key management tools; strong refinement, innovation, and integration, backed by excellent organizational-level analysis and sharing, are evident. The approach is fully integrated with your organizational needs identified in the other Criteria Categories.

2.1 Strategy Development. The organization has well-deployed, effective, systematic processes in place to do the following:

a. *Strategy Development Process*
  (1) Define the overall strategic planning process including key steps, key participants, short- and longer-term planning time horizons, and a description of these timing horizons, and the manner by which the strategic planning process addresses these timing horizons.
  (2) Collect and analyze data and information relevant to strategic planning and ensure that strategic planning addresses the key factors listed below:
    i.   Patient and customer and market needs, expectations, and opportunities
    ii.   Competitive environment and capabilities relative to competitors
    iii. Technological and other key innovations or changes that might affect products, services, and operations
    iv.   Internal strengths and weaknesses, including human and other resources
    v.   Opportunities to redirect resources to higher priority programs, offerings, services, or areas
    vi.   Financial, societal and ethical, regulatory, and other potential risks
    vii. Changes in the national or global economy
    viii. Factors unique to the organization, including partner and supply chain needs, strengths, and weaknesses

b. *Strategic Objectives*
  (1) Define key strategic objectives and the timetable for accomplishing them. Define the most important goals for these strategic objectives.
  (2) Ensure that strategic objectives—
    • Address the challenges identified in response to P.2 in the Organizational Profile.
    • Balance short-term and longer-term challenges and opportunities.
    • Balance the needs of all key stakeholders.

The approach is well deployed with no significant gaps. In addition, there is a systematic, fact-based process in place to evaluate and improve (a) and (b) above with clear evidence of innovation, learning, and organizational sharing, which results in refinements and improved integration.

Notes:

N1. "Strategy development" refers to your organization's approach (formal or informal) to preparing for the future. Strategy development *might* utilize various types of forecasts, projections, options, scenarios, and/or other approaches to envisioning the future for purposes of decision making and resource allocation.

N2. "Strategy" *should* be interpreted broadly. Strategy *might* be built around or lead to any or all of the following: new services and markets; revenue growth via various approaches, including acquisitions; and new partnerships and alliances. Strategy *might* be directed toward becoming a preferred supplier, a local supplier in each of your major patient and customers' markets, a low-cost producer, a market innovator, or a high-end or customized health care service provider.

N3. Strategies to address key challenges [2.1b(2)] *might* include rapid response, customization, rapid innovation, ISO 9000:2000 registration. Web-based supplier and patient- and customer-relationship management, and service quality. Responses to Item 2.1 *should* focus on your specific challenges—those most important to your health care success and to strengthening your organization's overall performance.

N4. Item 2.1 addresses your overall organizational strategy, which *might* include changes in services. However, the Item does not address health care service and program design; you *should* address these factors in Item 6.1, as appropriate.

2.2 Strategic Deployment	
Scoring Guidelines	**Expected Observations**
10%–20% The beginning of a systematic approach to the *basic* requirements of the Item is evident. Major gaps exist in deployment that would inhibit progress in achieving the basic requirements of the Item. Early stages of a transition from reacting to problems to a general improvement orientation are evident.	*2.2 Strategy Deployment.* The organization is in the beginning stages of developing its action plans to carry out the strategic objectives. *Major gaps exist where the action plans do not cover many elements essential to effective deployment of strategic objectives.*
30%–40% An effective, systematic approach, responsive to the *basic* requirements of the Item, is evident. The approach is deployed, although some areas or work units are in early stages of deployment. The beginning of a systematic approach to evaluation and improvement of key processes is evident.	*2.2 Strategy Deployment.* The organization has effective, systematic processes in place to convert its strategic objectives into action plans. *Action plans have been developed for most strategic objectives in most areas important to the organization.* *The organization is beginning to evaluate and make some improvements in the key elements of these processes.*
50%–60% An effective, systematic approach, responsive to the *overall* requirements of the Item and your key health care requirements, is evident. The approach is well deployed, although deployment may vary in some areas or work units. A fact-based, systematic evaluation and improvement process is in place for improving the efficiency and effectiveness of key processes. The approach is aligned with your basic organizational needs identified in the other Criteria Categories.	*2.2 Strategy Deployment.* The organization has effective, systematic processes in place to do the following: a. *Action Plan Development and Deployment.* Convert strategic objectives into action plans and related performance measures or indicators. b. *Performance Projection.* Project future performance levels for key measures or indicators. *Some relatively minor gaps may exist in these processes in some parts of the organization.* *However, there is a systematic, fact-based process in place to evaluate and improve the key elements of (a) and (b) above.*

Continued

2.2 Strategic Deployment		*Continued*
Scoring Guidelines	**Expected Observations**	

70%–80% An effective, systematic approach, responsive to the *multiple* requirements of the Item and your current and changing health care needs, is evident. The approach is well deployed, with no significant gaps. A fact-based, systematic evaluation and improvement process and organizational learning/sharing are key management tools; there is clear evidence of refinement, innovation, and improved integration as a result of organizational-level analysis and sharing. The approach is well integrated with organizational needs identified in the other Criteria Categories.

90%–100% An effective, systematic approach, fully responsive to *all* the requirements of the Item and all your current and changing health care needs, is evident. The approach is fully deployed without significant weaknesses or gaps in any areas or work units. A very strong, fact-based, systematic evaluation and improvement process and extensive organizational learning/sharing are key management tools; strong refinement, innovation, and integration, backed by excellent organizational-level analysis and sharing, are evident. The approach is fully integrated with your organizational needs identified in the other Criteria Categories.

2.2 Strategy Deployment. The organization has well-deployed, effective, systematic processes in place to do the following:

a. *Action Plan Development and Deployment*
  (1) Develop and deploy action plans to achieve key strategic objectives. Allocate resources to ensure accomplishment of action plans. Ensure that the key changes resulting from action plans can be sustained.
  (2) Define key short- and longer-term action plans. Define key changes, if any, in products and services, customers and markets, and in operations.
  (3) Define key staff plans that derive from short- and longer-term strategic objectives and action plans.
  (4) Define key performance measures or indicators for tracking progress with action plans. Ensure that the overall action plan measurement system reinforces organizational alignment and covers all key deployment areas and stakeholders.

b. *Performance Projection*
  Define both short- and longer-term time performance projections horizons for the key performance measures or indicators identified in 2.2a(4). Show how the organization's projected performance compares with competitors' projected performance, key benchmarks, goals, and past performance, as appropriate.

The approach is well deployed with no significant gaps. In addition, there is a systematic, fact-based process in place to evaluate and improve (a) and (b) above with clear evidence of innovation, learning, and organizational sharing, which results in refinements and improved integration.

Notes:

N1. Strategy and action plan development and deployment are closely linked to other Items in the Criteria. Examples of key linkages are:
  • Item 1.1 for how your senior leaders set and communicate directions
  • Category 3 for gathering patient and customer and market knowledge as input to your strategy and action plans and for deploying action plans;
  • Category 4 for information, analysis and knowledge management to support your key information needs; to support your development of strategy; to provide an effective basis for your performance measurements; and to track progress relative to your strategic objectives and action plans
  • Category 5 for your work system needs; staff education, training, and development needs; and related human resource factors resulting from action plans;
  • Category 6 for process requirements resulting from your action plans
  • Item 7.5 for specific accomplishments relative to your organizational strategy and action plans

N2. Measures and indicators of projected performance [2.2b] *might* include changes resulting from new health care ventures; health care acquisitions or mergers; new health care processes; market entry and shifts; and significant anticipated innovations in programs, services, and technology.

3.1 Patient, Other Customer, and Health Care Market Knowledge	
Scoring Guidelines	**Expected Observations**
10%–20% The beginning of a systematic approach to the *basic* requirements of the Item is evident. Major gaps exist in deployment that would inhibit progress in achieving the basic requirements of the item. Early stages of a transition from reacting to problems to a general improvement orientation are evident.	*3.1 Patient/Customer and Health Care Market Knowledge.* The organization is in the beginning stages of acquiring patient and customer and market knowledge to identify their requirements and/or expectations. *Major gaps exist where the listening and learning (knowledge acquisition) processes do not cover many customer segments or groups essential to effectively understand their requirements.*
30%–40% An effective, systematic approach, responsive to the *basic* requirements of the Item, is evident. The approach is deployed, although some areas or work units are in early stages of deployment. The beginning of a systematic approach to evaluation and improvement of key processes is evident.	*3.1 Patient/Customer and Health Care Market Knowledge.* The organization has effective, systematic processes in place to acquire (listen and learn about) patient and customer and market knowledge to identify their requirements and/or expectations for most key patient and customer and market segments. *The organization is beginning to evaluate and make some improvements in the key elements of these processes.*
50%–60% An effective, systematic approach, responsive to the *overall* requirements of the Item and your key health care requirements, is evident. The approach is well deployed, although deployment may vary in some areas or work units. A fact-based, systematic evaluation and improvement process is in place for improving the efficiency and effectiveness of key processes. The approach is aligned with your basic organizational needs identified in the other Criteria Categories.	*3.1 Patient/Customer and Health Care Market Knowledge.* The organization has effective, systematic processes in place to do the following: a. *Patient/Customer, and Health Care Market Knowledge.* Determine (target) market and patient and customer segments. Listen and learn about patient and customer requirements, expectations, and preferences to determine the relative value and ensure the continuing relevance of programs and services and develop new health care opportunities. *Some relatively minor gaps may exist in these processes in some parts of the organization, with some customer or market segments, or with some programs and services.* *However, there is a systematic, fact-based process in place to evaluate and improve the key elements of (a) above.*

Continued

3.1 Patient, Other Customer, and Health Care Market Knowledge   *Continued*

Scoring Guidelines

70%–80% An effective, systematic approach, responsive to the *multiple* requirements of the Item and your current and changing health care needs, is evident. The approach is well deployed, with no significant gaps. A fact-based, systematic evaluation and improvement process and organizational learning/sharing are key management tools; there is clear evidence of refinement, innovation, and improved integration as a result of organizational-level analysis and sharing. The approach is well integrated with organizational needs identified in the other Criteria Categories.

90%–100% An effective, systematic approach, fully responsive to *all* the requirements of the Item and all your current and changing health care needs, is evident. The approach is fully deployed without significant weaknesses or gaps in any areas or work units. A very strong, fact-based, systematic evaluation and improvement process and extensive organizational learning/sharing are key management tools; strong refinement, innovation, and integration, backed by excellent organizational-level analysis and sharing, are evident. The approach is fully integrated with your organizational needs identified in the other Criteria Categories.

Expected Observations

3.1 Patient/Customer and Health Care Market Knowledge. The organization has well-deployed, effective, systematic processes in place to do the following:

a. *Patient/Customer, and Health Care Market Knowledge.*
  (1) Determine or target patient and customers, patient and customer groups, and market segments after considering the requirements of patient and customers of competitors and other potential patient and customers and markets.
  (2) Determine key patient and customer requirements and expectations (including product and service features) and their relative importance to patient and customers purchasing decisions. To effectively determine patient and customer expectations and preferences—
  • Adjust the methods of determining patient and customer requirements and preferences according to the unique needs of these different groups.
  • Use relevant information from current and former patient and customers, including marketing and sales information, patient and customer loyalty and retention data, win/loss analysis, and complaints in the determination of patient and customer requirements and preferences.
  • Use this information for health care program and service planning, marketing, process improvements, and health care development.
  (3) Keep your listening and learning methods current with health care service needs and directions.

The approach is well deployed with no significant gaps. In addition, there is a systematic, fact-based process in place to evaluate and improve (a) above with clear evidence of innovation, learning, and organizational sharing, which results in refinements and improved integration.

Notes:

N1. Patients, as a key customer group, are frequently identified separately in the Criteria. Other customer groups could include patients' families, the community, insurers and other third-party payors, employers, health care providers, patient advocacy groups, Department of Health, and students. Generic references to customers include patients.

N2. Your responses to this Item *should* include the patient and customer groups and market segments identified in P.1b(2).

N3. "Health care service features" [3.1a(2)] refers to all the important characteristics of products and services and to their performance throughout their full life cycle and the full "consumption chain." This includes all patient and customers' purchase experiences and other interactions with your organization that influence purchase decisions. The focus *should* be on features that affect patient and customer preference and repeat health care—for example, those features that differentiate your products and services from competing offerings. Those features *might* include price, reliability, value, delivery requirements for hazardous materials use, disposal, patient and customer or technical support, and the sales relationship. Key program and service features and purchasing decisions (3.1a(2)] *might* take into account how transactions occur and factors, such as confidentiality and security.

N4. Listening and learning [3.1a(2)] *might* include gathering and integrating surveys, focus group findings, and Web-based and other data and information that bear upon patient and customers' purchasing decisions. Keeping your listening and learning methods current with health care service needs and directions [3.1a(3)] also *might* include use of newer technology, such as Web-based data gathering.

3.2 Patient and Other Customer Relationships and Satisfaction	
Scoring Guidelines	**Expected Observations**
10%–20% The beginning of a systematic approach to the *basic* requirements of the Item is evident. Major gaps exist in deployment that would inhibit progress in achieving the basic requirements of the Item. Early stages of a transition from reacting to problems to a general improvement orientation are evident.	*3.2 Patient and Other Customer Relationships and Satisfaction.* The organization is in the beginning stages of establishing good relationships with patients and customers and assessing their levels of satisfaction. *Major gaps exist where the relationship building and/or satisfaction determination processes do not cover many customer segments/groups and/or products and services.*
30%–40% An effective, systematic approach, responsive to the *basic* requirements of the Item, is evident. The approach is deployed, although some areas or work units are in early stages of deployment. The beginning of a systematic approach to evaluation and improvement of key processes is evident.	*3.2 Patient and Other Customer Relationships and Satisfaction.* The organization has effective, systematic processes in place to establish good relationships and assess the levels of satisfaction with most patient and customer groups/segments and most products/services. *The organization is beginning to evaluate and make some improvements in the key elements of these processes.*
50%–60% An effective, systematic approach, responsive to the *overall* requirements of the Item and your key health care requirements, is evident. The approach is well deployed, although deployment may vary in some areas or work units. A fact-based, systematic evaluation and improvement process is in place for improving the efficiency and effectiveness of key processes. The approach is aligned with your basic organizational needs identified in the other Criteria Categories.	*3.2 Patient and Other Customer Relationships and Satisfaction.* The organization has effective, systematic processes in place to do the following: a. *Patient/Customer Relationships.* Build relationships to acquire, satisfy, and retain patient and customers, increase loyalty, and develop new health care services. b. *Patient/Customer Satisfaction Determination.* Determine patient and customer satisfaction. *Some relatively minor gaps may exist in these processes in some parts of the organization, with some customer or market segments, or with some products and services* *However, there is a systematic, fact-based process in place to evaluate and improve the key elements of (a) and (b) above.*

Continued

3.2 Patient and Other Customer Relationships and Satisfaction	*Continued*
Scoring Guidelines	**Expected Observations**

70%–80% An effective, systematic approach, responsive to the *multiple* requirements of the Item and your current and changing health care needs, is evident. The approach is well deployed, with no significant gaps. A fact-based, systematic evaluation and improvement process and organizational learning/sharing are key management tools; there is clear evidence of refinement, innovation, and improved integration as a result of organizational-level analysis and sharing. The approach is well integrated with organizational needs identified in the other Criteria Categories.

90%–100% An effective, systematic approach, fully responsive to *all* the requirements of the Item and all your current and changing health care needs, is evident. The approach is fully deployed without significant weaknesses or gaps in any areas or work units. A very strong, fact-based, systematic evaluation and improvement process and extensive organizational learning/sharing are key management tools; strong refinement, innovation, and integration, backed by excellent organizational-level analysis and sharing, are evident. The approach is fully integrated with your organizational needs identified in the other Criteria Categories.

3.2 Patient and Other Customer Relationships and Satisfaction. The organization has well-deployed, effective, systematic processes in place to do the following:

a. *Patient and Other Customer Relationship Building*
   (1) Build relationships to acquire patients and customers, meet and exceed their expectations, increase loyalty and repeat health care business, and gain positive referrals.
   (2) Establish—
   • Access mechanisms to make it easy for patients and customers to seek information, conduct health care transactions, and make complaints.
   • Patient and customer contact requirements for each mode of patient and customer access and ensure that these contact requirements are deployed to all people and processes involved in the patient and customer response chain.
   (3) Establish an effective complaint management process to ensure that complaints are resolved effectively and promptly. Aggregate and analyze the complaints and use this information to drive improvements throughout the organization and to affected partners.
   (4) Keep approaches to building relationships and providing patient and customer access current with health care service needs and directions.

b. *Patient and Other Customer Satisfaction Determination*
   (1) Determine patient and customer satisfaction and dissatisfaction and adjust these determination methods according to the needs of differing patient and customer groups.
   • Ensure that measurements capture actionable information for use in exceeding your patient and customers' expectations, securing their future health care business, and gaining positive referrals.
   • Use patient and customer satisfaction and dissatisfaction information to drive improvements.
   (2) Follow up with patients and customers on programs, services, and transaction quality to receive prompt and actionable feedback.
   (3) Obtain and use information about your patient and customers' satisfaction relative to the patient and customers' satisfaction with competitors and/or industry benchmarks.
   (4) Keep your approaches to determining satisfaction current with health care service needs and directions.

The approach is well deployed with no significant gaps. In addition, there is a systematic, fact-based process in place to evaluate and improve (a) and (b) above with clear evidence of innovation, learning, and organizational sharing,which results in refinements and improved integration.

Notes:

N1. Patient and customer relationship building [3.2a] *might* include the development of partnerships or alliances with patient and customers.

N2. Determining patient and customer satisfaction and dissatisfaction [3.2b] *might* include use of any or all of the following: surveys, formal and informal feedback, patient and customer account histories, complaints, win/loss analysis, and transaction completion rates. Information *might* be gathered on the Internet, through personal contact or a third party, or by mail.

N3. Patient and customer satisfaction measurements *might* include both a numerical rating scale and descriptors for each unit in the scale. Actionable patient and customer satisfaction measurements provide useful information about specific program and service features, delivery, relationships, and transactions that bear upon the patient and customers' future actions—choice of health care provider and positive referral.

N4. Your patient and customer satisfaction and dissatisfaction results *should* be reported in Item 7.2.

4.1 Measurement and Analysis of Organizational Performance	
Scoring Guidelines	**Expected Observations**
10%–20 % The beginning of a systematic approach to the *basic* requirements of the Item is evident. Major gaps exist in deployment that would inhibit progress in achieving the basic requirements of the Item. Early stages of a transition from reacting to problems to a general improvement orientation are evident.	*4.1 Measurement and Analysis of Organizational Performance.* The organization is in the beginning stages of establishing effective performance management systems for measuring and analyzing organizational performance. *Major gaps exist where the measures and analyses do not cover many elements essential to effective organizational decision making.*
30%–40% An effective, systematic approach, responsive to the *basic* requirements of the Item, is evident. The approach is deployed, although some areas or work units are in early stages of deployment. The beginning of a systematic approach to evaluation and improvement of key processes is evident.	*4.1 Measurement and Analysis of Organizational Performance.* The organization has effective, systematic processes in place for measuring and analyzing organizational performance. *Measures and analyses cover most areas essential to effective organizational decision making. The organization is beginning to evaluate and make some improvements in the key elements of these processes.*
50%–60% An effective, systematic approach, responsive to the *overall* requirements of the Item and your key health care requirements, is evident. The approach is well deployed, although deployment may vary in some areas or work units. A fact-based, systematic evaluation and improvement process is in place for improving the efficiency and effectiveness of key processes. The approach is aligned with your basic organizational needs identified in the other Criteria Categories.	*4.1 Measurement and Analysis of Organizational Performance.* The organization has effective, systematic processes in place to do the following: a. *Performance Measurement.* Select the right measures to align and ensure effective decision making to improve performance at all levels and in all parts of the organization. b. *Performance Analysis.* Analyze data to support effective decision making to improve performance at all levels and in all parts of the organization. *Some relatively minor gaps may exist in the data measurement and analysis processes in some parts of the organization. However, there is a systematic, fact-based process in place to evaluate and improve the key elements of (a) and (b) above.*

Continued

4.1 Measurement and Analysis of Organizational Performance — *Continued*

Scoring Guidelines	Expected Observations
70%–80% An effective, systematic approach, responsive to the *multiple* requirements of the Item and your current and changing health care needs, is evident. The approach is well deployed, with no significant gaps. A fact-based, systematic evaluation and improvement process and organizational learning/sharing are key management tools; there is clear evidence of refinement, innovation, and improved integration as a result of organizational-level analysis and sharing. The approach is well integrated with organizational needs identified in the other Criteria Categories. **90%–100%** An effective, systematic approach, fully responsive to *all* the requirements of the Item and all your current and changing health care needs, is evident. The approach is fully deployed without significant weaknesses or gaps in any areas or work units. A very strong, fact-based, systematic evaluation and improvement process and extensive organizational learning/sharing are key management tools; strong refinement, innovation, and integration, backed by excellent organizational-level analysis and sharing, are evident. The approach is fully integrated with your organizational needs identified in the other Criteria Categories.	*4.1 Measurement and Analysis of Organizational Performance.* The organization has well-deployed, effective, systematic processes in place to do the following: a. *Performance Measurement* (1) Select, collect, align, and integrate data and information for tracking daily operations and for tracking overall organizational performance. Use these data and information to support organizational decision making and innovation. (2) Select and effectively use key comparative data and information to support operational and strategic decision making and innovation. (3) Keep the performance measurement system current with educational service needs and directions and ensure the system is sensitive to rapid or unexpected organizational or external changes. b. *Performance Analysis* (1) Perform appropriate analyses to support senior leaders' organizational performance review and organizational strategic planning. (2) Communicate the results of organizational-level analyses to work group and functional-level operations to enable effective support for their decision making. *The approach is well deployed with no significant gaps. In addition, there is a systematic, fact-based process in place to evaluate and improve (a) and (b) above with clear evidence of innovation, learning, and organizational sharing, which results in refinements and improved integration.*

Notes:

N1. Performance measurement is used in fact-based decision making for setting and aligning organizational directions and resource use at the work unit, key process, departmental, and whole organization levels.

N2. Comparative data and information [4.1a(2)] are obtained by benchmarking and by seeking competitive comparisons. "Benchmarking" refers to identifying processes and results that represent best practices and performance for similar activities, inside or outside your organization's industry. Competitive comparisons relate your organization's performance to that of competitors in your markets.

N3. Analysis includes examining trends; organizational, industry, and technology projections; and comparisons, cause-effect relationships, and correlations intended to support your performance reviews, help determine root causes, and help set priorities for resource use. Accordingly, analysis draws upon all types of data: patient and customer-related, financial and market, operational, and competitive/comparative.

N4. The results of organizational performance analysis *should* contribute to your senior leaders' organizational performance review in 1.1c and organizational strategic planning in Category 2.

N5. Your organizational performance results *should* be reported in Items 7.1-7.6.

4.2 Information and Knowledge Management	
Scoring Guidelines	**Expected Observations**
10%–20% The beginning of a systematic approach to the *basic* requirements of the Item is evident. Major gaps exist in deployment that would inhibit progress in achieving the basic requirements of the Item. Early stages of a transition from reacting to problems to a general improvement orientation are evident.	*4.2 Information and Knowledge Management.* The organization is in the beginning stages of ensuring that needed information and knowledge are available. *Major gaps exist where the needed information and/or knowledge are not available to support organizational decision making and/or learning.*
30%–40% An effective, systematic approach, responsive to the *basic* requirements of the Item, is evident. The approach is deployed, although some areas or work units are in early stages of deployment. The beginning of a systematic approach to evaluation and improvement of key processes is evident.	*4.2 Information and Knowledge Management.* The organization has effective, systematic processes in place to ensure that needed information and knowledge are available. *Information and knowledge cover most areas essential to effective organizational decision making and/or learning.* *The organization is beginning to evaluate and make some improvements in the key elements of these processes.*
50%–60% An effective, systematic approach, responsive to the *overall* requirements of the Item and your key health care requirements, is evident. The approach is well deployed, although deployment may vary in some areas or work units. A fact-based, systematic evaluation and improvement process is in place for improving the efficiency and effectiveness of key processes. The approach is aligned with your basic organizational needs identified in the other Criteria Categories.	*4.2 Information Management.* The organization has effective, systematic processes in place to do the following: a. *Data Availability.* Ensure needed data and information are available to appropriate staff, suppliers and partners, and patients and customers. b. *Organizational Knowledge.* (1) Build and manage knowledge assets to effectively transfer needed knowledge. (2) Ensure the quality (such as accuracy, reliability, timeliness) of needed data and information. *Some relatively minor gaps may exist in the data availability and knowledge management processes in some parts of the organization. However, there is a systematic, fact-based process in place to evaluate and improve the key elements of (a) and (b) above.*

Continued

4.2 Information and Knowledge Management	*Continued*
Scoring Guidelines	**Expected Observations**

70%–80% An effective, systematic approach, responsive to the *multiple* requirements of the Item and your current and changing health care needs, is evident. The approach is well deployed, with no significant gaps. A fact-based, systematic evaluation and improvement process and organizational learning/sharing are key management tools; there is clear evidence of refinement, innovation, and improved integration as a result of organizational-level analysis and sharing. The approach is well integrated with organizational needs identified in the other Criteria Categories.

90%–100% An effective, systematic approach, fully responsive to *all* the requirements of the Item and all your current and changing health care needs, is evident. The approach is fully deployed without significant weaknesses or gaps in any areas or work units. A very strong, fact-based, systematic evaluation and improvement process and extensive organizational learning/sharing are key management tools; strong refinement, innovation, and integration, backed by excellent organizational-level analysis and sharing, are evident. The approach is fully integrated with your organizational needs identified in the other Criteria Categories.

4.2 Information Management. The organization has well-deployed, effective, systematic processes in place to do the following:

a. *Data and Information Availability*
 (1) Make needed data and information available and accessible to appropriate staff, suppliers and partners, and patients and customers.
 (2) Ensure that hardware and software are reliable, secure, and user friendly.
 (3) Keep data and information availability mechanisms, including software and hardware systems, current with educational service needs and directions.

b. *Organizational Knowledge*
 (1) Manage organizational knowledge to accomplish:
  • The collection and transfer of staff knowledge
  • The transfer of relevant knowledge from patients and customers, suppliers, and partners
  • The identification and sharing of best practices
 (2) Ensure the following properties of data, information, and organizational knowledge:
  • Integrity (completeness) • Timeliness (available when needed)
  • Reliability (consistency • Security (free from tampering)
  • Accuracy (correctness) • Confidentiality (no inappropriate release)

The approach is well deployed with no significant gaps. In addition, there is a systematic, fact-based process in place to evaluate and improve (a) and (b) above with clear evidence of innovation, learning, and organizational sharing, which results in refinements and improved integration.

Notes:

N1. Data availability [4.2a] are of growing importance as the Internet, e-business, and e-commerce are used increasingly for health care-to-health care and health care-to-consumer interactions and intranets become more important as a major source of organizationwide communications.

N2. Data and information access [4.2a(1)] *might* be via electronic and other means.

5.1 Work Systems	
Scoring Guidelines	**Expected Observations**
10%–20% The beginning of a systematic approach to the *basic* requirements of the Item is evident. Major gaps exist in deployment that would inhibit progress in achieving the basic requirements of the Item. Early stages of a transition from reacting to problems to a general improvement orientation are evident.	*5.1 Work Systems.* The organization is in the beginning stages of ensuring work and jobs enabling staff and the organization to achieve high performance. *Major gaps exist where the work systems do not help most staff to achieve high performance objectives.*
30%–40% An effective, systematic approach, responsive to the *basic* requirements of the Item, is evident. The approach is deployed, although some areas or work units are in early stages of deployment. The beginning of a systematic approach to evaluation and improvement of key processes is evident.	*5.1 Work Systems.* The organization has effective, systematic processes in place to enable many staff in many parts of the organization to achieve high performance objectives. *Work and jobs in some parts of the organization do not support (or are just beginning to support) high performance work.* *The organization is beginning to evaluate and make some improvements in the key elements of these processes.*
50%–60% An effective, systematic approach, responsive to the *overall* requirements of the Item and your key health care requirements, is evident. The approach is well deployed, although deployment may vary in some areas or work units. A fact-based, systematic evaluation and improvement process is in place for improving the efficiency and effectiveness of key processes. The approach is aligned with your basic organizational needs identified in the other Criteria Categories.	*5.1 Work Systems.* The organization has effective, systematic processes in place to do the following: a. *Organization and Management of Work.* Organize and manage work and jobs and related workforce practices to motivate staff and managers to achieve high performance objectives. b. *Staff Performance Management System.* Ensure compensation practices align with and support the achievement of high performance objectives. c. *Recruitment and Career Progression.* Ensure career progression opportunities and related workforce practices align with and support the achievement of high performance objectives. *Some relatively minor gaps may exist in work systems in some parts of the organization that inhibit the achievement of high-performance objectives. However, there is a systematic, fact-based process in place to evaluate and improve the key elements of (a), (b), and (c) above.*

Continued

5.1 Work Systems	*Continued*
Scoring Guidelines	**Expected Observations**

70%–80% An effective, systematic approach, responsive to the *multiple* requirements of the Item and your current and changing health care needs, is evident. The approach is well deployed, with no significant gaps. A fact-based, systematic evaluation and improvement process and organizational learning/sharing are key management tools; there is clear evidence of refinement, innovation, and improved integration as a result of organizational-level analysis and sharing. The approach is well integrated with organizational needs identified in the other Criteria Categories.

90%–100% An effective, systematic approach, fully responsive to *all* the requirements of the item and all your current and changing health care needs, is evident. The approach is fully deployed without significant weaknesses or gaps in any areas or work units. A very strong, fact-based, systematic evaluation and improvement process and extensive organizational learning/sharing are key management tools; strong refinement, innovation, and integration, backed by excellent organizational-level analysis and sharing, are evident. The approach is fully integrated with your organizational needs identified in the other Criteria Categories.

5.1 Work Systems. The organization has well-deployed, effective, systematic processes in place to do the following:

a. *Organization and Management of Work*
   (1) Organize and manage work and jobs to achieve high performance
      • Promote cooperation, initiative, empowerment, innovation, and organizational culture.
      • Achieve the agility to keep current with health care service needs.
   (2) Ensure work systems capitalize on the diverse ideas, cultures, and thinking of staff and the communities with which you interact (your staff hiring and your patient and customer communities).
   (3) Achieve effective communication and skill sharing across work units, jobs, and locations.

b. *Staff Performance Management Systems*
   How does your staff performance management system, including feedback to staff—
      • Supports high performance work?
      • Supports a patient and customer and health care results focus?
      • Ensures compensation, recognition, and related reward and incentive practices reinforce high performance and a patient and customer and health care results focus?

c. *Hiring and Career Progression*
   (1) Identify characteristics and skills needed by potential staff.
   (2) Recruit, hire, and retain new staff and ensure the staff represent the diverse ideas, cultures, and thinking of your staff hiring community.
   (3) Accomplish effective succession planning for leadership and management positions, including senior leadership and manage effective career progression for all staff throughout the organization.

The approach is well deployed with no significant gaps. In addition, there is a systematic, fact-based process in place to evaluate and improve (a), (b), and (c) above with clear evidence of innovation, learning, and organizational sharing, which results in refinements and improved integration.

Notes:

N1. "Staff" refers to your organization's permanent, temporary, and part-time personnel, as well as any contract staff supervised by your organization. Staff includes team leaders, supervisors, and managers at all levels. Contract staff supervised by a contractor should be addressed in Category 6.

N2. "Your organization's work" refers to how your staff are organized or organize themselves in formal and informal, temporary, or longer-term units. This *might* include work teams, process teams, project teams, patient and customer action teams, problem-solving teams, centers of excellence, functional units, remote (e.g., at-home) workers, cross-functional teams, and departments—self-managed or managed by supervisors. "Jobs" refers to responsibilities, authorities, and tasks of individuals. In some work systems, jobs might be shared by a team.

N3. Compensation and recognition (5.1b) include promotions and bonuses that *might* be based upon performance, skills acquired, and other factors. Recognition includes monetary and nonmonetary, formal and informal, and individual and group mechanisms. Recognition systems for volunteers and independent practitioners who contribute to the work of the organization should be included, as appropriate.

5.2 Staff Learning and Motivation	
Scoring Guidelines	**Expected Observations**
10%–20% The beginning of a systematic approach to the *basic* requirements of the Item is evident. Major gaps exist in deployment that would inhibit progress in achieving the basic requirements of the Item. Early stages of a transition from reacting to problems to a general improvement orientation are evident.	*5.2 Staff Learning and Motivation.* The organization is in the beginning stages of establishing an effective education and training program to support staff learning and motivation to help staff achieve high performance objectives. *Major gaps exist where the education and training processes do not help most employees to achieve high performance.*
30%–40% An effective, systematic approach, responsive to the *basic* requirements of the Item, is evident. The approach is deployed, although some areas or work units are in early stages of deployment. The beginning of a systematic approach to evaluation and improvement of key processes is evident.	*5.2 Staff Learning and Motivation.* The organization has effective, systematic, education and training processes in place to support staff learning and motivation to help staff achieve high performance objectives. *Learning and motivation processes in some parts of the organization do not support (or are just beginning to support) high performance work. The organization is beginning to evaluate and make some improvements in the key elements of these processes.*
50%–60% An effective, systematic approach, responsive to the *overall* requirements of the Item and your key health care requirements, is evident. The approach is well deployed, although deployment may vary in some areas or work units. A fact-based, systematic evaluation and improvement process is in place for improving the efficiency and effectiveness of key processes. The approach is aligned with your basic organizational needs identified in the other Criteria Categories.	*5.2 Staff Learning and Motivation.* The organization has effective, systematic processes in place to do the following: a. *Staff Education, Training, and Development.* Build staff knowledge, skills, and capabilities through education and training to help them achieve overall organizational objectives and high performance. b. *Motivation and Career Development.* Build staff knowledge, skills, and capabilities through career development programs to help them achieve overall organizational objectives and high performance. *Some relatively minor gaps may exist in education, training, and career development in some parts of the organization that inhibit the achievement of overall objectives and high performance. However, there is a systematic, fact-based process in place to evaluate and improve the key elements of (a) and (b) above.*

Continued

5.2 Staff Learning and Motivation		*Continued*
Scoring Guidelines	**Expected Observations**	

70%–80% An effective, systematic approach, responsive to the *multiple* requirements of the Item and your current and changing health care needs, is evident. The approach is well deployed, with no significant gaps. A fact-based, systematic evaluation and improvement process and organizational learning/sharing are key management tools; there is clear evidence of refinement, innovation, and improved integration as a result of organizational-level analysis and sharing. The approach is well integrated with organizational needs identified in the other Criteria Categories.

90%–100% An effective, systematic approach, fully responsive to *all* the requirements of the Item and all your current and changing health care needs, is evident. The approach is fully deployed without significant weaknesses or gaps in any areas or work units. A very strong, fact-based, systematic evaluation and improvement process and extensive organizational learning/sharing are key management tools; strong refinement, innovation, and integration, backed by excellent organizational-level analysis and sharing, are evident. The approach is fully integrated with your organizational needs identified in the other Criteria Categories.

5.2 Staff Education, Training, and Development. The organization has well-deployed, effective, systematic processes in place to do the following:

a. *Staff Education, Training, and Development*
  (1) Ensure staff education and training—
     • Contribute to the achievement of action plans.
     • Address key needs associated with organizational performance measurement, performance improvement, and technological change.
     • Balance short- and longer-term organizational objectives with staff needs for development, learning, and career progression.
  (2) Ensure staff education, training, and development address key organizational needs associated with—
     • New staff orientation, diversity, ethical health care business practices, and management and leadership development.
     • Staff, workplace, and environmental safety.
  (3) Seek and use input from staff and their supervisors and managers to determine education and training need. Incorporate organizational learning and knowledge assets into your education and training.
  (4) Deliver education and training based on input from staff and their supervisors and managers regarding options for the delivery of education and training. Use both formal and informal delivery approaches, including mentoring and other approaches, as appropriate.
  (5) Reinforce the use of new knowledge and skills on the job.
  (6) Evaluate the effectiveness of education and training, taking into account individual and organizational performance.

b. *Motivation and Career Development*
  Motivate staff to develop and utilize their full potential. Use formal and informal mechanisms, with assistance from managers and supervisors, to help staff attain job- and career-related development and learning objectives.

The approach is well deployed with no significant gaps. In addition, there is a systematic, fact-based process in place to evaluate and improve (a) and (b) above with clear evidence of innovation, learning, and organizational sharing, which results in refinements and improved integration.

Note:

Education and training delivery [5.2a(4)] *might* occur inside or outside your organization and involve on- the-job, classroom, computer-based, distance learning, and other types of delivery (formal or informal).

	5.3 Staff Well-Being and Satisfaction
Scoring Guidelines	**Expected Observations**
10%–20% The beginning of a systematic approach to the *basic* requirements of the Item is evident. Major gaps exist in deployment that would inhibit progress in achieving the basic requirements of the Item. Early stages of a transition from reacting to problems to a general improvement orientation are evident.	*5.3 Staff Well-Being and Satisfaction.* The organization is in the beginning stages of establishing a work environment that contributes to the well-being and satisfaction of staff. *Major gaps exist where the organization has not created a work environment to promote employee well-being and satisfaction.*
30%–40% An effective, systematic approach, responsive to the *basic* requirements of the Item, is evident. The approach is deployed, although some areas or work units are in early stages of deployment. The beginning of a systematic approach to evaluation and improvement of key processes is evident.	*5.3 Staff Well-Being and Satisfaction.* The organization has effective, systematic processes in place to provide a work environment that contributes to the well-being and satisfaction of staff. *Processes in some parts of the organization do not support (or are just beginning to support) employee well-being and satisfaction. The organization is beginning to evaluate and make some improvements in the key elements of these processes.*
50%–60% An effective, systematic approach, responsive to the *overall* requirements of the Item and your key health care requirements, is evident. The approach is well deployed, although deployment may vary in some areas or work units. A fact-based, systematic evaluation and improvement process is in place for improving the efficiency and effectiveness of key processes. The approach is aligned with your basic organizational needs identified in the other Criteria Categories.	*5.3 Staff Well-Being and Satisfaction.* The organization has effective, systematic processes in place to do the following: a. *Work Environment.* Maintain a work environment that contributes to the well-being, satisfaction, and motivation of all staff. b. *Staff Support and Satisfaction.* Maintain a support climate that contributes to the well-being, satisfaction, and motivation of all staff. *Some relatively minor gaps may exist in some parts of the organization to maintain a work environment and support climate that inhibit the achievement of employee well-being, satisfaction, and motivation. However, there is a systematic, fact-based process in place to evaluate and improve the key elements of (a) and (b) above.*

Continued

	5.3 Staff Well-Being and Satisfaction	*Continued*
Scoring Guidelines	**Expected Observations**	

Scoring Guidelines	**Expected Observations**
70%–80% An effective, systematic approach, responsive to the *multiple* requirements of the Item and your current and changing health care needs, is evident. The approach is well deployed, with no significant gaps. A fact-based, systematic evaluation and improvement process and organizational learning/sharing are key management tools; there is clear evidence of refinement, innovation, and improved integration as a result of organizational-level analysis and sharing. The approach is well integrated with organizational needs identified in the other Criteria Categories. **90%–100%** An effective, systematic approach, fully responsive to *all* the requirements of the Item and all your current and changing health care needs, is evident. The approach is fully deployed without significant weaknesses or gaps in any areas or work units. A very strong, fact-based, systematic evaluation and improvement process and extensive organizational learning/sharing are key management tools; strong refinement, innovation, and integration, backed by excellent organizational-level analysis and sharing, are evident. The approach is fully integrated with your organizational needs identified in the other Criteria Categories.	*5.3 Staff Well-Being and Satisfaction.* The organization has well-deployed, effective, systematic processes in place to do the following: a. *Work Environment* (1) Improve workplace health, safety, security, and ergonomics. • Involve staff in workplace improvements. • Define performance measures or targets for each of key workplace factors (health, safety, security, and ergonomics). Define significant differences in workplace factors and performance measures or targets, if different staff groups and work units have different work environments. (2) Ensure workplace preparedness for emergencies or disasters and ensure health care service continuity for the benefit of your staff and patients and customers. b. *Staff Support and Satisfaction* (1) Determine the key factors that affect staff well-being, satisfaction, and motivation. Segment these factors, as appropriate, to consider the needs of a diverse workforce and different categories and types of staff. (2) Provide services, benefits, and policies to support staff and tailor these to the needs of a diverse workforce and different categories and types of staff. (3) Conduct formal and informal assessments to determine (measure) staff well-being, satisfaction, and motivation. Use different methods and measures as appropriate to capture accurate information about the well-being, satisfaction, and motivation across a diverse workforce and for different categories and types of staff. • Use these and other indicators, such as staff retention, absenteeism, grievances, safety, and productivity, to assess and improve staff well-being, satisfaction, and motivation. (4) Establish priorities for improving the work environment and staff support climate by relating assessment findings to key health care service results. *The approach is well deployed with no significant gaps. In addition, there is a systematic, fact-based process in place to evaluate and improve (a) and (b) above with clear evidence of innovation, learning, and organizational sharing, which results in refinements and improved integration.*

Notes:

N1. Specific factors that *might* affect your staff well-being, satisfaction, and motivation [5.3b(1)] include effective staff problem or grievance resolution; safety factors; staff views of management; staff training, development, and career opportunities; staff preparation for changes in technology or the work organization; the work environment and other work conditions; management's empowerment of staff; information sharing by management; workload; cooperation and teamwork; recognition; services and benefits; communications; job security; compensation; and equal opportunity.

N2. Approaches for staff support [5.3b(2)] *might* include providing counseling, career development and employability services, recreational or cultural activities, nonwork-related education, day care, job rotation or sharing, special leave for family responsibilities or community service, home safety training, flexible work hours and location, outplacement, and retirement benefits (including extended health care).

N3. Measures and indicators of well-being, satisfaction, and motivation (5.3b(3)] *might* include data on safety and absenteeism, the overall turnover rate, the turnover rate for patient and customer contact staff, staff charitable contributions, grievances, strikes, other job actions, insurance costs, worker's compensation claims, and results of surveys. Survey indicators of satisfaction *might* include staff knowledge of job roles, staff knowledge of organizational direction, and staff perception of empowerment and information sharing. Your results relative to such measures and indicators *should* be reported in Item 7.4.

N4. Setting priorities [5.3b(4)] *might* draw upon your human resource results presented in Item 7.4 and *might* involve addressing staff problems based on their impact on your health care results.

6.1 Health Care Processes	
Scoring Guidelines	**Expected Observations**
10%–20% The beginning of a systematic approach to the *basic* requirements of the Item is evident. Major gaps exist in deployment that would inhibit progress in achieving the basic requirements of the Item. Early stages of a transition from reacting to problems to a general improvement orientation are evident.	*6.1 Health Care Processes.* The organization is in the beginning stages of establishing key processes for patient health care services (such as designing core programs and services important to creating patient and customer value). *Major gaps exist where key value creation processes have not been developed that are essential to business success and growth.*
30%–40% An effective, systematic approach, responsive to the *basic* requirements of the Item, is evident. The approach is deployed, although some areas or work units are in early stages of deployment. The beginning of a systematic approach to evaluation and improvement of key processes is evident.	*6.1 Health Care Processes.* The organization has effective, systematic health care processes in place (such as designing and delivering core programs and services) important to creating patient and customer value. *However, in some parts of the organization effective systematic processes that are essential to value creation and business success and growth are just beginning to emerge.* *The organization is beginning to evaluate and make some improvements in the key elements of these processes.*
50%–60% An effective, systematic approach, responsive to the *overall* requirements of the Item and your key health care requirements, is evident. The approach is well deployed, although deployment may vary in some areas or work units. A fact-based, systematic evaluation and improvement process is in place for improving the efficiency and effectiveness of key processes. The approach is aligned with your basic organizational needs identified in the other Criteria Categories.	*6.1 Health Care Processes.* The organization has effective, systematic processes in place to do the following: a. *Health Care Processes.* Design and manage key processes to create patient and customer value and achieve health care success and growth. (Design activities for health care processes should ensure key patient and customer requirements are met. Management activities for these processes should ensure that process steps are effectively monitored and controlled to ensure required programs and services are consistently delivered.) *Some relatively minor gaps may exist in some value creation and business processes in parts of the organization. However, there is a systematic, fact-based process in place to evaluate and improve the key elements of (a) above.*

Continued

6.1 Health Care Processes		*Continued*
Scoring Guidelines	**Expected Observations**	

70%–80% An effective, systematic approach, responsive to the *multiple* requirements of the Item and your current and changing health care needs, is evident. The approach is well deployed, with no significant gaps. A fact-based, systematic evaluation and improvement process and organizational learning/sharing are key management tools; there is clear evidence of refinement, innovation, and improved integration as a result of organizational-level analysis and sharing. The approach is well integrated with organizational needs identified in the other Criteria Categories.

90%–100% An effective, systematic approach, fully responsive to *all* the requirements of the Item and all your current and changing health care needs, is evident. The approach is fully deployed without significant weaknesses or gaps in any areas or work units. A very strong, fact-based, systematic evaluation and improvement process and extensive organizational learning/sharing are key management tools; strong refinement, innovation, and integration, backed by excellent organizational-level analysis and sharing, are evident. The approach is fully integrated with your organizational needs identified in the other Criteria Categories.

6.1 Health Care Processes. The organization has well-deployed, effective, systematic processes in place to do the following:

a. *Health Care Processes*
 (1) Define key program, service, and health care processes used to—
  • Create or add value for the organization, its patients and customers, and other key stakeholders.
  • Contribute to profitability and health care success.
 (2) Determine and define (list) key health care process requirements, incorporating input from patients and customers, suppliers, and partners, as appropriate.
 (3) Design these processes to meet all the key requirements including the following:
  • Incorporate new technology and organizational knowledge into the design of these processes.
  • Incorporate cycle time, productivity, cost control, and other efficiency and effectiveness factors into the design of these processes.
  • Implement these processes to ensure they meet design requirements.
 (4) Define key performance measures or indicators used for the control and improvement of health care processes.
  • Ensure day-to-day operation of these processes consistently meet key process requirements.
  • Ensure in-process measures and appropriate patient and customer, supplier, and partner input are used to manage these processes.
 (5) Minimize overall costs associated with inspections, tests, and process or performance audits, as appropriate, while at the same time preventing errors and rework, and minimizing rework costs, as appropriate.
 (6) Improve value creation processes to—
  • Achieve better performance.
  • Reduce variability.
  • Improve programs and services.
  • Keep the processes current with health care service needs and directions and share improvements with other organizational units and processes.

The approach is well deployed with no significant gaps. In addition, there is a systematic, fact-based process in place to evaluate and improve (a) above with clear evidence of innovation, learning, and organizational sharing, which results in refinements and improved integration.

Notes:

N1. "Health care processes" refers to patient and community service processes for the purpose of prevention, maintenance, health promotion, screening, diagnosis, treatment/therapy, rehabilitation, recovery, palliative care, or supportive care. This includes services delivered to patients through other providers (e.g., laboratory or radiology studies). Responses to Item 6.1 *should* be based upon the most critical requirements for successful delivery of your services.

N2. Key processes for the conduct of health care research and/or a teaching mission *should* be reported in either Item 6.1 or 6.2, as appropriate to your organization's mission.

N3. Process requirements *should* include all appropriate components of health care service delivery. In a group practice, this *might* be the making of appointments, presentation, evaluation of risk factors, health education, and appointment closures. Depending upon the health care service, this *might* include a significant focus on technology and patient-specific considerations.

N4. To achieve better process performance and reduce variability, you *might* implement approaches, such as the PDSA process, six sigma methodology, use of ISO 9000:2000 standards, or other process improvement tools.

6.2 Support Processes	
Scoring Guidelines	**Expected Observations**
10%–20% The beginning of a systematic approach to the *basic* requirements of the Item is evident. Major gaps exist in deployment that would inhibit progress in achieving the basic requirements of the Item. Early stages of a transition from reacting to problems to a general improvement orientation are evident.	*6.2 Support Processes.* The organization is in the beginning stages of establishing key processes to support health care success and growth. *Major gaps exist where key value support processes have not been developed.*
30%–40% An effective, systematic approach, responsive to the *basic* requirements of the Item, is evident. The approach is deployed, although some areas or work units are in early stages of deployment. The beginning of a systematic approach to evaluation and improvement of key processes is evident.	*6.2 Support Processes.* The organization has effective, systematic processes in place to support health care success and growth. *However, these support processes are just beginning to emerge in some parts of the organization.* *The organization is beginning to evaluate and make some improvements in the key elements of these support processes.*
50%–60% An effective, systematic approach, responsive to the *overall* requirements of the Item and your key health care requirements, is evident. The approach is well deployed, although deployment may vary in some areas or work units. A fact-based, systematic evaluation and improvement process is in place for improving the efficiency and effectiveness of key processes. The approach is aligned with your basic organizational needs identified in the other Criteria Categories.	*6.2 Support Processes.* The organization has effective, systematic processes in place to do the following: a. *Business and Other Support Processes.* Design and manage key business processes that support patient and customer value and health care success and growth. (Design activities for key business and support processes should ensure key patient and customer requirements are met. Management activities for key business and support services should ensure that process steps are effectively monitored and controlled to ensure required programs and services are consistently delivered.) *Some relatively minor gaps may exist in some support processes in parts of the organization. However, there is a systematic, fact-based process in place to evaluate and improve the key elements of (a) above.*

Continued

	6.2 Support Processes *Continued*
Scoring Guidelines	**Expected Observations**

70%–80% An effective, systematic approach, responsive to the *multiple* requirements of the Item and your current and changing health care needs, is evident. The approach is well deployed, with no significant gaps. A fact-based, systematic evaluation and improvement process and organizational learning/sharing are key management tools; there is clear evidence of refinement, innovation, and improved integration as a result of organizational-level analysis and sharing. The approach is well integrated with organizational needs identified in the other Criteria Categories.

90%–100% An effective, systematic approach, fully responsive to *all* the requirements of the Item and all your current and changing health care needs, is evident. The approach is fully deployed without significant weaknesses or gaps in any areas or work units. A very strong, fact-based, systematic evaluation and improvement process and extensive organizational learning/sharing are key management tools; strong refinement, innovation, and integration, backed by excellent organizational-level analysis and sharing, are evident. The approach is fully integrated with your organizational needs identified in the other Criteria Categories.

6.2 Support Processes. The organization has well-deployed, effective, systematic processes in place to do the following:

a. *Business and Other Support Processes*
(1) Define key business and other support processes that support health care processes.
(2) Determine and define (list) key support process requirements, incorporating input from appropriate internal and external patients and customers, and suppliers and partners.
(3) Design support processes to meet all the key requirements including the following:
  • Incorporate new technology and organizational knowledge into the design of these processes.
  • Incorporate cycle time, productivity, cost control, and other efficiency and effectiveness factors into the design of these processes.
  • Implement these processes to ensure they meet design requirements.
(4) Define key performance measures or indicators used for the control and improvement of support processes.
  • Ensure day-to-day operation of these processes consistently meets key process requirements.
  • Ensure in-process measures and appropriate patient and customer, supplier, and partner input are used to manage these processes.
(5) Minimize overall costs associated with inspections, tests, and process or performance audits, while at the same time preventing defects and rework, and minimizing costs, as appropriate.
(6) Improve health care processes to—
  • Achieve better performance
  • Reduce variability
  • Improve programs and services
  • Keep the processes current with health care needs and directions and share improvements with other organizational units and processes

The approach is well deployed with no significant gaps. In addition, there is a systematic, fact-based process in place to evaluate and improve (a) above with clear evidence of innovation, learning, and organizational sharing, which results in refinements and improved integration.

Notes:

N1. Your key business processes are those non-health care service processes that are considered most important to business growth and success by your organization's senior leaders. These *might* include processes for innovation, technology acquisition, information and knowledge management, supply chain management, supplier partnering, outsourcing, mergers and acquisitions, project management, and sales and marketing. The key business processes to be included in Item 6.2 are distinctive to your organization and how you operate.

N2. Your other key support processes are those that are considered most important for support of your organization's health care service design and delivery processes, staff, and daily operations. These *might* include key patient support processes (e.g., housekeeping and medical records) and key administrative support processes (e.g., finance and accounting), facilities management, legal, human resource, and project management.

N3. The results of improvements in your key business and other support processes and their performance results should be reported in Item 7.5.

Category 7 Results

Category 7 uses different Scoring Guidelines than Categories 1-6. No additional clarification has been developed since the ambiguities in Approach/Deployment scoring are not present in Results scoring.

Self-Assessments of Organizations and Management Systems

Baldrige-based self-assessments of organization performance and management systems take several forms, ranging from rigorous and time intensive to simple and somewhat superficial. This section discusses the various approaches to organizational self-assessment and the pros and cons of each. Curt Reimann, the first director of the Malcolm Baldrige National Quality Award Office and the closing speaker for the 10th Quest for Excellence Conference, spoke of the need to streamline assessments to get a good sense of strengths, opportunities for improvement, and the vital few areas to focus leadership and drive organizational change. Three distinct types of self-assessment will be examined: the written narrative, the Likert scale survey, and the behaviorally anchored survey.

Full-Length Written Narrative

The Baldrige application development process is the most time-consuming organizational self-assessment process. To apply for the Baldrige Award, applicants must prepare a 50-page written narrative to address the requirements of the Performance Excellence Criteria. In the written self-assessment, the applicant is expected to describe the processes and programs it has in place to drive performance excellence. The Baldrige application process serves as the vehicle for self-assessment in most state-level quality awards. The process has not changed since the national quality award program was created in 1987 (except for reducing the maximum page limit from 85 to 50 pages). *Author's Note: The CD attached to the back cover of this book contains a document designed to facilitate the collection of information within an organization to serve as a basis for a complete and thorough written application.*

Over the years, three methods have been used to prepare the full-length, comprehensive written narrative self-assessment:

1. The most widely used technique involves gathering a team of people to prepare the application. The team members are usually assigned one of the seven Categories and asked to develop a narrative to address the Criteria requirements of that Category. The Category writing teams are frequently subdivided to prepare responses Item by Item. After the initial draft is complete, an oversight team consolidates the narrative and tries to ensure processes are linked and integrated throughout. Finally, top leaders review and scrub the written narrative to put the best spin on the systems, processes, and results reported.

2. Another technique is similar to that described above. However, instead of subdividing the writing team according to the Baldrige Categories, the team remains together to write the entire application. In this way, the application may be more coherent and the linkages between health care service processes are easier to understand. This approach also helps to ensure consistency and integrity of the review processes. However, with fewer people involved, the natural "blind spots" of the team may prevent a full and accurate analysis of the management system. Finally, as with the method described above, top leaders review and scrub the written narrative.

3. The third method for preparing the written narrative is the least common and involves one person writing for several days to produce the application. Considering the immense amount of knowledge and work involved, it is easy to

understand why the third method is used so rarely.

With all three methods, external experts are usually involved. Baldrige Award recipients usually reported that they hired consultants to help them finalize their application by sharpening its focus and clarifying linkages.

Pros:

- Baldrige-winning organizations report that the discipline of producing a full-length written narrative self-assessment (Baldrige application) helped them learn about their organization and identify opportunities for improvement before the site-visit team arrived. The written self-assessment process clearly helped focus leaders on their organization's strengths and opportunities for improvement—provided that a complete and honest assessment was made.

- The written narrative self-assessment also provides rich information to help examiners conduct a site visit (the purpose of which is to verify and clarify the information contained in the written self-assessment).

Cons:

- Written narrative self-assessments are extremely time- and labor-intensive. Organizations that use this approach for Baldrige or state applications or for internal organizational review report that it requires between approximately 2,000 and 4,000 person-hours of effort—sometimes much more. People working on the self-assessment are diverted from other tasks during this period.

- Because the application is closely scrutinized and carefully scrubbed, and because of page limits, it may not fully and accurately describe the actual management processes and systems of the organization. Decisions based on misleading or incomplete information may take the organization down the wrong path.

- Although the written self-assessment provides information to help guide a site visit, examiners cannot determine the depth of deployment because only a few points of view are represented in the narrative.

- Finally, and perhaps most importantly, the discipline and knowledge required to write a meaningful narrative self-assessment is usually far greater than that possessed within the vast majority of organizations. Even the four 1997 Baldrige winners hired expert consultants to help them prepare and refine their written narrative.

Short Written Narrative

Two of the most significant obstacles to writing a useful full-length written narrative self-assessment are poor knowledge of the Performance Excellence Criteria and the time required to produce a meaningful assessment. If people do not understand the Criteria, it takes significantly longer to prepare a written self-assessment. In fact, the amount of time required to write an application/assessment is inversely related to the knowledge of the Criteria possessed by the writers. The difficulty associated with writing a full-length narrative has prevented many organizations from participating in state, local, or school award programs.

To encourage more organizations to begin the performance improvement journey, many state award programs developed progressively higher levels of recognition, ranging from "commitment" at the low end, through "demonstrated progress," to "achieving excellence" at the top of the range. However, even with progressive levels of recognition, the obstacle of preparing a 50-page written narrative prevented many from engaging in the process. To help resolve this problem, several state programs permit applicants who seek recognition at the lower levels to submit a 7- to 20-page "short" written narrative self-assessment. The short form ranges from requiring a one-page description per Category to one page per Item (hence the 7- to 20-page range in length).

Pros:

- It clearly takes less time to prepare the short form.

- Because of the reduced effort required to complete the self-assessment, more organizations are beginning the process of assessing and improving their performance.

Cons:

- The short form provides significantly less information to help examiners prepare for the site visit. Although it does take less time to prepare than the full-length version, the short form still requires several hundred hours of team preparation.

- The short form is usually closely scrutinized and carefully scrubbed just as its full-length cousin. This reduces accuracy and value to both the organization and examiners.

- The knowledge required to write even a short narrative prevents organizations in the beginning stages from preparing an accurate and meaningful assessment.

- Finally, there is not enough information presented in the short form to understand the extent of deployment of the systems and processes covered by the Criteria.

The Survey Approach

Just about everyone is familiar with a Likert-scale survey. These surveys typically ask respondents to rate, on a scale of 1 to 5, the extent to which they strongly disagree or strongly agree with a comment. The following is an example of a simple Likert-scale survey item:

Senior leaders effectively communicate values and patient and customer focus.
1   2   3   4   5
Strongly Disagree   Strongly Agree

A variation on the simple Likert-scale survey item has been developed in an attempt to improve consistency among respondents. Brief descriptors have been added at each level as shown below in the descriptive Likert-scale survey item:

Senior leaders effectively communicate values and patient and customer focus.
1   2   3   4   5
None   Few   Some   Many   Most

Pros:

- The Likert-scale survey is quick and easy to administer. People from all functions and levels within the organization can provide input.

Cons:

- Both the simple and the descriptive Likert-scale survey items are subject to wide ranges of interpretation. One person's rating of "2" and another person's rating of "4" may actually describe the same systems or behaviors. This problem of scoring reliability raises questions about the accuracy and usefulness of both the simple and the descriptive survey techniques for conducting organizational self-assessments. After all, a quick and easy survey that produces inaccurate data still has low value. That is the main reason why states have not adopted the Likert-scale survey as a tool for conducting the self-assessments, even for organizations in the beginning stages of the quality journey.

The Behaviorally Anchored Survey

A behaviorally anchored survey contains elements of a written narrative and a survey approach to conducting a self-assessment. The method is simple. Instead of brief descriptors, such as "strongly agree/strongly disagree" or "none-few-some-many-most," a more complete behavioral description is presented for each level of the survey scale. Respondents simply identify the behavioral description that most closely fits the activities in the organization. In addition, by asking the respondent to describe briefly the processes used by the organization to do what the Baldrige Criteria require, we can simulate the kind of information collected on a site visit, checking deployment and process integration. A sample is shown on the next page.

Improving Leadership Effectiveness Throughout the Organization [1.1c(4)]	
How well do senior administrative and health care leaders, at all levels, evaluate and improve their effectiveness?	
1 **Not Evident** ☐	Leaders *do not* systematically check their own effectiveness or bother to become more effective.
2 **Beginning** ✔	A *few* leaders use financial and budget results to check their own effectiveness, but do not make improvements based on this information.
3 **Basically Effective** ☐	*Some* leaders effectively use financial and budget results to check their own effectiveness. They use this information to set personal improvement goals, but do not consistently make improvements.
4 **Mature** ☐	*Many* leaders effectively use performance results information to set personal improvement goals. *Some* have improved their own effectiveness.
5 **Advanced** ☐	*Most* leaders effectively use health care and staff results, financial and other key performance results to evaluate their own effectiveness. They use this information to set personal improvement goals. *Many* have improved their own effectiveness. The system to evaluate and improve leadership effectiveness is routinely checked and *some* refinements have been made.
6 **Role Model** ☐	*Nearly all* leaders effectively use key performance results and staff feedback to evaluate their own effectiveness. They use this information to set personal improvement goals. *Most* have improved their own effectiveness. The system to evaluate and improve leadership effectiveness is routinely checked and *ongoing* refinements have been made.
? or Not Applicable ☐	I do not have enough information to answer this question or it is not applicable to my organization.
Describe how senior administrative and health care leaders at all levels use performance data to improve their own effectiveness. List the usual measures that are used to assess leadership effectiveness. How widely is this done in the organization? Suggest ways to improve this process.	

Since the behavioral descriptions in the survey combine the requirements of the Criteria with the standards from the Scoring Guidelines, it is possible to produce accurate Baldrige-based scores for Items and Categories for the entire organization and for any subgroup or division.

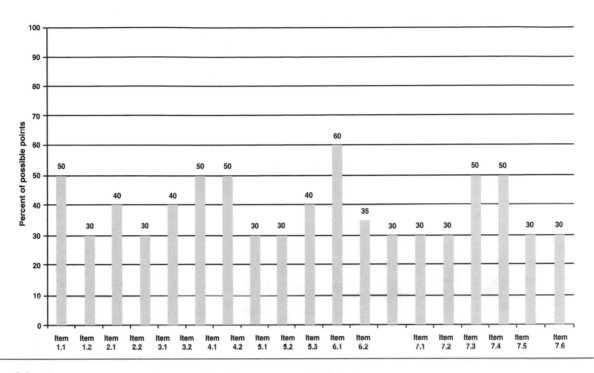

Figure 33 Sample organization overall percent scores by item.

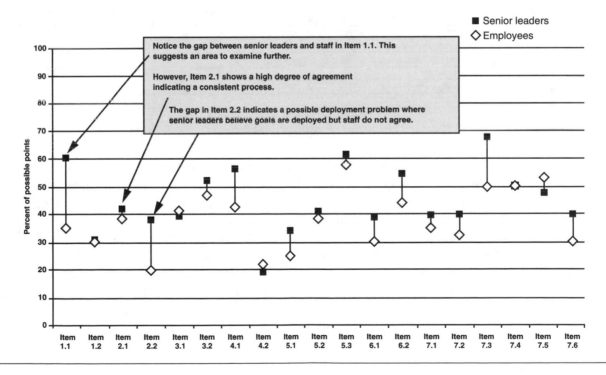

Figure 34 Item level scores by position.

Figure 34 provides sample scores for the entire organization and for two job classifications. Figure 33 shows the percent scores, on a 0 to 100 scale, for each Item. This helps users determine, at a glance, the relative strengths and weaknesses.

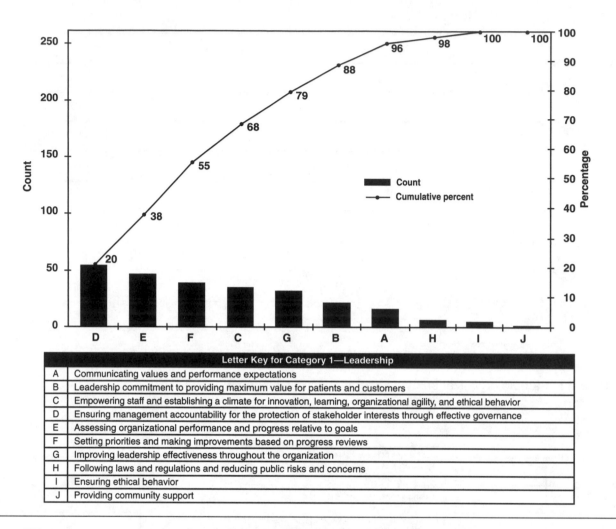

Letter Key for Category 1—Leadership	
A	Communicating values and performance expectations
B	Leadership commitment to providing maximum value for patients and customers
C	Empowering staff and establishing a climate for innovation, learning, organizational agility, and ethical behavior
D	Ensuring management accountability for the protection of stakeholder interests through effective governance
E	Assessing organizational performance and progress relative to goals
F	Setting priorities and making improvements based on progress reviews
G	Improving leadership effectiveness throughout the organization
H	Following laws and regulations and reducing public risks and concerns
I	Ensuring ethical behavior
J	Providing community support

Figure 35 Category 1—Leadership: Analysis of areas most needing improvement.

Figure 35 shows the ratings by subgroup, in this case, position of senior leaders and employees/staff. On the previous graph, Item 1.1, Leadership System, reflected a rating of 50 percent. However, according to the breakout, senior leaders believe the processes are much stronger (over 60 percent) than staff (less than 35 percent). This typically indicates incomplete systems development or poor deployment of existing systems and processes required by the Item.

The Pareto diagram in Figure 36 presents data reflecting the areas respondents believed were most in need of improvement. Continuing with the leadership example, it is clear that respondents believe that leaders need to do a better job of ensuring management accountability and the protection of stakeholder interests through effective governance (Theme D), assessing organizational performance and progress relative to goals (Theme E), and setting priorities and making improvements based on progress reviews (Theme F). This helps examiners focus on which areas in the leadership category may be the most important opportunities for improvement.

1. Leadership

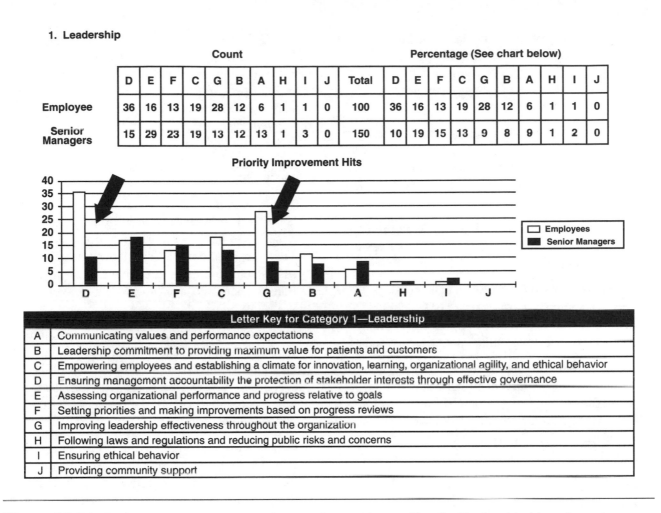

	Count											Percentage (See chart below)									
	D	E	F	C	G	B	A	H	I	J	Total	D	E	F	C	G	B	A	H	I	J
Employee	36	16	13	19	28	12	6	1	1	0	100	36	16	13	19	28	12	6	1	1	0
Senior Managers	15	29	23	19	13	12	13	1	3	0	150	10	19	15	13	9	8	9	1	2	0

Priority Improvement Hits

	Letter Key for Category 1—Leadership
A	Communicating values and performance expectations
B	Leadership commitment to providing maximum value for patients and customers
C	Empowering employees and establishing a climate for innovation, learning, organizational agility, and ethical behavior
D	Ensuring management accountability the protection of stakeholder interests through effective governance
E	Assessing organizational performance and progress relative to goals
F	Setting priorities and making improvements based on progress reviews
G	Improving leadership effectiveness throughout the organization
H	Following laws and regulations and reducing public risks and concerns
I	Ensuring ethical behavior
J	Providing community support

Figure 36 Priority improvement counts and percentages—by position for the leadership category.

Figure 36 allows examiners to determine management and staff identification of the various improvement priorities. Look at "D" and "G" and you will see that staff identified the need to improve these areas by a more than 2 to 1 margin over senior managers. This tends to indicate a deployment gap and suggests that senior managers are not perceived to be as effective as they believe themselves to be.

Finally, a complete report of the comments and explanations of the respondents can be prepared and used by examiners and organization leaders for improvement planning.

Pros:

- Descriptive behavioral anchors increase the consistency of rating. That is, one respondent's rating of "2" is likely to reflect the same observed behaviors as another respondent's rating of "2."

- Although completing a behaviorally anchored survey requires more reading than a Likert-scale survey, the amount of time and cost required to complete it is still less than 10 percent of the time and cost required to prepare a written narrative.

- Because it is easy and simple to use, the behaviorally anchored survey does not impose a barrier to participation as does the written narrative. States and companies that use surveys with properly written behavioral anchors find the accuracy of the assessment to be as good and in many cases better than that achieved by the full-length narrative self-assessment, and significantly better than Likert-scale or short narrative assessments. By obtaining input from a cross-section of functions, locations, and grade levels throughout the organization, a performance profile can be developed that not only identifies strengths and opportunities for improvement, but deployment gaps as well—something the written narrative assessments rarely provide.

- For organizations doing health care service throughout the world, the behaviorally anchored survey—translated into the native language of respondents—permits far greater input than the written narrative.

- Modern techniques involving surveying through Internet access created an easy way to survey a large, global company.

- Accurate survey data, based on behavioral anchors, can be used to compare or benchmark organizations within and among industries, and can also support longitudinal performance studies.

- Finally, examiners report that the effort required to analyze survey data and plan a site visit is about 50 percent less than the amount of effort required to analyze and prepare for a site visit based on a written narrative. Moreover, they report better information regarding deployment.

Cons:

- Organizations with highly developed performance-management systems that seek to apply for top state or national recognition may prefer to practice developing the full-length narrative self-assessment because it is usually required.

- Examiners who are comfortable with the Baldrige application review process, which requires 25 or more hours to conduct an individual review of a full-length narrative self-assessment, initially find it disconcerting to develop comments and plan a site visit based on data gathered from a survey. Different training for examiners is required to develop skills at using survey data to prepare feedback and plan site visits.

Note: The preceding report summary of a behaviorally anchored self-assessment survey written by Mark L. Blazey is administered only by the National Council for Performance Excellence, Winooski, VT. Readers may contact them by calling Wendy Steager, 802-655-1922, or by writing

to NCPE, 1 Main Street, Winooski, VT 05404. Several state quality awards and many private sector organizations are using this type of assessment instead of the written narrative form of evaluation. NCPE is the only organization authorized to administer this assessment tool. Any other use is not permitted.

In conclusion:

- The full-length written narrative self-assessment is costly. It provides useful information both to examiners and the organizations completing it. The process of completing the written self-assessment can help more advanced organizations to focus and work together as a team.

- The usefulness of the short-form written self-assessment is marginal, especially for beginning organizations; little useful information is provided to examiners and managers/staff of the organization. However, because it takes less time to complete, one of the barriers to participation is lowered.

- Concerns over the accuracy and inter-rater reliability of the simple and descriptive Likert scales make their use in conducting effective organizational assessments of management systems marginal.

- The behaviorally anchored survey with comments from respondents combines the benefits of survey speed with the accuracy and completeness of a well-developed written narrative self-assessment. In addition, the behaviorally anchored survey can identify gaps in deployment unlike the written narrative self-assessment and is less costly and faster to administer than the written narrative.

A complete copy of many health care service, education, and health care surveys can be obtained from the National Council for Performance Excellence, 1 Main Street, Winooski, VT 05404 (802-655-1922).
Their Web site is: www.PerformanceExcellence.com.

Following is a sample of a behaviorally anchored survey.

2003
Baldrige Health Care
Sample Organizational Self-Assessment, Behaviorally Anchored Version

Customized Demographic Profile

Each participating organization completes a customized demographic profile (a generic sample follows). In this way, survey data can be analyzed by these variables to help pinpoint specific areas needing improvement. This allows the extent of use (deployment) of management systems to be examined.

Please circle one selection from EACH column below to indicate your position within the organization.

Position	Location	Function	Org.	Years of Service
- Nurse - Physician - Supervisor - Medical Staff - Administrator - Other	- North - South - East - West - HQ	- Medical Support - Clinical - Human Resources - Finance - Public Relations - Supply - Info Technology - Other	- 1 - 2 - 3 - 4 - 5 - Other	- 0 < 1 - 1 < 3 - 3 < 5 - 5 < 10 - 10 +

BALDRIGE IN-DEPTH INSTRUCTIONS

The full survey consists of *62* themes or questions that relate to the 2003 Baldrige Performance Excellence Criteria. It is organized into seven "sections," one for each of the seven Performance Excellence Criteria Categories.

- To the best of your knowledge, select a rating (1 to 6) that describes the level of development in your organization. Note that *all* of the elements of a statement must be true before you can select that level. If one or more is not true, you must go to a lower level. After you have selected the rating level, please enter the value in the empty box to the right of the row of statements.

■ **Accuracy Tip:** The rating scale involves your assessment about the extent of use of the required management processes. The following definitions should help you rate this consistently:

- ✦ Few — up to 15 percent
- ✦ Some — more than 15 percent up to 30 percent
- ✦ Many — more than 30 percent up to 50 percent
- ✦ Most — more than 50 percent up to 80 percent
- ✦ Nearly All — more than 80 percent up to 99 percent
- ✦ All — 100 percent

■ **Time-Saving Tip**: Start reading at level 3. If all parts of the statement are true, go to level 4, if not, drop back to read level 2. After a few answers, save even more time by starting at the number you select most often. Don't waste time by reading from row 1 each time (unless most of your answers are 1).

- If you do not know an answer, enter NA (Not Applicable/Does Not Apply) or ? (Don't Know). If you are unsure of the meaning of a word or phrase, please check the glossary at the end of this booklet.

- After all statements in the first category (Leadership) have been rated, go to the last page in the Leadership Category. Follow the directions and identify two areas you believe most need improvement in your organization now. Then, go back to the space below each row of statements you identified as vital to improve. Describe briefly the activities your organization conducts that relate to the topic. Also, please suggest steps that your organization or its leaders could take to improve the processes. Your thoughtful comments are as helpful as the rating itself. If you want to comment on more themes, please do so.

- Continue in the same way to complete all seven Categories.

SUMMARY OF CATEGORY 1: LEADERSHIP

This sample assessment looks at one question in the Leadership Category (Figure 37). The full-length assessment of Leadership contains 10 themes.

The first part (seven questions, 1A through 1G) looks at how senior leaders guide the organization by setting directions and monitoring performance to help assure the long-term success of the organization. Senior leaders should express clear values and set high performance expectations that address the needs of patients and other customers and stakeholders. In addition, an effective governance structure must be in place to ensure management accountability and the protection of stockholder and stakeholder interests.

- You are asked to comment on the extent to which senior leaders set directions, communicate, and deploy values and performance expectations, and take into account the expectations of patients and customers and other stakeholders. This includes how leaders create an environment for empowerment, innovation, safety, and organizational agility.

- You are asked how the organizational governance structure ensures accountability for fiscal and management integrity as well as the protection of stockholder and stakeholder interests. You also are asked how senior leaders review organizational performance, what key performance measures they regularly review, and how review findings are used to drive improvement and change, including improving leaders' effectiveness.

The second part (three questions, 1H through 1J) looks at how well the organization meets its responsibilities to the public, ensures ethical behavior, and practices good citizenship.

- You are asked how the organization addresses current and future impacts on society in a proactive manner and how it ensures ethical health care service practices in all stakeholder interactions. The impacts and practices are expected to cover all relevant and important areas—programs, offerings, services, and operations. You also are asked how the organization, senior leaders, and staff identify, support, and strengthen key communities as part of good citizenship practices.

Leadership Commitment to Providing Maximum Value for Patients and Other Customers and Stakeholders [Baldrige reference: 1.1a(1)]

1B. How serious are top leaders about providing maximum value to patients and stakeholders? Do they make it clear that producing value for all patients and other customers and stakeholders is critical for success?

Not Evident
1. Leaders focus on short-term health care service issues, not on value for patients and other stakeholders.

Beginning
2. A few leaders are just beginning to focus on value for patients and other stakeholders.

Basically Effective
3. Some leaders effectively focus occasionally on value for patients and other customers and stakeholders based on their written and verbal communication.

Mature
4. Many leaders and supervisors effectively focus on providing maximum value to many patient and other customer and stakeholder groups. They sometimes check on the effectiveness of these activities.

Advanced
5. Most leaders and supervisors effectively focus on providing maximum value to most types of patients and other customers and stakeholders. They regularly check on the effectiveness of these activities. They sometimes make improvements.

Role Model
6. Nearly all leaders and supervisors effectively focus on providing maximum value to all types of patients and other customers and stakeholders. They regularly check on the effectiveness of these activities. They make ongoing improvements.

NA. Not Applicable
I do not have enough information to answer this question.

Figure 37 Sample leadership question.

SUMMARY OF CATEGORY 2: STRATEGIC PLANNING

This sample assessment looks at one question in the Strategic Planning Category (Figure 38). The full-length assessment of Strategic Planning contains seven themes.

The first part (three questions, 2A through 2C) looks at how the organization develops its strategic plans. The Category stresses that patient, other customer, health care market and overall performance excellence are key strategic issues that need to be integral parts of the organization's overall planning. Specifically:

- Patient, other customer, and health care market-driven quality is a strategic view of quality. The focus is on the drivers of patient and other customer, and health care market needs and expectations—key factors in competitiveness, innovation, and health care service success.

- Operational performance improvement contributes to short-term and longer-term productivity, growth, and competitiveness. Building operational capability—including speed, responsiveness, and flexibility—represents an investment in strengthening your competitive fitness.

The second part (four questions, 2D through 2G) looks at the way work processes support the organization's strategic directions, to help make sure that priorities are carried out.

- The organization must translate its strategic objectives into action plans to accomplish the objectives. The organization must also be able to assess the progress of action plans. The aim is to ensure that strategies are understood and followed by everyone in the organization to help achieve goals.

Developing and Deploying Action Plans Based on Strategic Objectives [Baldrige Reference: 2.2a(1)]

2D. How well do the organization's action plans support its strategic objectives? Do the action plans help all parts of the organization pull together (align) to carry out its strategic objectives? Are appropriate resources allocated to carry out the actions?

Not Evident
1. The organization does not systematically develop action plans to support strategic objectives.

Beginning
2. The organization has developed action plans to support a few strategic objectives. Resources are not effectively allocated to achieve desired actions.

Basically Effective
3. The organization has developed action plans to support some strategic objectives. Resources are generally allocated to achieve desired actions.

Mature
4. The organization has developed action plans to support many strategic objectives. Resources are effectively allocated to achieve desired actions. The action plans and resources are sometimes checked to make sure the work of some staff is focused on actions needed to carry out strategic objectives.

Advanced
5. The organization has developed action plans to support most strategic objectives. Resources are effectively allocated to achieve desired actions. The action plans and resources are sometimes improved to make sure the work of most staff is focused on actions needed to carry out strategic objectives.

Role Model
6. The organization has developed action plans to support all strategic objectives. Resources are effectively allocated to achieve desired actions. The action plans and resources are regularly checked to see how well they support objectives. Improvements resulting from the action plans are maintained. Action plans are consistently improved to make sure the work of nearly all staff is focused on actions needed to carry out strategic objectives.

NA. Not Applicable
I do not have enough information to answer this question.

Figure 38 Sample strategic planning question.

SUMMARY OF CATEGORY 3: FOCUS ON PATIENTS, OTHER CUSTOMERS, AND MARKETS

This sample assessment looks at one question in the Patient and Other Customer and Market Focus Category (Figure 39). The full-length assessment of Focus on Patients, Other Customers, and Markets contains 10 themes:

The first part (four questions, 3A through 3D) looks at how the organization tries to understand what the patients, other customers, and the marketplace wants. The organization must learn about patients, other customers, and markets to help make sure it understands new requirements, offers the right health care services, and keeps pace with changing patient, other customer, and marketplace demand, as well as increasing competition.

- You are asked how the organization determines key patient and other customer groups, and how it segments the markets.

- You are asked how the organization determines the most important health care service features.

- Also, you are asked how the organization improves the way it listens and learns from patients and other customers so that it keeps current with changing health care service needs and directions.

The second part (six questions, 3E through 3J) looks at how well the organization builds good relationships with patients, and other customers to increase loyalty, develop new opportunities, and get positive referrals. You are also asked how the organization gets data on patient and other customer satisfaction and dissatisfaction for itself and for its own and competitors' patients and other customers.

- You are asked how the organization makes it easy for patients, other customers and potential patients to get information or assistance and/or to comment and complain.

- You are asked how the organization gathers, analyzes, and learns from complaint information to increase patient and other customer satisfaction and loyalty.

- You are asked how the organization builds relationships with patients and other customers since success depends on maintaining close relationships.

- You are asked how the organization determines the satisfaction and dissatisfaction for different patient and other customer groups necessary for loyalty, repeat health care service, and positive referrals.

- Finally, you are asked how the organization follows up with patients and other customers, and how it determines their satisfaction relative to competitors so that it may improve future performance.

Understanding What Patients/Customers Value Most in Health Care Services [Baldrige Reference: 3.1a(2)]

3D. How well does the organization determine the most important requirements and preferences of its various patient/customer groups and market segments that drive their purchasing decisions?

Not Evident
1.   The organization does not have an effective process to learn about the priorities of its patient/customers.

Beginning
2.   The organization has just started to determine what is most important to a few patient/customer groups or segments for a few health care services.

Basically Effective
3.   An effective system is in place to determine what is most important to some patient/customer groups or segments for some health care services.

Mature
4.   An effective system is in place to determine what is most important to many patient/customer groups or segments for many health care services. These processes are sometimes checked for accuracy and completeness.

Advanced
5.   An effective system is in place to determine what is most important to most patient/customer groups or segments for most health care services. These processes are regularly checked for accuracy and completeness and sometimes improved.

Role Model
6.   An effective system is in place to determine what is most important to all patient/customer groups or segments for nearly all health care services for the entire service life cycle. These processes are regularly checked for accuracy and completeness and consistently improved.

NA. Not Applicable
I do not have enough information to answer this question.

Figure 39   Sample patient and other customer and market focus question.

SUMMARY OF CATEGORY 4: MEASUREMENT, ANALYSIS, AND KNOWLEDGE MANAGEMENT

This sample assessment looks at one question in the Measurement, Analysis, and Knowledge Management Category (Figure 40).

Measurement, Analysis, and Knowledge Management is the "brain center" of an effective management system. Appropriate information and analysis are used to improve decision making at all levels to achieve high levels of performance. Effective measures, properly deployed, help align the organization's operations to achieve its strategic goals as well as protect organizational knowledge. The first part (five questions, 4A through 4E) looks at the selection, collection, alignment and integration of data and information to support effective decision making at all levels. Data and information guide decision making to help the organization achieve key health care service results and strategic objectives. Measurement, Analysis, and Knowledge systems serve as a key foundation for achieving innovation and sustaining peak performance.

- The organization must build an effective performance-measurement system. It must select, align, and integrate the right measures for tracking daily operations and use those measures for monitoring overall organizational performance. The organization must also make sure that data and information are accurate and reliable.

- Competitive comparisons and benchmarking (best practices) information should be used to help drive innovation and performance improvement.

- The organization should evaluate and improve the performance-measurement system to keep it current with changing health care service needs and able to respond to rapid changes.

- Data and information concerning processes and results (outcomes) from all parts of the organization must be analyzed to support the senior leaders' assessment of overall organizational health, organizational planning, and daily operations.

- Analyses must be communicated to support decision making and strategic planning at all levels of the organization.

The second part (four questions, 4F through 4I) looks at how the organization ensures the quality and availability of data and information to support effective decision making for staff and appropriate suppliers, partners, patients, and other customers. It also examines building and managing knowledge assets.

- The organization must ensure integrity (completeness) of data and information and ensure they are available, accessible, reliable, accurate, timely, confidential, and secure.

- The organization must identify, manage, collect, and transfer relevant knowledge and best practices.

- For data that are captured, stored, analyzed, and/or accessed through electronic means, the organization must ensure hardware and software reliability, security, and user friendliness.

All of these systems must be evaluated and enhanced to ensure they remain current with changing health care service needs and directions.

Selecting Measures to Track Daily Operations and Overall Organizational Performance [Baldrige Reference: 4.1a(1 and 3)]

4B. How well does the organization select and align appropriate measures throughout the organization to effectively track daily operations and overall organizational performance?

Not Evident

1. The organization does not systematically collect data to track how well it performs.

Beginning

2. The organization collects data to track health care service results, but very few other areas.

Basically Effective

3. The organization collects data to understand some areas of organizational performance, such as health care, patient and other customer, financial, market, staff and work systems.

Mature

4. Effective processes are in place to select and collect data to understand organizational performance in many of the following areas: patient and other customer, financial and market, staff and work systems, operational effectiveness, and governance and social responsibility. The organization sometimes checks how well the data enable tracking at the different levels.

Advanced

5. Effective processes are in place to select, collect, and align data to understand organizational performance in most of the following areas: health care, patient and other customer, financial and market, staff and work systems, operational effectiveness, and governance and social responsibility. The organization regularly checks how well the data enable tracking and promote alignment at the different levels and sometimes makes improvements.

Role Model

6. Effective processes are in place to select, collect, align, and integrate data to understand organizational performance in nearly all of the following areas: health care, patient and other customer, financial and market, staff and work systems, operational effectiveness, and governance and social responsibility. The organization regularly checks how well the data enable tracking and promote alignment throughout the organization and makes ongoing improvements.

NA. Not Applicable

I do not have enough information to answer this question.

Figure 40 Sample measurement, analysis, and knowledge management question.

SUMMARY OF CATEGORY 5: STAFF FOCUS

This sample assessment looks at one question in the Staff Focus Category (Figure 41). The full-length assessment of Staff Focus contains 13 themes.

The first part (six questions, 5A through 5F) looks at how well the organization's systems for work and job design, compensation, motivation, recognition, and hiring help all staff reach peak performance.

- You are asked how the organization designs work and jobs to empower staff to exercise initiative, innovation, and decision making, resulting in high performance.

- You are asked how the organization compensates, recognizes, and rewards staff to support its high performance objectives (strategic objectives) as well as ensuring a patient/customer and health care service focus.

- Finally, you are asked how the organization recruits and hires staff that will meet its expectations and needs. The right workforce is an enabler of high performance.

The second part (three questions, 5G through 5I) looks at how well education, training, and career development support high performance.

- You are asked how education and training are designed, delivered, reinforced on the job, and evaluated.

- You are also asked about how well the organization provides training in different areas of performance excellence, which includes leadership development.

- In addition, you are asked how staff are motivated to reach their full potential.

The third part (four questions, 5J through 5M) looks at the organization's work environment, its staff support climate, and how the organization determines staff satisfaction, with the aim of fostering the well-being, satisfaction, and motivation of all staff.

- You are asked how the organization's work environment for all staff is safe, secure, and healthful.

- You are also asked how well the organization is prepared to deal with emergencies and disasters to ensure the organization continues to function.

- You are asked how the organization enhances well-being, satisfaction, and motivation for all staff groups.

- Finally, you are asked how the organization assesses staff well-being, satisfaction, and motivation, and how it relates assessment findings to key health care service results to set improvement priorities.

2003 Baldrige Health Care

Providing Feedback, Compensation, and Recognition to Support High Performance Goals and a Patient/Customer and Health Care Service Focus [Baldrige Reference: 5.1b]

5D. How well do leaders and supervisors at all levels provide feedback to staff and make sure pay, reward, and recognition support high performance and a patient/customer and health care service focus? [Note that compensation and recognition might include promotions and bonuses based on performance, skills acquired, and other factors contributing to high performance goals. Recognition may be provided to individuals and/or groups and includes monetary and non-monetary and formal and informal techniques.]

Not Evident

1. The organization does not systematically provide effective feedback to staff, or tie pay or recognition to performance.

Beginning

2. The organization provides effective feedback about performance to a few staff. It rarely ties pay and recognition to performance.

Basically Effective

3. The organization provides effective feedback about performance to some staff. It ties pay and recognition to some high performance.

Mature

4. The organization provides effective feedback about performance to many staff. It ties pay and recognition to many high performance goals. The organization sometimes checks its processes.

Advanced

5. The organization provides effective feedback about performance to most staff. It ties pay and recognition to most high performance, patient/customer and health care service goals and strategies. The organization regularly checks its feedback and compensation processes, and improvements are sometimes made.

Role Model

6. The organization provides effective feedback about performance to nearly all staff. It ties pay and recognition to nearly all high performance, patient/customer and health care service goals and strategies. The organization regularly checks its feedback and compensation processes and makes ongoing improvements.

NA. Not Applicable

I do not have enough information to answer this question.

Figure 41 Sample staff focus question.

SUMMARY OF CATEGORY 6: PROCESS MANAGEMENT

This sample assessment looks at one question in the Process Management Category (Figure 42). The full-length assessment of Process Management contains seven themes. Process Management is the focal point for all key work processes.

The first part (four questions, 6A through 6D) looks at the organization's key processes for delivering patient health care services.

- You are asked how key health care services and service delivery processes are determined using input from patient, other customers, stakeholders, and suppliers/partners as appropriate.

- You are asked how all key requirements are addressed in the design process. You are also asked how patient safety, regulatory accreditation, payor requirements, productivity, cost control, new technology, and efficiency and effectiveness are considered during the design phase. You should make sure that design processes actually work as expected.

- You are asked how the organization makes sure that health care services and service delivery processes work consistently and how performance measures are used to get an early alert of potential problems so you can take prompt corrective action.

- You are asked how patients' expectations, preferences, and decision making are addressed and how delivery processes and outcomes are explained.

- You are asked how measures and indicators are used to control and improve key health care services and service delivery processes.

- In addition, you are asked how the organization improves its health care services and service delivery processes to achieve better performance, and how it shares these improvements and keeps processes current with changing health care needs and directions.

The second part (three questions, 6E through 6G) examines the organization's key business and other support processes, with the aim of improving overall performance.

- You are asked how key support processes are designed to meet all the requirements of internal and external patients.

- The day-to-day operation of key support processes should meet the key requirements. In-process measures and internal patients and stakeholder feedback should be used to get an early alert of problems.

- Finally, you are asked how the organization improves its key support processes to achieve better performance.

Defining Key Health Care Process Requirements [Baldrige reference: 6.1a(1, 2, and 7)]

6A. How does the organization determine key health care service and related delivery process requirements using input from patients/customers, stakeholders, and suppliers/partners as appropriate? [Note that key health care service processes are those considered most important to creating value for the organization, patients and other customers, and stakeholders.]

Not Evident
1.   The organization does not systematically define key health care service processes or identify key process requirements.

Beginning
2.   The organization defines a few of the basic health care service processes. Performance requirements are not well defined.

Basically Effective
3.   Effective processes are in place to identify performance requirements based on patient input for some health care service processes.

Mature
4.   Effective processes are in place to accurately and completely identify performance requirements in measurable terms based on patient and stakeholder input for many health care service processes. The organization sometimes checks the effectiveness of these processes.

Advanced
5.   Effective processes are in place to accurately and completely identify performance requirements in measurable terms based on patient, other customer, stakeholder, and appropriate supplier and partner input for most health care service processes. The organization regularly checks the effectiveness of these processes, sometimes makes improvements, and sometimes shares the improvements with other organizational units.

Role Model
6.   Effective processes are in place to accurately and completely identify performance requirements in measurable terms based on patient, other customer, stakeholder, and appropriate supplier and partner input for nearly all health care service processes. The organization regularly checks the effectiveness of these processes, makes ongoing improvements, and nearly always shares the improvements with other organizational units.

NA. Not Applicable
I do not have enough information to answer this question.

Figure 42 Sample process management question.

SUMMARY OF CATEGORY 7: ORGANIZATIONAL PERFORMANCE RESULTS

This sample assessment looks at one theme in the Organizational Performance Results Category (Figure 43). The full-length assessment contains six themes.

The Organizational Performance Results Category looks for the results produced by the management systems described in Categories 1 through 6. Results range from lagging performance outcomes, such as health care results, patient- and other customer-focused satisfaction, to predictive outcomes, such as internal operating measures and staff and work system results. Together, these lagging and leading results create a set of balanced indicators of organizational health, commonly called a "balanced scorecard."

- Question 7A looks at key health care results.

- Question 7B looks at how well the organization has been satisfying patients and customers.

- Question 7C looks at the strength of the organization's financial and market results.

- Question 7D looks at how well the organization has been creating and maintaining a positive, productive, learning, and caring work environment.

- Question 7E looks at the organization's key operational (internal) performance results with the aim of achieving organizational effectiveness.

- Question 7F looks at key results in the areas of the organization's social responsibilities, fiscal accountability, citizenship, ethical behavior, and compliance with applicable laws and regulations.

Patient and Customer-Focused Results [Baldrige Reference: 7.2a (1 and 2)]

What are the trends and results for patient and other customer satisfaction and dissatisfaction? These include measures of perceived value, patient- and other-customer relationship building, loyalty, retention, and positive referral. [Results data may include internal measures, such as gains and losses of patients. It may also include information from independent organizations and key stakeholders such as surveys, awards, recognition, and ratings.]

Not Evident
1. No results or poor results exist.

Beginning
2. Performance levels are good in very few areas that are important to health care service.

Basically Effective
3. Performance levels are good in some areas important to health care service. The organization is beginning to demonstrate improvement trends and to get comparison data.

Mature
4. Performance levels are good in many areas of importance to the organization's key health care service requirements (such as patient and other customer satisfaction, dissatisfaction, and loyalty indicators, measures of patient- and other customer-perceived value, retention, and positive referral) when compared to industry average. Some trends in areas of importance to the organization's key health care service requirements show growth.

Advanced
5. Performance levels are good to very good in many to most areas of importance to the organization's key health care service requirements (such as patient and other customer satisfaction, dissatisfaction, and loyalty indicators, measures of patient- and other customer-perceived value, retention, and positive referral) when compared to top-performing competitors or benchmarks. Unless the actual level of performance is already at the top levels, many to most trends in areas of importance to the organization's key health care service requirements continue to improve and show sustained growth. No pattern of adverse trends and no poor performance levels are evident in areas of importance to the organization's key health care service requirements.

Role Model
6. Performance levels are good to excellent in many to most areas of importance to the organization's key health care service requirements (such as patient and other customer satisfaction, dissatisfaction, and loyalty indicators, measures of patient- and other customer-perceived value, retention, and positive referral) when compared to top-performing competitors or benchmarks. Unless the actual level of performance is already at the top levels, most trends in areas of importance to the organization's key health care service requirements continue to improve and show sustained growth. No pattern of adverse trends and no poor performance levels are evident in areas of importance to the organization's key health care service requirements.

NA. Not Applicable
I do not have enough information to answer this question.

Figure 43 Sample process management question.

The Site Visit

INTRODUCTION

Many people and organizations have asked about how to prepare for site visits. This section is intended to help answer those questions and prepare the organization for an on-site examination. It includes rules of the game for examiners and what they are taught to look for. As we all know, the best preparation for this type of examination is to see things through the eyes of the trained examiner.

Before an organization can be recommended to receive the Malcolm Baldrige National Quality Award, it must receive a visit from a team of health care service assessment experts from the National Board of Examiners. Approximately 25 percent to 30 percent of organizations' applying for the Baldrige Award in recent years have received these site visits.

The Baldrige Award site-visit team usually includes at least two senior Examiners—one of whom is designated as team leader—and three to eight other Examiners. In addition, the team is accompanied by a representative of the National Quality Award Office and a representative of the American Society for Quality (ASQ), which provides administrative services to the Baldrige Award Office under contract.

The site-visit team usually gathers at a hotel near the organization's headquarters on the Sunday morning immediately preceding the site visit. During the day, the team makes final preparations and plans for the visit.

Each team member is assigned lead responsibility for one or more Categories of the Award Criteria. Each Examiner is usually teamed with one other Examiner during the site visit. These Examiners usually conduct the visit in pairs to ensure the accurate recording of information.

Site visits usually begin on a Monday morning and last one week. By Wednesday or Thursday, most site-visit teams will have completed their on-site review. They retire to the nearby hotel to confer and write their reports. By the end of the week, the team must reach consensus on the findings and prepare a final report for the panel of judges.

Purpose of Site Visits

Site visits help clarify uncertain points and verify self-assessment (that is, application) accuracy. During the site visit, examiners investigate areas most difficult to understand from self-assessments, such as the following:

- Deployment: How widely a process is used throughout the organization

- Integration: Whether processes fit together to support Performance Excellence

- Process ownership: Whether processes are broadly owned, simply directed, or micromanaged

- Staff involvement: Whether the extent to which staff participation in managing processes of all types is optimized

- Continuous improvement maturity: The number and extent of improvement cycles and resulting refinements in all areas of the organization and at all levels

Characteristics of Site Visit Issues

Examiners look at issues that are an essential component of scoring and role model determination. They have a responsibility to:

- Clarify information that is missing or vague, and verify significant strengths identified from the self-assessment

- Verify deployment of the practices described in the self-assessment

  Examiners will:

- Concentrate on cross-cutting issues

- Examine data, reports, and documents

- Interview individuals and teams

- Receive presentations from the applicant organization

Examiners may not conduct their own focus groups or surveys with patients and customers, suppliers, or dealers. Conducting focus groups or surveys would violate confidentiality agreements and be statistically unsound.

Discussions with the Applicant Prior to the Site Visit

Prior to the official Baldrige Award site visit, all communication between the applicant organization and its team must be routed through their respective single points of contact. Only the team leader may contact the applicant on behalf of the site-visit team prior to the site visit. This helps ensure consistency of message and communication for both parties. It prevents confusion and misunderstandings. The team leader should provide the applicant organization with basic information about the process. This includes schedules, arrival times, and equipment and meeting room needs.

Applicant organizations usually provide the following information prior to the site-visit team's final planning meeting at the hotel on the day before the site visit starts:

- List of key contacts

- Organization chart

- Facility layout

- Performance data requested by Examiners

Typically Important Site Visit Issues

- Role of senior leaders in leading and serving as a role model
- Independence of governance system to protect stakeholder interests and hold management accountable
- Degree of involvement and self-direction of staff below upper management
- Comprehensiveness and accessibility of the information system
- Extent that facts and data are used in decision making
- Degree of emphasis on patient and customer satisfaction
- Extent of systematic approaches to work processes
- Training effectiveness
- Use of compensation, recognition, and rewards to promote key values
- Extent that strategic plans align organizational work
- Extent of the use of measurable goals at all levels in the organization
- Evidence of evaluation and improvement cycles in all work processes and in system effectiveness
- Improvements in cycle times and other operating processes
- Extent of integration of all processes—operational and support
- Extent of benchmarking effort
- Uncovering improvements since the submission of the application (self-assessment) and receiving up-to-date health care service results

The team leader, on behalf of team members, will ask for supplementary documentation to be compiled (such as results data brought up to date) to avoid placing an undue burden on the organization at the time of the site visit. The site-visit team will select sites that allow them to examine key issues and check deployment in key areas. This information may or may not be discussed with the applicant prior to the site visit. Examiners will need access to all areas of the organization.

Conduct of Site-Visit Team Members (Examiners)

Examiners are not allowed to discuss findings with anyone but team members. Examiners may not disclose the following to the applicant:

- Personal or team observations and findings

- Conclusions and decisions

- Observations about the applicant's performance systems, whether in a complimentary or critical way

Examiners may not discuss the following with anyone:

- Observations about other applicants

- Names of other award program applicants

Examiners may not accept trinkets, gifts, or gratuities of any kind (coffee, cookies, rolls, breakfast, and lunch are OK), so applicant organizations should not offer them. At the conclusion of the site visit, Examiners are not permitted to leave with any of the applicant's materials including logo items or catalogs—not even items usually given to visitors. Examiners will dress in appropriate business service attire unless instructed otherwise by the applicant organization.

Opening Meeting

An opening meeting will be scheduled to introduce all parties and set the structure for the site visit. The meeting is usually attended by senior executives and the self-assessment writing team. The opening meeting usually is scheduled on the initial day of the site visit (8:30 or 9:00 a.m.). The team leader generally starts the meeting, introduces the team, and opens the site visit. Overhead slides and formal presentations are usually unnecessary.

The applicant organization usually has one hour to present any information it believes important for the Examiners to know. This includes time for a tour, if necessary.

Immediately after the meeting, Examiners usually meet with senior leaders and those responsible for preparing sections of the self-assessment (application) since those people are likely to be at the opening meeting.

Conducting the Site Visit

The team will follow the site-visit plan, subject to periodic adjustments according to its findings. The site-visit team will need a private room to conduct frequent caucuses. Applicant representatives are not present at these caucuses. The team will also conduct evening meetings at the hotel to review the findings of the day, reach consensus, write comments, and revise the site-visit report.

If, during the course of the site visit, someone from the applicant organization believes the team or any of its members are missing the point, the designated point of contact should inform the team leader or the Baldrige Award office monitor. Also, someone who believes an Examiner behaved inappropriately should inform the designated point of contact, who will inform the team leader or the award office monitor.

Staff should be instructed to mark every document given to Examiners with the name and work location of the person providing the document. This will ensure that it is returned to the proper person. Records should be made of all material given to team members. Organizational personnel may not ask Examiners for opinions and advice. Examiners are not permitted to provide any information of this type during the site visit.

GENERIC SITE VISIT QUESTIONS

Examiners must verify or clarify the information contained in an application, whether they have determined a process to be a strength or an opportunity for improvement. Examiners must verify the existence of strengths as well as clarify the nature of each opportunity for improvement in the final feedback report.

Before and during the site visit review process, Examiners formulate a series of questions based on the Baldrige Criteria. It is possible to identify a series of generic questions that examiners are likely to ask during the site visit process, based only on the Baldrige Criteria. Of course, all questions should be tailored to the specific key factors of the organization to be most relevant. The questions in the following section are presented to help prepare applicants and Examiners for the site-visit process.

Category 1—Leadership

1. (To top leaders) How do you set direction and guide the organization? Please share with us the values of your organization.

   - What are your top priorities?

   - How do you ensure that all your staff know these priorities?

   - How do you know how effective you are at communicating these values?

   - How do you know your messages to staff are understood as intended?

2. What are your key patient, other customer, or stakeholder segments?

   - Pick one and ask: What does this patient, customer/stakeholder group value? How do you know?

   - Arc the requirements or value expected of this customer group different from any other group? If so, what are the differences, and how have you ensured that the different or competing interests of these groups is addressed by your organization?

3. What are the ways you communicate throughout the organization and to key partners and suppliers?

   - What kinds of communication or feedback do you receive from staff and partners/suppliers? What do you do with this information? How well do these processes work? How do you know? What has been done to improve them?

4. What is your role in supporting processes to ensure performance excellence?

   - What are the behaviors you want your managers and other staff to emulate? Give me some examples of what you do personally to model these behaviors to staff and managers throughout the organization.

   - How do you encourage innovation and staff empowerment? Give me some examples of improved innovation throughout the organization as a result of your efforts. (Follow up on these examples with other staff.)

   - How do you ensure that middle managers and other subordinates promote staff empowerment and innovation throughout the organization?

   - What does organizational agility mean to you? What are the barriers to this agility you have identified in the organization? Pick some barriers and ask: What have you done to overcome this barrier?

   - What processes have you put in place to ensure that innovations and other knowledge are effectively shared throughout the organization to appropriate managers and staff? How well do these processes work? How do you know? What has been done to improve them?

5. What policies and principles exist in the organization to promote or require ethical and legal behavior?

   - What are some of the most important ethical principles? What processes have you put in place to achieve the desired ethical behavior?

How well do these processes work? How do you know? What has been done to improve them?

6. How independent is your board of directors?

- What percentage of the board is not affiliated with your organization in any way (other than being a board member)?

- How does your audit function ensure objectivity and independence?

- Have problems existed in the past where stakeholder interests were threatened? If so, what was done to prevent the possibility of those problems recurring?

- How does the board make sure managers behave properly and account for their actions in the organization?

- How would you rate the board's climate of trust? To what extent is dissension and disagreement among board members tolerated? Encouraged?

- What policies are in place to ensure the board remains alert to management problems in the organization?

- What type of fiscal oversight does the board provide? What problems or issues have emerged in the past three to five years? Pick some and ask: What was the board's reaction to this issue? How was it resolved? What steps were taken to prevent the problem from happening again?

- What processes have you put in place to ensure the board effectively protects stockholder and shareholder value? How well do these processes work? How do you know? What has been done to improve them?

7. What is the process used to monitor the performance of your organization? How does it relate to the organization's strategic health care service plan?

- What measurable goals exist? How are they monitored? How often? How well do these

processes work? How do you know? What has been done to improve them?

- What are the key success factors (or key result areas, critical success factors, key health care service drivers) for your organization, and how do you use them to drive Performance Excellence?

- What percentage of your time is spent on performance review and improvement activities? How do you review performance to assess the organization's health, competitive performance, and progress against key objectives? What key performance measures do you and other senior leaders regularly review?

- How do top priorities and opportunities for innovation reflect organizational review findings? Have you set or changed priorities for innovation and resource allocation? Please give examples of how this is done.

- How do you ensure that these priorities and opportunities for innovation are understood and used throughout the organization to align work? (After you identify a top priority for innovation, ask the leader to provide specific examples of how he or she ensures these priorities are implemented and aligned throughout the organization, as appropriate.) To what extent do these priorities and innovation opportunities involve support from key suppliers and/or partners? (Pick one example of a priority and ask the leader to help you understand how the organization works with affected suppliers or partners.)

8. What is your process for evaluating the effectiveness of the leadership system?

- How do you include or use staff feedback in the evaluation?

- Please identify specific examples where senior leadership improved the leadership system as a result of these evaluations. How do managers evaluate and improve their personal leadership effectiveness? How are data from organizational performance reviews used here?

9. What are the criteria for promoting and rewarding managers within the organization?

   • How are you making managers accountable for performance improvement, staff involvement, and customer satisfaction objectives? (Look at some samples of managers' evaluations [chosen at random] and check to see if they reflect refinements based on organizational performance-review findings and staff feedback.)

   • How have you improved the process of evaluating managers over the years?

   • What processes have been put in place to evaluate and improve the effectiveness of the board of directors as a whole and individual board members? How well do these processes work? How do you know? What has been done to improve them?

10. What do you do to anticipate public concerns over the possible impact of your organization? How do you determine what risks the public faces because of your programs, products, services, and operations? What are some examples of risks you have identified? Pick some risks at random and ask: What have you done to reduce the risk or threat to the public? How do you know you are successful in these areas? How do you measure progress?

   • What goals have been developed to identify and reduce risks?

   • What are the biggest environmental issues your organization faces? As a corporate citizen, what is your process for contributing to and improving the environment and society?

   • How do you know that your processes for protecting the public from risks associated with your programs, services, and programs are effective? How have you improved these processes?

11. What are some ways your organization ensures that staff and key partners act in an ethical manner in all health care service and stakeholder transactions? How is this measured and monitored to ensure compliance?

12. What support does your organization provide to local communities? Why do you provide this support?

   • How do you know that the processes you have in place for identifying and supporting key communities are appropriate?

   • How do you know the resource issues allocated for these purposes are appropriately used? Have you always provided this type of support?

   • What has been done to improve your efforts to support these communities?

Category 2—Strategic Planning

1. When was the last time the strategic plan was updated? Were you involved in the strategic planning process? What was your role? Who else was involved and what did each contribute?

   • How far out does your planning look? Why? Why not shorter or longer?

   • How does the overall process for developing strategy work? (If the person was involved in the planning process, ask them to recite how the process works without referring to written documentation. We must determine whether a consistent planning process is in place that meets the requirements of the criteria; we are not testing the ability of senior leaders to read a written document.)

2. What data, information, and other factors did you consider in the development of your strategic plan?

   • Does your organization depend on key suppliers or partners to be successful? If so, which ones? Pick some from their list and ask: How did you consider the needs and capabilities of these suppliers/partners during the process of developing your strategic plan?

- Does your organization have key competitors that affect your ability to be successful? Which ones? Pick some and ask: What abilities does this competitor possess that may create a problem for your organization? How did you consider the threats posed by this key competitor during the process of developing your strategic plan? How has your plan addressed these potential problems or threats?

- Is your organization helped or hurt by new technologies? Which ones? Pick some and ask: How did you consider these new technologies during the process of developing your strategic plan?

- How do you consider the needs of key patients and customers (or other appropriate stakeholders) in the development of the strategic plan? How do you balance the requirements and preferences of these patients and customers when they are conflicting? Please give some examples.

- What future regulatory, legal, financial, economic, or ethical risks does your organization face? Pick some and ask: How did you determine this was a risk? How did your planning process consider the potential problems presented by this risk when developing your plan?

- Were you or are you likely to be affected by changes in national or global economy? If so, in what ways? Help me understand how you considered the likely impact of these problems in your planning process.

- How has your planning process helped you identify opportunities to redirect resources to more productive uses, such as higher priority services or programs? Please give some examples of new opportunities and describe how you capitalized on them, as a result of your planning.

- What have you done to check the accuracy of planning assumptions and projections you used in the past to develop your strategic plan? How accurate have your past planning assumptions been? What have you done to improve the accuracy and effectiveness of your planning process? What refinements have you made during the past few years?

3. How often do you review progress of your key strategic objectives? Please show me the timelines or projections for achieving each objective. How did you develop the projected or expected levels of future performance for each strategic objective (also called timelines)?

   - Can you tell from this information where you expect to be on each objective next quarter? Next year? In two years? (Note: the frequency of review should be consistent with the review processes described in Item 1.1c(1). For example, if progress toward achieving the patient- and customer-satisfaction objectives is reviewed quarterly by the senior leadership team, then quarterly milestones should be defined to permit effective review. In addition, the timelines reported under 2.1b(1) should identify the measurable levels of performance that are expected during these reviews.)

   - How did you determine the appropriate frequency or period to review progress for these objectives?

   - How did you determine the appropriate frequency or period to review progress for these objectives?

4. What is the process you use to identify the actions that need to be taken throughout the organization in order to meet your goals or strategic objectives?

   - How do you break the strategic objectives up into actions that drive work at all levels of the organization?

   - How do you make sure that every staff member knows what work he or she must do to achieve his or her part of the plan?

   - What process is used to figure out what resources are needed to do this work? How are resources allocated to make sure the actions can be completed on schedule? How effective are these processes? How do you know? What improvements in the processes of converting plans to actions and assigning resources have been made in the past few years?

- How do you determine what people and skills you will need to carry out your strategic objectives and related action plans? What changes have been made in your staffing plans during the past few years to help you achieve your strategic objectives and related action plans? How effective and accurate have your human resource plans been?

5. Another way of examining the issues outlined in the question above is as follows: How do you make sure that goals, objectives, and action plans are understood and used throughout the organization to drive and align work?

- How do you ensure that organizational, work unit, and individual actions and resources are aligned at all levels? (Pick a strategy that the leader has indicated is important to organizational success. Then ask the leader what actions he or she has determined are critical to achieve the strategy. From the list of actions, pick one or two and ask the leader to explain specifically how resources were allocated to ensure these plans would be accomplished. Then ask how the leader checks to determine if appropriate resources were allocated. Ask if any improvements have been made in this process over the past few years. Repeat this line of questioning at different levels in the organization to check alignment.)

6. Describe your long- and short-term plans to meet the recruitment, recognition, safety and security, motivation, development, education, and training needs of the organization that are necessary to carry out the strategic plans. What are the measures of progress to meet these staffing plans?

- Summarize the organization's human resource plans that are needed to carry out the strategic objectives and related action plans. How do these human resource plans ensure sufficient staff?

- What are examples of changes to the human resource plans based on inputs from the

strategic planning in the following areas: recruitment, training, compensation, rewards, incentives, fringe benefits, and other programs, as appropriate?

7. What is (summarize) your process for evaluation and improvement of the strategic planning and plan deployment process, including human resource planning?

- What are examples of improvements made as a result of these evaluation processes? Where and when did they occur?

- Why did you decide to focus on these improvements? What facts helped with your decisions on what to improve and how to improve the planning process?

8. How did you determine that the goals or objectives you set were appropriate?

- Show how the strategic objectives address each of the challenges you said were important in the Organizational Profile (P.2).

9. Who do you consider to be your top competitors, and how does your planned performance (goals) compare to theirs and/or similar providers? How did you determine who your top competitors are?

- At what level do you expect your key competitors or other similar providers to perform during the same period as your plan covers?

- How did you figure this out?

- How accurate have your past estimates of competitor's future performance been? What have you done to make these projections more accurate?

Category 3—Patient, Other Customer and Market Focus

1. Who are your key patients and customers, customer groups, or market segments?

- What was your reason for grouping them this way?

- How did you determine what your patients and customers expect of you?

- How does your organization determine short- and long-term patient and customer requirements for each of the groups or segments? Do you use the same techniques for all patient and customer groups? Why or why not?

- How do you know what the patients and customers of your competitors (your potential patients and customers) are getting or want? How have you used this knowledge?

- How do you use information you learned from patients and customers, including data such as retention rates, complaints, and loyalty, to plan programs and services, market them, make improvements in them, or develop new health care services?

2. What are the key requirements of your patients and customers (break out by segment or group)? Are the requirements of potential patients and customers different from the requirements of the patients and customers you presently serve?

- What is most important or valuable to the different groups you serve or want to serve? What features of programs and services are most important to getting them and keeping them happy? How do you separate the most important patient and customer requirements from less important requirements?

- How do you anticipate new or emerging customer requirements? What do you do with this information?

- How do you evaluate and improve processes for determining customer requirements? What role has new technology or changing health care service needs played in deciding what improvements to make? Provide some examples of improvements that you have made in the past few years.

3. How do you make it easy for your patients and customers to contact you, get information and assistance, or complain? What do you expect to

learn from patient and customer complaints? What have you learned? Please provide examples.

- What is your process for handling patient and customer complaints? What do you do with the complaint or comment data? (Ask to see some sample complaints and follow the data trail. Determine how the data are analyzed and used to drive improvements.)

- What does "prompt and effective resolution of a complaint" mean to your organization? What processes do you have in place to ensure complaints are resolved by the first person in your organization to receive the complaint? What skills and authority do your patient- and customer-contact staff need to resolve complaints promptly and effectively? How do you check to determine if your complaint resolution processes are effective or not? What improvements have you made in these processes over the past few years?

- What are the patient- and customer-contact requirements or service standards? How were they determined? How do you make sure that every staff that comes in contact with patients and customers understands and works to these standards? How do you know the contact requirements (standards) are consistently met for all patients and customers throughout the organization?

- Describe your process for follow-up with patients and customers after the patients and customers have had contact with the organization or used its services? What do you do with feedback you solicit from patients and customers regarding services? What triggers follow-up action?

- How do you evaluate and improve the patient- and customer-relationship process? What are some improvements you have made to the way you strengthen patient and customer relationships and loyalty? How did you decide they were important to make and when were they made?

4. What are your key measures for patient and customer satisfaction and dissatisfaction? How do

these measures provide information on likely future market behavior, such as loyalty, future business, and referrals?

- What tools and techniques do you use to measure patient and customer satisfaction and dissatisfaction?

- Do you measure satisfaction/dissatisfaction for all key patient and customer groups/segments? What do you do with the information?

- What patient and customer satisfaction information do you have about your competitors or benchmarks? What do you do with this information? How do staff use this information in their regular work? What action do they take as a result? Please provide some examples.

- How do you know appropriate action is taken in response to patient and customer satisfaction data at all levels of the organization?

- How do you know you are asking patients and customers the right questions when trying to determine satisfaction and dissatisfaction?

- How do you go about improving the way you determine patient and customer satisfaction and dissatisfaction? Please provide some examples of how you have improved these techniques over the past several years.

Category 4—Measurement and Analysis of Organizational Performance

1. What are the major performance indicators critical to running your organization?

2. How do you determine whether the information you collect and use for decision making is appropriate for tracking your daily work and the performance of the entire organization?

   - What criteria do you use for data selection? How do you ensure that all data collected meet these criteria?

3. What is the process you use to determine the relevance of the information to organizational goals and action plans?

   - Describe how you obtain feedback from the users of the information, the staff, suppliers, and patients and customers who use this information to support their decision making. How is this feedback used to make improvements in the data and information you collect and analyze?

4. You have told us what your top priorities are. How do you benchmark against these? Please describe how needs and priorities for selecting comparisons and benchmarking are determined. Show us samples of comparative studies and how the resulting information was used to support or lead to better and innovation throughout the organization. Picking some at random, determine:

   - Why was the area selected for benchmarking?

   - How did you use competitive or comparative performance data?

   - How are the results of your benchmarking efforts used to set appropriate goals, make better decisions about work, set priorities for improvement or innovation?

   - How are the results of your benchmarking efforts used to improve work processes?

   - How do you evaluate and improve your benchmarking processes to make them more efficient and useful?

5. Please share with us an example of analysis of information important to organizational performance review and strategic planning:

   - How are data analyzed to determine relationships between patient and customer information and financial performance; operational data and financial performance; or operational data and staff requirements and/or performance?

   - What data and analyses do you use to understand your staff, your patients and customers, and your market to help with strategic planning?

- How widely are these analyses used for decision making throughout the organization at both functional or workgroup levels?

- What are you doing to improve the analysis process and make it more useful for organizational and operational decision making?

6. How do you make sure that the analysis needed to support decision making at all levels of the organization is effectively communicated (made available)? Show how the following types of analyses are used to support decision making and innovation or improvements:

- Technology projections

- Cause-effect relationships

- Root cause analysis

- Descriptive analyses, such as statistical process control, central tendencies, Pareto analysis, histograms

- Other statistical tools, such as correlation analysis, regression and factor analyses, and tests of significance (t-tests, f-tests)

7. How do you make sure that data, information, and analysis needed to support decision making at all levels of the organization are available, timely, and accurate?

- What do you do to make sure the data that support decision making are compete, tell the whole story (data integrity)?

- What are the data security requirements you believe are critical to your system? (For example, certain statutes and regulations, such as Rights to Privacy, may require certain levels of security and data protection.) How do you guarantee data and system security and confidentiality?

- How do you make sure that your hardware and software systems meet the needs of all users? How do you determine whether the software and hardware are "user-friendly?"

(Ask what groups use the hardware/software system. Randomly pick a group and ask how the organization makes sure these people can easily use the hardware and software. Then randomly ask some people in a group how their "user-friendliness" requirements were identified and met.)

- What kind of reliability problems have you experienced with your hardware and software? How have you resolved them? What have you done to prevent these types of problems from happening again?

- Please show how you make sure software and hardware are up to date. What drives decisions to change or upgrade systems?

8. How do you make sure relevant knowledge and information is appropriately shared throughout the organization and with appropriate suppliers, partners, and patients and customers?

- How are worthy processes and work practices shared among all appropriate staff quickly and effectively? (These processes and practices are also known as best practices, exemplary practices, role model practices or, in Minnesota, pretty good practices.)

Category 5—Staff Focus

1. What authority does staff have to direct their own actions and make decisions about their work?

- (To staff) What authority do you have to make decisions about your work, such as resolving problems, improving work processes, and communicating across departments? What have managers done to encourage innovation within the workforce?

- (To all) To what extent do leaders, managers, and supervisors make it easy to change and keep pace with changing health care service and patient and customer requirements? If extremely agile and flexible were a 10, and slow moving, bureaucratic, and bound in "red tape" were a 1, where would you rate the organization as a whole? Where would you rate your unit?

- (To managers) How do you empower staff? What do you do to encourage initiative and self-directed responsibility among staff in their regular work and jobs? What are some examples of processes you have used to evaluate and enhance opportunities for staff to take individual initiative and demonstrate self-directed responsibility in designing and managing their work? What have you done to increase staff innovation—where staff actually make improvements, not just suggestions? Show examples of actions taken and improvements made. When were they made?

2. What have you done to draw out and use ideas and thinking of diverse cultures and types of staff?

3. What do you do to ensure effective communication and knowledge sharing among staff and work units?

   - How do you break down barriers to effective sharing and communication?

4. Describe your approach to staff recognition and compensation.

   - What specific reward and recognition programs are in place? Is the reward and recognition the same for all staff? Why are they the same (or different)?

   - How does the organization link recognition, reward, and compensation to achieve high-performance objectives (which are usually stated as strategic objectives or goals)?

   - How do compensation, recognition, and related reward and incentive systems reinforce, strengthen, or support patient- and customer-focus objectives (for example, patient and customer satisfaction)?

   - (General question for staff) What do you get rewarded for around here? What recognition is offered and why? Are the reward and recognition systems consistent? Fair?

5. How do you figure out what skills will be needed by future (potential) staff?

   - How do you attract staff with the right skills your organization needs to be successful? How do you make sure that staff represent the diversity of the general community from which you hire? What diverse staff do you recruit and why? How does this recruitment help you get the right mix of diverse ideas, culture, and thinking?

   - How do you make sure these skills, diverse ideas, and cultures are used to maximum advantage within your organization?

6. What replacement strategy or process do you have in place for key leaders and staff groups throughout the organization? (For example, if the organization knows key senior leaders or a group of technicians are scheduled to retire, determine what it is doing to fill the gap this retirement will make?)

7. What training is provided for your staff?

   - From the action plans identified in 2.2, pick some and ask: What training and education is provided to support the achievement of (the selected action plan)?

   - How is your training curriculum designed and delivered? What methods are used to determine what training should be offered and how it should be delivered?

   - How do you integrate staff, supervisor, and manager feedback into the design and delivery of your training program? (Ask related follow-up questions to supervisors, managers, and staff to determine the extent their needs for development, learning, and career progression were identified and considered when designing the education and training approach.)

   - How does your training program affect operational performance goals? How do you know your training improves your health care service results? Show examples.

   - After you determine the key groups or segments of staff within the organization, ask the following question: What training and education do you provide to ensure that you meet the needs of all categories of staff?

- What training does new staff receive to obtain the knowledge and skills necessary for success and high performance, including leadership development?

- How do you address key training needs, such as new staff orientation, environmental safety, ethical health care service practices, and diversity?

- If applicable, how do staff in remote locations participate in training programs?

- How do you make sure that the knowledge and skills acquired during training are actually used and reinforced on the job? Provide some examples (then select from this list and follow-up with staff and their supervisors to determine how skills are reinforced on the job).

- What is your system for improving training? Please give us some examples of improvements made and when they were made.

- To what extent is training provided to enhance staff motivation and career development and progression? What do you (senior leaders, managers, and supervisors) do to develop the full potential of staff?

8. What are your standards and performance measures and targets for staff health, ergonomics, security, and safety?

- How were they derived?

- How do you make sure that your approach to health and safety address the needs of all staff groups?

9. How do you determine that you have a safe and healthy work environment? How do you measure this?

- What are your procedures for systematic evaluation and improvement of workplace health, safety, and ergonomics?

- What have you done to improve workplace health, safety, and ergonomics?

10. What processes or systems have you put in place to prepare for emergencies or disasters that may affect your workplace?

- How do you know these systems work as intended? What kinds of disruptions have you faced in the past? What was the impact on the workplace and your patients, customers, and staff? What have you put in place to reduce the possible impact of such disasters or emergencies?

11. What services, facilities, activities, and benefits are most important to your workforce?

- How did you determine these were the most important? Are they the same for all groups or segments of the workforce? If not, how have the services and benefits been modified or tailored to meet the needs of different groups or categories of staff?

12. What are the key elements, conditions, or factors that help or hurt staff well-being, satisfaction, and motivation?

- How did do you determine that these were the key elements? Are the elements the same for all groups of staff? If not, how do they differ?

13. What are the benefits and services you provide for staff to enhance motivation and satisfaction?

- To what extent are these customized for different staff types or groups? How did you determine what changes in the benefits and services should be offered?

14. How is staff satisfaction measured? (If a survey is used, ask how they know they are asking the right questions on the survey. Unless they have already told you, ask for some specific examples about how they use other information, such as staff retention, absenteeism, grievances, safety, and productivity data, to assess and improve staff well-being, satisfaction, and motivation.)

- What do you do with the information? Provide examples.

- Please show me how your staff assessment tools (for example, surveys) reflect the key factors you identified that affect staff well-being, satisfaction and motivation.

15. What do you do to actually improve staff well-being, satisfaction, and motivation systematically?

   • Describe the process you use to analyze staff satisfaction data and other indicators to determine what problems exist that may disrupt or hurt staff well-being, satisfaction, and motivation?

   • How quickly or effectively do you use this information to drive improvements to staff well-being, satisfaction, and motivation?

16. When you identify the priorities for improving the work environment to promote staff well-being, satisfaction, and motivation, what factors do you consider?

   • What are the top three or four improvement priorities? Pick one and ask the leader: What specific finding from the staff satisfaction survey or other assessment tool did the organization use to identify this priority action? How is this priority for improving the work environment likely to affect key health care service results?

17. How do you ensure that managers throughout the organization work to improve the climate for staff well-being, satisfaction, and motivation? [Links to 1.1a(2)]

18. What improvements have you made to the work climate after assessing staff satisfaction, well-being, and motivation?

Category 6—Process Management

1. What new program or service have you designed in the past few years? Pick one from their list and ask: What is your process for designing this new or revised program or service to ensure that patient and customer requirements are met and value is created for the patients and customers, the organization, or other stakeholders? Please walk me through the steps.

   • What new design technologies, including e-technology, have you used in recent health care programs or services?

   • How do you test new programs or services before they are introduced to be sure they perform as expected and meet all patient and customer and operational requirements? What have you done to prevent errors in the design process? What kinds of problems or troubles have you had with past introductions of new programs and services? Provide examples of how you have learned from these problems and prevented them in subsequent service designs.

   • How do you evaluate and improve the process for designing new patient health care services that will make improvements in cycle time, cost control, productivity, and other effectiveness or efficiency factors? Please provide some examples of improvements and when they were made.

   • What process do you have in place to make sure that lessons learned in one part of the organization (or from past improvement efforts) are transferred to others in the organization to save time and prevent rework?

2. What are your key delivery processes and their requirements for creating value, including quality and performance indicators?

   • What steps have you taken to improve the effectiveness/efficiency of key work processes, including cycle time?

   • What are the processes by which you develop and deliver these programs and services to ensure that patient and customer expectations are met or exceeded?

   • Once you determine that a process may not be meeting measurement goals or performing according to expectations, what process do you use to determine root cause and bring about process improvement?

   • Please give an example of how a patient and customer request or complaint resulted in an improvement of a current process or the establishment of a new process. How often do patients and customers change their requirements? How do you respond to these changes? How has this process been refined to respond more quickly, especially when patient and customer requirements change more often?

3. Please share with us your list of key health care service processes, requirements, and associated performance measures, including in-process measures. (Remember that key health care service processes include critical processes that support value for patients and customers and are necessary for health care service growth and success.) For example, if supply chain management is designated as a key health care service process, the following series of questions may be useful: What process is in place for managing your supplier chain? Who are your most important [key] suppliers? How do you establish and communicate to your key suppliers the key requirements they must meet so that your needs are met? What are the key performance requirements? Please explain how you measure your suppliers' performance and provide feedback to help them improve.

- What are the steps you have taken to design your key health care service processes to ensure they meet all performance requirements? How do you determine the types of services and outputs needed? How do your key health care service processes enhance health care service growth and success?

4. Please share with us your list of key support processes, requirements, and associated process measures, including in-process measures:

- How is performance of support services systematically evaluated and refined? Please provide some examples.

- What are the steps you have taken to design your key support processes? How do you determine the types of services needed? How do your support services interact with and add value to your operational processes?

- How does your organization maintain the performance of key support services? Share

some examples of processes used to determine root causes of support problems and how you prevent recurrence of problems. How do you monitor costs of these processes? How have you reduced costs? Please give examples.

Category 7—Organizational Performance Results

The Performance Excellence Criteria require organizations to report performance results in the areas of health care results (7.1), patient and customer-focused results (7.2), financial and market results (7.3), staff and work system results (7.4), organizational effectiveness results (7.5), and governance and social responsibility results (7.6). Normally, applicants are careful to display "good" results and sometimes neglect to report results that are not as good. The Scoring Guidelines penalize applicants for failing to provide results for "most areas of importance to the organization's key health care service requirements."

To score accurately, Examiners must be able to determine what results should be reported in the application that are important to the organization's success. To evaluate Category 7 properly, Examiners first develop a list of the results that they "expect" to be provided in Category 7, based on what the organization reported was important to its success. Then, they compare the list of "expected" results to the results actually provided in the application and note any differences.

Usually a description of important results can be found either in the Organizational Profile, strategic goals [Item 2.1b], the list of actions required to achieve strategic objectives [Item 2.2a(1)], the priority customer requirements [Item 3.1a(2)], or other places in the application. The following is an example of the table of expected results. The first three columns identify, by Item, what results are expected and the location in the application of information that created the expectation for results. The last two columns identify where the results were displayed in the application and provide notations about whether the performance was improving and whether comparison data were provided to help judge the strength or goodness of the performance.

Examiners should prepare this analysis in table format as Figure 44 shows.

Table of expected results				
Item reference	**Expected result**	**Reference**	**Actual result**	**Comparison data**
Identify the area in Category 7 where the result should appear (i.e., 7.2a).	Provide a name or label for the expected result.	List the source in the application where you learned about the importance of the result to the organization.	Indicate if the resource data were provided (yes/no) and whether the results show improvement (+) or not (-).	Indicate whether the organization has provided comparison data from other relevant organizations (yes/no) and whether results are good relative to those organizations (+) or not (-).
Sample				
Completed prior to analyzing Category 7				**Completed based on Category 7 data provided**
7.2a	Patient and Customer Satisfaction			
7.2a	Cost	Org Profile (OP), p ii; and 2.1b, p. 11	Data were provided in Figure 7.1-1 and show 7% improvement (+)	Comparison data were provided (yes-industry mean) and they do better than average (+)
7.2a	Service	OP p. iii; and 2.1b, p. 12	Data were provided in Fig. 7.1-2 and show 5-8% improvement (+)	Comparison data were provided (yes-industry best competitor) and they do better. (++)
7.2a	Courtesy	OP p. iii; and 2.1b, p. 12	Data were provided in Fig. 7.1-2 and show flat performance (~)	No comparative data provided (no)

Figure 44 Table of expected results.

Most of the site-visit work for Category 7 involves studying reports containing raw data as well as trend and comparison data. All relevant results that were reported in the application should be updated to reflect current conditions.

Comparison data, and the rationale for offering the comparison data, should be examined to determine if the comparisons are appropriate and relevant. Comparisons are relevant if the applicant is able to present a plausible explanation or link between the comparison data and the data the applicant has reported.

1. What are the health care outcome levels at this time? [Links to P.1b and Items 6.1, 6.2]

   - Please show a breakout of data by patient and customer group or segment.

   - What are your current levels and trends for how patients and customers perceive your performance?

   - How do these patient and customer satisfaction/dissatisfaction trends and levels compare with those of your competitors or similar providers?

   - What are the performance results for key services that are most critical to patient and customer satisfaction?

   - Please bring your results up to date and close any information gaps that may have been noted in your application.

   - How do these trends and levels compare with those of your competitors or similar providers?

2. What are the patient and customer satisfaction/dissatisfaction trends at this time? [Links to P.1b and Items 3.1, 3.2]

   - Please show a breakout of data by patient and customer group or segment.

   - What are your current levels and trends for patient and customer loyalty, positive referral, customer-perceived value, and relationship building?

   - Please bring your patient and customer satisfaction, dissatisfaction, and related results up to date and close any information gaps that may have been noted in your application.

3. What are the current levels and trends showing financial and marketplace performance or economic value?

   - Please provide data on key financial measures, such as return on investment (ROI), operating profits (or budget reductions, as appropriate), or economic value added.

   - Please provide data on market share or health care service growth, as appropriate. Identify new markets entered and the level of performance in those markets.

   - Please show a breakout of data by patient and customer and market group or segment.

   - Please bring your financial and marketplace performance results up to date and close any information gaps that may have been noted in your application.

   - Show how these trends and levels compare with those of your competitors or similar providers?

4. What are the current levels and trends showing the effectiveness of your staff practices? [Links to processes in Category 5]

   - Please provide data on key indicators, such as safety/accident record, absenteeism, turnover by category and type of staff/manager, and grievances and related litigation.

   - Please bring your staff results up to date and close any information gaps that may have been noted in your application.

   - How does performance on these key indicators compare to your competitors, other providers, or benchmarks?

5. What are the current levels and trends showing the effectiveness of your health care and support processes? [Links to Items 6.1 and 6.2]

- What are current levels and trends for key design and delivery, and health care service process performance?

- What are current levels and trends for production and cycle time for design, delivery, and production?

- Please show us your supplier/partner performance data trends and current levels for each key indicator, such as on-time delivery, error rate, and reducing costs. [Links to supply chain issues in Item 6.1 or 6.2 as appropriate]

- Please show us Results data that demonstrate the extent to which you accomplished your organizational strategy or strategic objectives? [Links to 2.1b(1) and 2.2a]

- Please bring your data about organizational effectiveness up to date and close any information gaps that may have been noted in your application.

- How does your performance on these key indicators compare to your competitors, other providers, or benchmarks?

6. What are the current levels and trends showing the effectiveness of your governance and social responsibility processes? [Links to processes in P.1, P.2, and Items 1.1b and 1.2]

- Please show us your performance data related to fiscal accountability, such as financial statement issues and risks, questioned accounting practices, auditor findings and recommendations, and management's response to these issues. [Links to Item 1.2a(1)]

- Please show us your performance data related to effective governance, management accountability, and ethical behavior, such as percentage of independent members on the board of directors and results of ethics reviews and audits. [Links to Item 1.2a(2)]

- What are your results for regulatory/legal compliance? [Links to Item 1.2a(3)]

- What are your results for organizational citizenship? [Links to Item 1.2c]

- Please bring your governance and social responsibility results up to date and close any information gaps that may have been noted in your application.

- How does your performance on these key indicators compare to your competitors, other providers, or benchmarks?

General Cross-Cutting Questions to Ask Staff

- Who are your patients and customers?

- What are the organization's mission, vision, and values?

- What is the strategic plan for the organization? What are the organization's goals, and what role do you play in helping to achieve the goals?

- What kind of training have you received? Was it useful? Who decided what training you should receive? What kind of on-the-job support did you get for using the new skills you learned during training?

- What kinds of decisions do you usually make about your work and the work of the organization? What data or information do you use to help make these decisions? Is this information easily available to help make decisions easier?

- What activities or work are recognized or rewarded? Is achieving patient and customer satisfaction a critical part of your job? Are your rewards and/or recognition determined in part on achieving certain patient and customer satisfaction levels? If so, explain how this works.

Glossary

This glossary of key terms defines and briefly describes terms used throughout the health care criteria booklet that are important to performance management. As you may have noted, key terms are more easily identified in this version of the Criteria than when they appear in the Categories and Scoring Guidelines sections. In these sections, key terms are presented in small caps/sans serif to indicate that more information is available in the glossary.

Action Plans—The term "action plans" refers to specific actions that respond to short- and longer-term strategic objectives. Action plans include details of resource commitments and time horizons for accomplishment. Action plan development represents the critical stage in planning when strategic objectives and goals are made specific so that effective, organizationwide understanding and deployment are possible. In the Criteria, deployment of action plans includes creation of aligned measures for all departments and work units. Deployment might also require specialized training for some staff or recruitment of personnel.

An example of a strategic objective for a health system in an area with an active business alliance focusing on cost and quality of health care might be to become the low-cost provider. Action plans likely would entail design of efficient processes to minimize length of hospital stays, analysis of resource and asset use, and analysis of the most commonly encountered Diagnosis Related Groups (DRGs) with a focus on preventive health in those areas. Performance requirements might include staff training in setting priorities based upon costs and benefits. Organizational-level analysis and review likely would emphasize process efficiency, cost per member, and health care quality.

Alignment—The term "alignment" refers to consistency of plans, processes, information, resource decisions, actions, results, analysis, and learning to support key organizationwide goals. Effective alignment requires a common understanding of purposes and goals, and the use of complementary measures and information for planning, tracking, analysis, and improvement at three levels: the organizational level, the key process level, and the department and work unit level.

Analysis—The term "analysis" refers to an examination of facts and data to provide a basis for effective decisions. Analysis often involves the determination of cause-effect relationships. Overall organizational analysis guides process management toward achieving key organizational-performance results and toward attaining strategic objectives.

Despite their importance, individual facts and data do not usually provide an effective basis for actions or setting priorities. Actions depend on an understanding of relationships derived from analysis of facts and data.

Anecdotal—The term "anecdotal" refers to process information that lacks specific methods, measures, deployment mechanisms, and evaluation/improvement/learning factors. Anecdotal information frequently uses examples and describes individual activities rather than systematic processes.

An anecdotal response to how senior leaders deploy performance expectations might describe a specific occasion when a senior leader visited all facilities. On the other hand, a systematic approach might describe the communication methods used by all senior leaders to deliver performance expectations on a regular basis, the measures used to assess effectiveness of the methods, and tools and techniques used to evaluate and improve the communication methods.

Approach—The term "approach" refers to how an organization addresses the Baldrige Criteria Item requirements, that is, the methods and processes used by the organization. Approaches are evaluated on the basis of the appropriateness of the methods and processes to the Item requirements, the effectiveness of their use, and their alignment with organizational needs. For further description, see the Scoring System chapter.

Basic Requirements—The term "basic requirements" refers to the most central concept of an Item. Basic requirements are the fundamental theme of that Item. *In the Criteria, the basic requirements of each Item are presented as the Item title.* See the chapter that discusses and defines basic-, overall-, and multiple-requirements.

Benchmarks—The term "benchmarks" refers to processes and results that represent best practices and performance for similar activities, inside or outside an organization's industry. Organizations engage in benchmarking as a process to understand the current dimensions of world-class performance and to achieve discontinuous (nonincremental) or breakthrough improvement.

Benchmarks are one form of comparative data. Other comparative data might include information obtained from other organizations through sharing or contributing to external reference databases; information obtained from the open literature (for example, outcomes of research studies and practice guidelines), data gathering and evaluation by independent organizations (for example, Health Care Finance Administration, accrediting organizations, and commercial organizations) regarding industry data (frequently industry averages), performance of competitors, and comparisons with other organizations providing similar health care services.

Customer—The term "customer" refers to actual and potential users of the organization's services. Patients are the primary customers of health care organizations. Other customers could include patients' families, the community, insurers/third-party payors, employers, health care providers, patient advocacy groups, Departments of Health, and students. The Criteria address customers broadly, in referencing current customers, future customers, as well as customers of competitors and other organizations providing similar health care services.

Patient-focused excellence is a Baldrige Core Value embedded in the beliefs and behaviors of high-performance organizations. Customer focus impacts and integrates an organization's strategic directions, its health care processes, and its organizational performance results.

Cycle Time—The term "cycle time" refers to the time required to fulfill commitments or to complete tasks. Time measurements play a major role in the Criteria because of the great importance of time performance to improving overall performance. "Cycle time" refers to all aspects of time performance. Cycle time improvement might include test results reporting time, time to introduce new health care technology, order fulfillment time, length of stay, billing time, and other key measures of time.

Deployment—The term "deployment" refers to the extent to which an organization's approach is applied to the requirements of a Baldrige Criteria Item. Deployment is evaluated on the basis of the breadth and depth of application of the approach to relevant processes and departments and work units throughout the organization.

Effective—The term "effective" refers to how well an approach, a process, or a measure addresses its intended purpose. Determining effectiveness requires the evaluation of how well a need is met by the approach taken, its deployment, or the measure used.

Empowerment—The term "empowerment" refers to giving staff the authority and responsibility to make decisions and take appropriate actions. Empowerment results in decisions being made closest to the patient or the business "front line," where patient/customer needs and work-related knowledge and understanding reside.

Empowerment is aimed at enabling staff to satisfy patients/customers on first contact, to improve processes and increase productivity, and to better the organization's health care and other performance results. Empowered staff require information to make appropriate decisions; thus, an organizational requirement is to provide that information in a timely and useful way.

Goals—The term "goals" refers to a future condition or performance level that one intends to attain. Goals can be both short-term and longer-term.

Goals are ends that guide actions. Quantitative goals frequently referred to as "targets," include a numerical point or range. Targets might be projections based on comparative and/or competitive data. The term "stretch goals" refers to desired major, discontinuous (nonincremental) or breakthrough improvements, usually in areas most critical to the organization's future success.

Goals can serve many purposes, including the following:

- Clarifying strategic objectives and action plans to indicate how success will be measured

- Fostering teamwork by focusing on a common end

- Encouraging "out-of-the-box" thinking to achieve a stretch goal

- Providing a basis for measuring and accelerating progress

Governance—The term "governance" refers to the system of management and controls exercised in the stewardship of the organization. It includes the responsibilities of the organization's owners/shareholders, board of directors, and administrative and health care leaders. Corporate charters, by-laws, and policies document the rights and responsibilities of each of the parties and describe how the organization will be directed and controlled to ensure the following:

- Accountability to all stakeholders, including owners/shareholders

- Transparency of operations

- Fair treatment of all stake-holders

Governance processes may include approving strategic direction, monitoring and evaluating senior leader performance, succession planning, financial auditing, establishing executive compensation and benefits, managing risk, disclosure, and shareholder reporting. Ensuring effective governance is important to stakeholders' and the larger society's trust, and to organizational effectiveness.

Health Care Services—The term "health care services" refers to all services delivered by the organization that involve professional clinical/medical judgment, including those delivered to patients and those delivered to the community.

High-Performance Work—The term "high-performance work" refers to work approaches used to systematically pursue ever-higher levels of overall organizational and individual performance, including quality, productivity, innovation rate, and cycle time performance. High-performance work results in improved service for patients/customers and other stakeholders.

Approaches to high-performance work vary in form, function, and incentive systems. Effective approaches frequently include cooperation between administration/management and the staff, which may involve workforce bargaining units; cooperation among work units, often involving teams; self-directed responsibility/staff empowerment; staff input to planning; individual and organizational skill building and learning; learning from other organizations; flexibility in job design and work assignments; a flattened organizational structure, where decision making is decentralized and decisions are made closest to the patient or the business "front line"; and effective use of performance measures, including comparisons. Many high-performance work systems use monetary and nonmonetary incentives based upon factors such as organizational performance, team and/or individual contributions, and skill building. Also, high-performance work approaches usually seek to align the organization's structure, work, jobs, staff development, and incentives.

Ho—The term "how" refers to the processes that an organization uses to accomplish its mission requirements. In responding to "how" questions in the Approach/Deployment Item requirements, process descriptions should include information such as methods, measures, deployment, and evaluation/improvement/learning factors.

Innovation—The term "innovation" refers to making meaningful change to improve services and/or processes and create new value for stakeholders. Innovation involves the adoption of an idea, process, technology, or product that is either new or new to its proposed application.

Successful organizational innovation is a multi-step process that involves development and knowledge sharing, a decision to implement, implementation, evaluation, and learning. Although innovation is often associated with health care research and technological innovation, it is applicable to all key organizational processes that would benefit from change, whether through breakthrough improvement or change in approach or outputs.

Integration—The term "integration" refers to the harmonization of plans, processes, information, resource decisions, actions, results, analysis, and learning to support key organizationwide goals. Effective integration is achieved when the individual components of a performance-management system operate as a fully interconnected unit.

Key—The term "key" refers to the major or most important elements or factors, those that are critical to achieving the organization's intended outcomes. The Baldrige Criteria, for example, refer to key challenges, key patient/customer groups, key plans, key processes, and key measures—those that are most important to the organization's success. They are the essential elements for pursuing or monitoring a desired outcome.

Knowledge Assets—The term "knowledge assets" refers to the accumulated intellectual resources of the organization. It is the knowledge possessed by the organization and its staff in the form of information, ideas, learning, understanding, memory, insights, cognitive and technical skills, and capabilities. Staff, databases, documents, guides, policies and procedures, and software and patents are repositories of an organization's knowledge assets.

Knowledge assets are held not only by an organization, but reside within its patients and other customers, suppliers, and partners as well. Knowledge assets are the "know how" that the organization has available to use, to invest, and to grow. Building and managing its knowledge assets are key components for the organization to create value for its stakeholders.

Leadership System—The term "leadership system" refers to how leadership is exercised, formally and informally, throughout the organization—the basis for and the way key decisions are made, communicated, and carried out. It includes structures and mechanisms for decision making; selection and development of leaders and managers; and reinforcement of values, directions, and performance

expectations. In health care organizations with separate administrative/operational and health care provider leadership, the leadership system also includes the relationships among those leaders.

An effective leadership system respects the capabilities and requirements of staff and other stakeholders, and it sets high expectations for performance and performance improvement. It builds loyalties and teamwork based on the organization's values and the pursuit of shared goals. It encourages and supports initiative and appropriate risk taking, subordinates organization to purpose and function, and avoids chains of command that require long decision paths. An effective leadership system includes mechanisms for the leaders to conduct self-examination, receive feedback, and improve.

Levels—The term "levels" refers to numerical information that places or positions an organization's results and performance on a meaningful measurement scale. Performance levels permit evaluation relative to past performance, projections, goals, and appropriate comparisons.

Measures and Indicators—The term "measures and indicators" refers to numerical information that quantifies input, output, and performance dimensions of processes, products, services, and the overall organization (outcomes). The Health Care Criteria place particular focus on measures of health care outcomes, health care service delivery, and patients' functional status. Measures and indicators might be simple (derived from one measurement) or composite.

The Criteria do not make a distinction between measures and indicators. However, some users of these terms prefer the term "indicator" when: (1) The measurement relates to performance, but is not a direct measure of such performance (for example, the number of complaints is an indicator of dissatisfaction, but not a direct measure of it) or (2) The measurement is a predictor ("leading indicator") of some more significant performance (for example, increased patient satisfaction might be a leading indicator of a gain in HMO member retention).

Mission—The term "mission" refers to the overall function of an organization. The mission answers the question, "What is this organization attempting to accomplish?" The mission might define patients, other customers, or markets served; distinctive competencies; or technologies used.

Multiple Requirements—The term "multiple requirements" refers to the individual questions Criteria users need to answer within each Area to Address. These questions constitute the details of an Item's requirements. They are presented in black text under each Item's Area(s) to Address. See the chapter that discusses and defines basic-, overall-, and multiple-requirements.

Overall Requirements—The term "overall requirements" refers to the topics Criteria users need to address when responding to the central theme of an Item. Overall requirements address the most significant features of the Item requirements. In the Criteria, the overall requirements of each Item are presented as an introductory sentence(s) printed in bold. See the chapter that discusses and defines basic-, overall-, and multiple-requirements.

Patient—The term "patient" refers to the person receiving health care, including preventive, promotion, acute, chronic, rehabilitative, and all other services in the continuum of care. Other terms organizations use for "patient" include member, consumer, client, or resident.

Performance—The term "performance" refers to output results and their outcomes obtained from processes and services that permit evaluation and comparison relative to goals, standards, past results, and other organizations. Performance might be expressed in nonfinancial and financial terms. The Baldrige Health Care Criteria address four types of performance: (1) health care; (2) patient- and other customer-focused; (3) financial and marketplace; and (4) operational.

"Health care" refers to performance relative to measures and indicators of health care service important to patients and other customers. Examples of health care performance include reductions in hospital admission rates, mortality and morbidity rates, nosocomial infection rates, length of stay and increases in outside-the-hospital treatment of chronic illnesses, lifestyle changes, patient compliance and adherence, and patient experienced error level. Health care performance

might be measured at the organizational level and at the DRG-specific level.

"Patient- and other customer-focused performance" refers to measures and indicators of patients' and other customers' perceptions, reactions, and behaviors. Examples of patient- and other customer-focused performance include patient loyalty, customer retention, complaints, customer survey results, and service response time.

"Financial and marketplace performance" refers to performance using measures of cost, revenue, and market position, including asset utilization, asset growth, and market share. Examples include returns on investments, value added per staff member, bond ratings, debt-to-equity ratio, returns on assets, operating margins, other profitability and liquidity measures, and market gains.

"Operational performance" refers to organizational, staff, and ethical performance relative to effectiveness, efficiency, and accountability measures and indicators. Examples include cycle time, productivity, waste reduction, staff turnover, staff cross-training rates, accreditation results, legal/regulatory compliance, fiscal accountability, community involvement, and contributions to community health. Operational performance might be measured at the department and work-unit level, key process level, and organizational level.

Performance Excellence—The term "performance excellence" refers to an integrated approach to organizational performance management that results in: (1) Delivery of ever-improving value to patients and other customers, contributing to improved health care quality; (2) Improvement of overall organizational effectiveness and capabilities as a health care provider; and (3) Organizational and personal learning.

The Baldrige Health Care Criteria for Performance Excellence provide a framework and an assessment tool for understanding organizational strengths and opportunities for improvement and thus for guiding planning efforts.

Performance Projections—The term "performance projections" refers to estimates of future performance or goals for future results. Projections may be inferred from past performance, may be based on competitors' performance or the performance of other organizations providing similar health care services, or may be predicted based on changes in a dynamic health care marketplace. Projections integrate estimates of the organization's rate of improvement and change, and they may be used to indicate where breakthrough improvement or change is needed. Thus, performance projections serve as a key planning management tool.

Process—The term "process" refers to linked activities with the purpose of producing a product or service for patients and other customers (users) within or outside the organization. Generally, processes involve combinations of people, machines, tools, techniques, and materials in a systematic series of steps or actions. In some situations, processes might require adherence to a specific sequence of steps, with documentation (sometimes formal) of procedures and requirements, including well-defined measurement and control steps.

In many service situations, such as health care treatment, particularly when customers are directly involved in the service, process is used in a more general way, that is, to spell out what must be done, possibly including a preferred or expected sequence. If a sequence is critical, the service needs to include information to help customers understand and follow the sequence. Service processes involving customers also require guidance to the providers of those services on handling contingencies related to customers' likely or possible actions or behaviors.

In knowledge work, such as health care assessment and diagnosis, strategic planning, research, development, and analysis, process does not necessarily imply formal sequences of steps. Rather, process implies general understandings regarding competent performance, such as timing, options to be included, evaluation, and reporting. Sequences might arise as part of these understandings.

Productivity—The term "productivity" refers to measures of the efficiency of resource use. Although the term often is applied to single factors, such as staffing (labor productivity), machines, materials, energy, and capital, the productivity concept applies as well to the total resources used in producing outputs. The use of an aggregate measure of overall productivity allows a determination of whether the net effect of overall changes in a process—possibly involving resource tradeoffs—is beneficial.

Purpose—The term "purpose" refers to the fundamental reason that an organization exists. The primary role of purpose is to inspire an organization and to guide its setting of values. Purpose is generally broad and enduring. Two organizations providing different health care services could have similar purposes, and two organizations providing similar health care services could have different purposes.

Results—The term "results" refers to outputs and outcomes achieved by an organization in addressing the purposes of a Baldrige Criteria Item. Results are evaluated on the basis of current performance; performance relative to appropriate comparisons; the rate, breadth, and importance of performance improvements; and the relationship of results measures to key organizational performance requirements. For further description, see the Scoring System chapter.

Senior Leaders—The term "senior leaders" refers to an organization's senior management group or team. In many organizations, this consists of the head of the organization and his or her direct reports. In health care organizations with separate administrative/operational and health care provider leadership, "senior leaders" refers to both sets of leaders and the relationships among those leaders.

Staff—The term "staff" refers to all people who contribute to the delivery of an organization's services, including paid staff (for example, permanent, part-time, temporary, and contract employees supervised by the organization), independent practitioners (for example, physicians, physician assistants, nurse practitioners, acupuncturists, and nutritionists not paid by the organization), volunteers, and health profession students (for example, medical, nursing, and ancillary).

Stakeholders—The term "stakeholders" refers to all groups that are or might be affected by an organization's services, actions, and success. Examples of key stakeholders include patients and other customers (for example, patients' families, insurers/third-party payors, employers, health care providers, and patient advocacy groups,

Departments of Health, and students), staff, partners, investors, and local/professional communities.

Strategic Challenges—The term "strategic challenges" refers to those pressures that exert a decisive influence on an organization's likelihood of future success. These challenges frequently are driven by an organization's future collaborative environment and/or competitive position relative to other providers of similar health care services. While not exclusively so, strategic challenges generally are externally driven. However, in responding to externally driven strategic challenges, an organization may face internal strategic challenges. External strategic challenges may relate to patient/customer or health care market needs/expectations; health care service or technological changes; or financial, societal, and other risks. Internal strategic challenges may relate to an organization's capabilities and its human and other resources.

Strategic Objectives—The term "strategic objectives" refers to an organization's articulated aims or responses to address major change or improvement, competitiveness issues, and/or health care advantages. Strategic objectives generally are focused externally and relate to significant patient/customer, market, service, or technological opportunities and challenges (strategic challenges). Broadly stated, they are what an organization must achieve to remain or become competitive. Strategic objectives set an organization's longer-term directions and guide resource allocations and redistributions.

Systematic—The term "systematic" refers to approaches that are repeatable and use data and information so that improvement and learning are possible. In other words, approaches are systematic if they build in the opportunity for evaluation and learning and thereby permit a gain in maturity. For use of the term, see the Scoring Guidelines.

Trends—The term "trends" refers to numerical information that shows the direction and rate of change for an organization's results. Trends provide a time sequence of organizational performance.

A minimum of three data points generally is needed to begin to ascertain a trend. The time period for a trend is determined by the cycle time of the process being measured. Shorter cycle times demand more frequent measurement, while longer cycle times might require longer periods before a meaningful trend can be determined.

Examples of trends called for by the Criteria include data related to patient/customer and staff satisfaction and dissatisfaction results, health care outcomes and other health care service results, financial performance, health care marketplace performance, and operational performance, such as cycle time and productivity.

Value—The term "value" refers to the perceived worth of a product, service, process, asset, or function relative to cost and relative to possible alternatives. Organizations frequently use value considerations to determine the benefits of various options relative to their costs, such as the value of various product and service combinations to customers. Organizations need to understand what different stakeholder groups value and then deliver value to each group. This frequently requires balancing value for customers and other stakeholders, such as patients, third-party payors, investors, staff, and the community.

Values—The term "values" refers to the guiding principles and/or behaviors that embody how the organization and its people are expected to operate. Values reflect and reinforce the desired culture of an organization. Values support and guide the decision making of every staff member, helping the organization to accomplish its mission and attain its vision in an appropriate manner.

Vision—The term "vision" refers to the desired future state of the organization. The vision describes where the organization is headed, what it intends to be, or how it wishes to be perceived.

Work Systems—The term "work systems" refers to how the staff is organized into formal or informal units to accomplish the organization's mission and strategic objectives; how job responsibilities and processes for compensation, staff-performance management, recognition, communication, hiring, and succession planning are managed. Organizations design work systems to align their components to enable and encourage all staff to contribute effectively and to the best of their ability.

Clarifying Confusing Terms

Comparative Information vs. Benchmarking

Comparative information includes benchmarking and competitive comparisons. Benchmarking refers to collecting information and data about processes and performance results that represent the best practices and performance for similar activities inside or outside the organization's health care or industry. Competitive comparisons refer to collecting information and data on performance relative to direct competitors or similar providers.

For example, a personal computer manufacturer, ABC Micro, must store, retrieve, pack, and ship computers and replacement parts. ABC Micro is concerned about shipping response time, errors in shipping, and damage during shipping. To determine the level of performance of its competitors in these areas, and to set reasonable improvement goals, ABC Micro would gather competitive comparison data from similar providers (competitors). However, these performance levels may not reflect best practices for storage, retrieval, packing, and shipping. Benchmarking would require ABC Micro to find organizations that carry out these processes better than anyone else and examine both their processes and performance levels, such as the catalog company L.L. Bean.

Benchmarking seeks best-practices information. Competitive comparisons look at competitors, whether or not they are the best.

Patient- and Customer-Contact Staff

Patient- and customer-contact staff are any staff who are in direct contact with patients and customers. They may be direct service providers or answer complaint calls. Whenever a patient and customer makes contact with an organization, either in person or by phone or other electronic means, that patient and customer forms an opinion about the organization and its staff based on this initial interaction. Staff who come in contact with patients and customers are in a critical position to influence patients and customers for the good of the organization, or to its detriment.

Patient and Customer Satisfaction vs. Patient and Customer Dissatisfaction

One is not the inverse of the other. The lack of complaints does not indicate satisfaction although the presence of complaints can be a partial indicator of dissatisfaction. Measures of patient and customer dissatisfaction can include direct measures through surveys as well as complaints, product returns, and warranty claims.

Patient and customer satisfaction and dissatisfaction are complex areas to assess. Patients and customers are rarely "thoroughly" dissatisfied, although they may dislike a feature of a product or an aspect of service. There are usually degrees of satisfaction and dissatisfaction.

Data vs. Information

Information can be qualitative and quantitative. Data lend themselves to quantification and statistical analysis. For example, an incoming inspection might produce a count of the number of units accepted, rejected, and total shipped. This count is considered *data*. These counts add to the base of *information* about supplier quality.

Education vs. Training

Training refers to learning about and acquiring job-specific skills and knowledge. Education refers to the general development of individuals. An organization might provide training in equipment maintenance for its workers, as well as support the education of workers through an associate degree program at a local community college.

Empowerment and Involvement

Empowerment generally refers to processes and procedures designed to provide individuals and teams the tools, skills, and authority to make decisions that affect their work—decisions traditionally reserved for managers and supervisors.

Empowerment as a concept has been misused in many organizations. For example, managers may appear to extend decision-making authority under the guise of chartering teams and individuals to make recommendations about their work, while continuing to reserve decision-making authority for themselves.

This practice has given rise to another term—involvement—that describes the role of staff who are asked to become involved in decision making, without necessarily making decisions. Involvement is a practice that many agree is better than not involving staff at all, but still does not optimize their contribution to initiative, flexibility, and fast response.

Measures and Indicators

The Award Criteria do not make a distinction between measures and indicators. However, some users of these terms prefer the term indicator when the measurement:

* Relates to performance, but is not a direct or exclusive measure of such performance. For example, the number of complaints is an indicator of dissatisfaction, but not a direct or exclusive measure of it.

* Is a predictor (leading indicator) of some more significant performance. For example, a gain in patient and customer satisfaction might be a leading indicator of market share gain.

Operational Performance and Predictors of Patient and Customer Satisfaction

Operational performance processes and predictors of patient and customer satisfaction are related, but not always the same. Operational performance measures can reflect issues that concern patients and customers as well as those that do not. Operational performance measures are used by the organization to assess effectiveness and efficiency, and to predict patient and customer satisfaction.

In the example of the coffee shop, freshness is a key patient and customer requirement. One predictor of patient and customer satisfaction might be the length of time, in minutes, between brewing and serving to guarantee freshness and good aroma. The standard might be 10 minutes or less to ensure satisfaction. Coffee more than 10 minutes old would be discarded.

A measure of operational effectiveness might be how many cups were discarded (waste) because the coffee was too old. The patient and customer does not care if the coffee shop pours out stale coffee, and therefore, that measure is not a predictor of satisfaction. However, pouring out coffee does affect profitability and should be measured and minimized.

Ideally, an organization should be able to identify enough measures of product and service quality to predict patient and customer satisfaction accurately and monitor operating effectiveness and efficiency.

Performance Requirements vs. Performance Measures

Performance requirements are an expression of patient and customer requirements and expectations. Sometimes performance requirements are expressed as design requirements or engineering requirements. They are viewed as a basis for developing measures to enable the organization to determine, generally without asking the patient and customer, whether the patient and customer is likely to be satisfied.

Performance measures can also be used to assess efficiency, effectiveness, and productivity of a work process. Process performance measures might include cycle time, error rate, or throughput.

Support Services

Support services are those services that support the organization's product and service delivery core operating processes. Support services might include finance and accounting, management information services, software support, marketing, public relations, personnel administration (job posting, recruitment, and payroll), facilities maintenance and management, secretarial support, and other administration services.

In the staff area (Category 5), the Criteria require organizations to manage their staff assets to optimize performance. However, many staff support services might also exist, such as payroll, travel, position control, recruitment, and staff services. These processes must be designed, delivered, and refined systematically according to the requirements of Item 6.2.

Teams and Natural Work Units

Natural work units reflect the people that normally work together because they are a part of a formal work unit. For example, on an assembly line, three or four people may naturally work together to install a motor in a new car. Hotel staff who prepare food in the kitchen might constitute another natural work unit. Teams may be formed of people within a natural work unit, or may cross existing (natural) organization boundaries. To improve room service in a hotel, for example, some members of several natural work units, such as the switchboard, kitchen workers, and waiters, may form a special team. This team would not be considered a natural work unit. It might be called a cross-functional work team because its members come from different functions within the organization.

About the Authors

Mark L. Blazey, Ed.D.

Mark Blazey is the president of Quantum Performance Group, Inc.—a management consulting and training firm specializing in organization assessment and high-performance systems development. Dr. Blazey has an extensive background in quality systems. For five years he served as a Senior Examiner for the Malcolm Baldrige National Quality Award. He also served as the lead judge for the quality awards for New York, Vermont, and Aruba, and a judge for the Wisconsin Forward Award and Delaware Quality Award. Dr. Blazey has participated on and led numerous site-visit teams for national, state, and private quality awards and audits over the past 15 years.

Dr. Blazey has trained thousands of quality award examiners and judges for state and national quality programs including the Alabama Quality Award, Delaware Quality Award, Illinois Lincoln Award for Health Care Excellence, Kentucky Quality Award, Minnesota Quality Award, New York State Quality Award, Pennsylvania Quality Leadership Award, Nebraska Quality Award, Vermont Quality Award, Wisconsin Forward Award, Aruba Quality Award, Costa Rica Quality Award, and the national Workforce Excellence Network Award. He has also trained managers and examiners for schools, health care organizations, major businesses, and government agencies. He has set up numerous Baldrige-based programs to enhance and assess performance excellence for all sectors and types of organizations—many of which have subsequently received State and Baldrige recognition.

Dr. Blazey is a member and Certified Quality Auditor of the American Society for Quality. He earned an Ed.D. from the State University of New York at Albany in education policy, curriculum, and instruction; an MS from SUNY Albany in educational psychology and statistics; an MS from SUNY Albany in education, and a AB degree from Syracuse University. He received post graduate certificates in management from the Kennedy School of Government at Harvard University, George Washington University, Institute for Educational Leadership, and Rochester Institute of Technology.

Dr. Blazey may be contacted via email at Blazey@QuantumPerformance.com or by telephone, 315-986-9200. He encourages feedback, recommendations, and questions about this book.

Joel H. Ettinger

Joel H. Ettinger is a principal in Pugh, Ettinger, McCarthy, and Associates, advisors to the health care industry focusing on performance excellence and strategy. Mr. Ettinger has held executive positions in several world-renown health care organizations and has lectured nationally and internationally on the applications of performance excellence methods in health care.

He is an alumni member of the Board of Examiners for The Malcolm Baldrige National Quality Award and is the most tenured and experienced examiner from the health care industry.

For eleven years, Mr. Ettinger served as the first president and CEO of VHA Pennsylvania, a regional health care system of VHA, Inc., a national alliance of over 1,300 health care organizations. He has served on the executive staffs of The Mayo Clinic, Memorial Sloan-Kettering Cancer Center, and University Health Center of Pittsburgh and, Allegheny-University Hospitals. He has also served as chairman of the Executive Committee of the Quality Management

Network and Forum Co-Chairman for the Institute for Health Care Improvement located in Boston, Massachusetts.

He is an adjunct associate professor at the School of Public Health, University of Pittsburgh.

Mr. Ettinger is a cum laude graduate of City University of New York, Queens College, where he earned his BA degree in communications theory. He received his master's degree in Health Administration from the University of Minnesota.

He is the founder and permanent vice chairman of Family House, a home away from home for patients and their families undergoing treatment for life-threatening illness. Family House is considered to be one of the nation's most successful charities.

Paul L. Grizzell

Paul L. Grizzell is business excellence manager at Medtronic Cardiac Surgery. He has helped a variety of companies implement quality initiatives based on the Malcolm Baldrige Criteria for Performance Excellence, both in leadership and consulting roles. He has also implemented a Lean and Six Sigma program based on a Baldrige management system foundation.

Paul has served for four years as an Examiner and Senior Examiner for the Malcolm Baldrige National Quality Award. He also serves on the Board of Directors of the Minnesota Council for Quality, where he is also a Judge and a Senior Evaluator. He is a member of the Juran Fellows Selection Board for the Juran Center for Leadership in Quality at the University of Minnesota's Carlson School of Management.

Paul is an active community volunteer, helping to implement Baldrige-based initiatives in his children's school and his church. He lives in Woodbury, MN, with his wife, Janice, and his children, Ashley and Nicholas.

Linda M. Janczak

Linda M. Janczak is the president/CEO of F.F. Thompson Health System, Inc., a recent recipient of the New York Governor's Award for quality. Health System delivers integrated health care through seven corporate entities comprising acute hospital care, continuing care, advanced life support, preferred provider organization, medical office real estate, foundation/ development, and independent and enriched senior living.

Ms. Janczak is the 1993 winner of the Athena Award. She serves on boards of directors for the NYS Excellence at Work (formerly The New York State Excelsior Award), the Rochester Regional Health Care Association, Seagate Alliance, and the Canandaigua Chamber of Commerce. Ms. Janczak is a diplomat of the American College of Health Care Executives and serves on the Ontario County Commission for Total Quality Management.

Ms. Janczak serves on various health care committees including Quality Health Care Reform, and Rural Health, as well as the Partnership for Community Health Task Force. She has been appointed by the governor of New York State to the Rural State Health Council. She is married with two children.

Index